Hugh M. Shingleton
MD FACS FACOG
Professor of Obstetrics and Gynecology; Associate Professor
of Pathology, Division of Gynecologic Oncology, University
of Alabama Medical Center, Birmingham, Alabama

James W. Orr Jr
MD
Assistant Professor, Obstetrics and Gynecology, Division of
Gynecologic Oncology, University of Alabama Medical Center,
Birmingham, Alabama

Cancer of the Cervix

Diagnosis and Treatment

Series Editors
ALBERT SINGER AND JOE JORDAN

Churchill Livingstone
EDINBURGH LONDON MELBOURNE AND NEW YORK 1983

CHURCHILL LIVINGSTONE
Medical Division of Longman Group Limited

Distributed in the United States of America by Churchill
Livingstone Inc., 1560 Broadway, New York, N.Y. 10036, and
by associated companies, branches and representatives
throughout the world.

© Longman Group Limited 1983

First published 1983

ISBN 0 443 02614 9

British Library Cataloguing in Publication Data
Shingleton, Hugh M.
    Cancer of the cervix. —— (Current reviews in
    obstetrics and gynaecology)
    1. Cervix uteri —— Cancer
    I. Title II. Orr, James W. III. Series
    616.99′466   RC280.U8

Library of Congress Catalog Card Number
Shingleton, Hugh M.
    Cancer of the cervix.
    (Current reviews in obstetrics
    and gynaecology)
    Includes index.
    1. Cervix uteri —— Cancer —— Addresses,
    essays, lectures.
I. Orr, James W. II. Title III. Series. [DNLM: 1. Cervix
neoplasms. W1 CU8093M / WP 480 S556c]
RC280.U8S48 1983   616.99′466   83-7258

Printed in Great Britain by
Butler & Tanner Ltd, Frome and London

£9.95

Cancer of the Cervix
Diagnosis and Treatment

CURRENT REVIEWS IN OBSTETRICS AND GYNAECOLOGY

OBSTETRICS

Series Editor
Tom Lind MB BS DSc PhD MRCPath MRCOG
MRC Human Reproduction Group, Princess Mary Maternity Hospital, Newcastle upon Tyne

Volumes published
Obstetric Analgesia and Anaesthesia *J. Selwyn Crawford*
Early Diagnosis of Fetal Defects *D. J. H. Brock*
Early Teenage Pregnancy *J. K. Russell*

Volumes in preparation
Coagulation Problem in Pregnancy *E. A. Letsky*
Drugs in Pregnancy *B. Krauer, F. Krauer and F. Hytten*
Immunology of Pregnancy *W. Page Faulk and H. Fox*
Hypertension and Related Problems in Pregnancy *W. A. W. Walters*
Ultrasound in Obstetrics *W. J. Garrett and P. S. Warren*
Fetoscopy *C. H. Rodeck*
Diabetic Pregnancy *M. Brudenell and M. Dodderidge*
Spontaneous Abortion *H. J. Huisjes*

GYNAECOLOGY

Series Editors
Albert Singer DPhil PhD FRCOG
Whittington Hospital, London
Joe A. Jordan MD DObst FRCOG
Birmingham Maternity Hospital, Queen Elizabeth Medical Centre, Birmingham

Volume published
Ovarian Malignancies *M. S. Piver*

Volumes in preparation
Therapeutic Abortion *A. A. Calder*
Male Infertility *A. M. Jequier*
Gynaecological Premalignant Disease *A. Singer, F. Sharp and J. Jordan*
The Menopause *M. Thom*
Urinary Incontinence *S. L. R. Stanton, L. Cardozo and P. Hilton*
Endometriosis *D. O'Connor*
Endocrine Aspects of Female Infertility *M. Hull*

Dedication

To our wives, Lucy and Sandy,
for their patience and support

Foreword

The aim of this series of books is to present to the reader the personal views of one or two authors about one specific topic. The readers are primarily doctors training for the membership examination of the Royal College of Obstetricians and Gynaecologists or similar examinations and practising clinicians who wish to keep up-to-date.

In this volume, Professor Hugh Shingleton, together with his colleague Dr Orr, have produced an extremely comprehensive text relating to cancer of the cervix. Comprehensive it may be, but long and tedious it is not. It is a relatively short book which is well illustrated, easy to read, and more up-to-date than textbooks usually are by the time they are published.

They start with a detailed chronological history of the subject quoting references from as early as 2000 BC. They then give a review of the epidemiology of the subject ending with a quotation from Kessler who said that 'several decades of clinical observations and epidemiological investigations have confirmed that squamous carcinoma of the cervix behaves as a venereal disease'. The chapter dealing with pathology serves to highlight the importance of the pathologist in the modern oncology team: no longer is it enough for the pathologist to say simply that the lesion is either invasive or non-invasive! This chapter deals with the various parameters which need to be assessed by the pathologist and, in particular, highlights the current problem of microinvasive carcinoma.

In the section dealing with diagnosis, staging and selection of treatment they emphasize the importance of proper staging and make special reference to the presence or absence of para-aortic lymph node involvement. They stress that since some patients with microscopic metastatic disease in the aortic nodes can be salvaged by extended field irradiation it seems important to surgically stage those patients who are at high risk for affected aortic nodes, especially young patients.

Selection of therapy is therefore important and has to recognize the relevance of preservation of sexual function, the age of the patient, tumour volume, and demonstrating extra pelvic disease.

They also cover the subject of primary surgical and combined treatment and describe in detail how patients are selected for various modalities, stressing that treatment selection depends not only on age and extent of tumour but on tumour type.

During Hugh Shingleton's description of his technique for radical hysterectomy he quotes his personal experiences and preferences and this section is a marvellous example of one of the strengths of this series of books, namely that each is a personal appraisal of a topic in which the author is a recognized expert.

The section on radiation is introduced by a description of the fundamentals of radiation in a manner easily understandable by simple gynaecologists: it goes on to explain the rationale of radiotherapy and how this can be put to best advantage by the radiotherapist either alone or as an adjunct to surgery.

The management of the patient does not of course end immediately after surgery or radiotherapy and the book includes an excellent chapter on post-treatment surveyance stressing that those who treat cervical cancer will be faced with a persistence or recurrence in about half of all patients treated. Management of recurrent disease is always difficult but this too is dealt with in a logical and thorough fashion.

Cancer of the cervix is, thankfully, an uncommon condition but provides a major headache for the gynaecologist. The authors have had more experience than most people in dealing with this particular problem and their thoughts are particularly valid and most welcome. As one might expect from these two doctors the total welfare of the patient is paramount and they end their book with a chapter on an aspect of management which is often sadly neglected, namely the social, psychological and sexual aspects of cancer of the cervix. This final chapter completes what we believe to be one of the best texts ever written on the subject of cancer of the cervix, and we are confident that the knowledge which they share with the reader will be of advantage to every practising gynaecologist.

J.J.
A.S.

Preface

Extensive application of cervical cytological screening has been associated with a decreasing incidence of invasive carcinoma and could potentially eradicate it. However, advanced cervical cancer still confronts the gynaecologist in many countries around the world. Radiotherapeutic control of central pelvic tumour has increased with use of linear accelerators and afterloading applicators. More recently, techniques for surgical staging and fine needle aspiration cytology have allowed identification of extrapelvic disease which can be treated by extended field radiation.

Increasing numbers of young women with early stage disease allow use of the primary radical hysterectomy and pelvic lymphadenectomy developed by such pioneers as Wertheim, Bonney and Meigs. For those women with recurrent or persistent carcinoma, refinements in Brunschwig's pelvic exenteration operation have allowed salvage of many women in whom the disease would otherwise have been fatal.

This monograph is intended to provide both physicians in training and those practising gynaecology with precise guidelines for diagnosis and treatment. The authors' opinions reflect widespread clinical experience as well as a review of the recent literature.

We are indebted to a number of people who have assisted with the preparation of the monograph: Josephine Allen, for the preparation of tables, figures, photographs and assistance with the historical material; Judith Hubbard MSN, for assistance with the psychological material; Maxie Davis PhD MD, for his assistance with radiation physics, and Richard Kerr-Wilson FRCS(Ed) MRCOG, for his suggestions in regard to syntax and vocabulary. We thank Jean Elliott and Katherine Raley for their untiring efforts in organizing the reference material and in typing the monograph.

We are particularly indebted to our colleague, Kenneth D. Hatch MD for his devotion to the care of our patients with cervix cancer and for his many contributions to our understanding of this disease. We are also grateful to Peyton T. Taylor MD, J. Max Austin Jr MD, Edward E. Partridge MD and William J Mann Jr MD for their collaboration in past years. We are especially indebted to Hazel Gore MB BS for maintaining such a high standard of gynaecological pathology, and for her overall support of our efforts.

Finally, we wish to thank Charles E. Flowers MD, our Departmental Chairman, for his support, and for his dedication to excellence in the medical care of women.

Birmingham, Alabama, 1983   H.M.S.
                                                             J.W.O.

Contents

1

Carcinoma of the uterine cervix: historical aspects and epidemiology

The first reference to gynaecology as a recognised and practised field of medicine was by the ancient Egyptians. The Kahun papyrus (2000 BC), was devoted in large part to gynaecological medicine. As with other papyri, descriptions of surgical techniques were absent, and there was no specific reference to cancer. The writing of Hippocrates (approximately 450 BC), included a description of diseases of women. It was this work that first mentioned cancer of the uterus and described a gloomy prognosis. The Hindus (5th century BC) were thought to have excelled at surgical technique, and existing texts suggest that they performed procedures for the removal of tumours. One of these texts included a chapter devoted to the diseases of the generative organs, describing tumours of the vagina and cervix. The Romans also practised gynaecology and it is thought that their knowledge was largely gained from Greece and Alexandria. The works of Galen and Celsus suggest that vaginal specula were used as early as the 1st century AD. Two specula were found in Pompeii and Herculaneum, cities which had been destroyed by an eruption of Mt Vesuvius in 79 AD. Cancer of the uterus was described by Galen in his work *De morbis mulierum*, and his prognosis was similar to that of Hippocrates.

Aetius of Amida, a physician who practised in Alexandria in the 6th century AD, is said to have had dissecting rooms. He published four books collectively known as *Medici graeci tetrabiblos*. In the fourth discourse of the fourth book, 'On the rationale of conception and parturition and diseases of women, especially those of the uterus and mamma . . .' he describes the structure and function of the uterus and ovaries with a degree of accuracy that indicates an in depth knowledge of anatomy and physiology. One chapter, 'De Cancris Uteri', written by Archigenes, includes descriptions of the appearance of the cervix, the symptoms of pain, discharge and bleeding, and categorises uterine cancer into ulcerative and non-ulcerative types.

Little was written about cervical cancer until the time of the Renaissance. *The medieval woman's guide to health* (early 15th century) includes this information, 'cancers and festerings of the womb come

1

from old injuries of the womb that have not healed well, but that kind of sickness we will hardly mention because doctors say that, with regard to hidden cancers, it is better that they should be uncured rather than cured or treated. Nevertheless, this ointment is good for such things and for itching and blisters in the uterus.' A recipe for ointment follows, with which the patient was to be anointed 'inside'. Ambroïse Paré (1510–1590), eminent in the history of both gynaecology and surgery, recommended use of the vaginal speculum to expose and evaluate the malignant cervix. Astruc (1762) in *A treatise on the diseases of women* described uterine cancer and recommended methods of treatment. In 1793, Baillie, in his textbook of morbid anatomy included descriptions of diseases of the uterus and cervix, and gave a detailed account of cancer of the cervix. An excerpt from his text included this description, 'There is no enlargement of the uterus; ulceration continues until a great part of the uterus is destroyed. The disease begins in the cervix, and when it has made a great progress, the contiguous parts, as the rectum and the urinary bladder, are often involved in it'.

John Clarke in 1812 reported a peculiar degeneration of the cervix which he labelled 'cauliflower execrescence'. Although this condition had been described by other physicians, there remained doubt as to the nature of the tumour and its correct classification. Observations were based on macroscopic appearance and used nomenclature such as 'schirrous enlargement' and 'cervical ulceration'. Although Rudolf Virchow was said to have been the first to make the association between these conditions and cervical cancer, R. Hooper (1832) first published it. J. H. Bennett further described the differentiation between benign and malignant cervical changes in 1845. Sarcomatous lesions were distinguished from epithelial lesions, and a classification of cervical diseases evolved. The advent of the technique for light microscopic examination of tissues led to the publication of a more precise classification of cervical cancer by T. Gaillard (1872).

In addition to the recognition and classification of cervical cancer at this time, some observations were also made regarding its incidence. In 1844, Samuel Ashwell (Guy's Hospital, London) observed that the majority of the patients with cervical cancer were 'dark complexioned.' In 1872, the deaths from cervical cancer in black and white women in South Carolina (USA) were reported. It was apparent that the mortality rates were higher in black women.

Theories concerning the possible causes of cervical cancer were also recorded. Many physicians in the early 19th century shared the opinion that the disease was stress related, however others suggested that injuries, particularly those related to parturition, preceded cancer. Von Scanzoni (1861) who shared the beliefs of the latter group, was the first to observe that the disease was more frequent in city dwellers, and thus possibly related to the manner of living. His ideas concerning the 'excessive sexual excitation', which he considered a feature of women with the disease, coincided with Victorian moral ideas of the time. Other factors included cervical inflammation, the abuse of alcohol, the abuse of purgative medicines and the presence of haemorrhoids. Thomas (1872), C. H. Moore and Robin believed in a constitutional factor, but others regarded the disease as dependent on local factors.

By the beginning of the 20th century, it was a widely held opinion that untreated cervical lacerations were an important aetiological factor in development of cervical cancer. This theory was supported by the observations of many gynaecologists who noted cervical cancer to be rare in nulliparous women. It was thought that heredity, injury, irritation, occupation, stress and race were predisposing factors and that cervicitis, erosions and unhealed lacerations were precancerous conditions. Many physicians advocated prompt treatment of these conditions to prevent the development of cancer. The importance of early diagnosis was recognised and the investigation of early symptoms such as abnormal bleeding and discharge was advocated. J. H. Carstens advocated the education of women to recognize symptoms and to seek advice promptly. While some physicians recognised the importance of light microscopy as an aid to diagnosis, others felt that this technique was unreliable. During the first half of the 20th century, there developed an increasing awareness of the various forms of pelvic cancer and their histological diagnosis and classification. Emil Novak made a major contribution to the subject of tumour pathology with publications on the diagnosis of early cervical cancer and its differentiation from pseudomalignant inflammatory lesions.

The regular examination of those women considered to be in a high-risk category was advocated at this time. The Schiller test and microscopic examination of biopsy specimens from suspicious areas of epithelium were employed. The technique of colposcopy, first introduced by Von Hinselmann in 1925, subsequently developed into a widely used tool for the diagnosis of cervical cancer in Europe. The cytological smear, first described in 1943 by Papanicolaou & Traut, provided an economical method to screen large numbers of women for cervical cancer. These two methods of detection developed on opposite sides of the Atlantic Ocean and the benefits of combined use were not appreciated for a quarter of a century.

TREATMENT

The earliest specific reference to treatment of uterine cancer is recorded in the works of Hippocrates. Advanced disease was recognised as incurable, and the only treatment was one of local fumigation for symptomatic relief. Aetius indicated that the disease could be 'mitigated and alleviated' by utilising baths, poultices and irrigations consisting of various herbs and other concoctions.

Advocacy of surgical treatment began in the 16th century, when Ambroïse Paré recommended amputation of the cancerous cervix as treatment. This procedure was first successfully performed by Tulpius of Amsterdam in 1552. Astruc's treatise of 1762 describes non-surgical methods of treatment; blood letting, purging, control of the diet and direct injection into the tumour with such things as an extract of nightshade were recommended. Narcotics, such as opium, were given internally or injected directly into the uterus for relief of pain. Some of these techniques, though ineffective and potentially harmful, persisted into the 19th century. In 1837, Duparcque advocated the application of leeches to the cervix. At this same time, some physicians favoured the application of red hot irons or other powerful caustics. In the latter part of the 19th century local applications of gold and zinc chloride, creosote and nitric acid were advocated as therapy. Injections of silver nitrate, mercuric chloride and pure alcohol into the parametrial tissues were also used.

Advocates of surgical procedures in the latter part of the 18th century and the early part of the 19th century reported techniques of two basic types, amputation of the cervix and vaginal hysterectomy. Between 1801–1808 Osiander performed excision of the cervix in eight patients. L. H. Struve, a pupil of Osiander, presented a dissertation in 1802, outlining the procedure and advocating its use as a treatment for cervical malignancy. Between 1810 and 1840, many reports of cervical amputation using specially designed instruments appeared, some of these claiming cures. However, the survival rate was so poor that in 1846 C. D. Meigs commented, 'If the cervix was cut off and the woman recovered, it affords the most uncontestable proof that the operation was unnecessary'.

In 1813 C. J. M. Langenbeck performed a vaginal hysterectomy for malignancy. Sauter performed the same operation in 1821. In 1856, Charles West reviewed the literature and reported 25 authentic cases of vaginal hysterectomy for cervical malignancy. Twenty-two of these patients died postoperatively from shock, haemorrhage and peritonitis. The high mortality rate led one surgeon, Colombat de L'Isere, to comment, 'This statistical and funereal record of extirpations of the uterus is fitter than any course of reasoning to deter the practitioner from so redoubtable an attempt'. Because of the high mortality, surgical treatment temporarily fell into disfavour.

The 1870s saw the resumption of surgical treatment for cervical carcinoma. In 1878, W. A. Freund performed a total abdominal hysterectomy, using anaesthesia and antiseptic measures while paying careful attention to hemostasis. By 1882, 95 patients treated by this surgical procedure had been reported. Of the 95 cases, 65 died as a result of the surgery, while 30 survived to die later from recurrence of the disease. These results and those of McGraw in 1849, who reported the effects of limited surgery, strongly suggested that more extensive surgical procedures were necessary if the disease was to be completely extirpated. Investigators at this time also described local and lymphatic spread of the disease, and following experimental studies E. Ries in 1895 suggested the feasibility of total hysterectomy combined with the removal of the iliac lymph nodes and part of the broad ligament as a primary surgical procedure. However, he performed this operation only on cadavers and animals. In the same year such procedures were first performed on living patients in Germany by C. Rumpf and in America by J. G. Clark, a resident physician at Johns Hopkins Hospital. During a 12-month period, Clark performed 12 such operations, each with some technical variation. Lymph nodes were removed in some cases, while in others he widely excised the vaginal cuff, removing as much parametrium as possible. The technical difficulties associated with the operation, the resultant high urinary fistula and postoperative mortality rates led to the temporary abandonment of this technique in the United States. A radical resection of cervical cancer was first performed in 1898 by Ernst Wertheim, who reported his technique in 1900.

Wilhelm Roentgen discovered X-rays in 1895, and they were immediately applied to diagnosis of fractures and other medical uses. Therapeutic use of X-rays began with treatment of dermatoses and, in 1899, skin cancer. The discovery of radium in 1898 by the Curies was followed by its first use in treatment of cancer by Danysz in 1903. The first radium hospital, The Radiumhemmet, opened in 1910. In 1912, Wertheim published the results of 500 radical hysterectomy operations. His operative mortality rate was 18.6% and 31.5% of his patients had significant surgical complications. Wertheim's procedure emphasized removal of the uterus and the medial portion of the parametrium and paracolpos. The pelvic lymph nodes were removed only if enlarged and suspicious for metastases. The next year, Wertheim was to have presented his operative experience at a meeting in Halle an der Saale, but after the radium therapy results were presented, the less morbid technique appeared so superior that Wertheim withdrew his paper.

Schauta (1908) described a vaginal approach for radical extirpation of the uterus and parametrium, an operation he devised in 1901. This operation remained popular in Europe, but never gained widespread use in the United States, possibly because of the inability to dissect pelvic nodes by this route. The advantage of this technique over the abdominal approach was a lower (3–4%) operative mortality rate.

In J. G. Clark's report of 1913, he acknowledged that Wertheim should receive the credit for proceeding with and simplifying the radical abdominal operation. Clark presented a comparison of the results of the different surgical procedures, including Wertheim's abdominal hysterectomy, and the simple and radical vaginal hysterectomy techniques. While radical abdominal surgery resulted in the highest cure rate, it also had the highest mortality rate. In his concluding remarks, Clark expressed concern over the technical difficulties and high mortality rate associated with radical abdominal surgery. He was optimistic, however, that future developments in technique would lead to more satisfactory results.

When compared with the results of radiation therapy, radical surgery did not seem to be a safe and effective form of treatment until the reports of Bonney in 1935 and Meigs in 1944. Between 1907 and 1935, Bonney performed 483 radical operations. His operative mortality was 20% for his first 100 operations, but fell to 9.5% for his last 200 cases. His 5-year cure rate was only 20%; however these rates were higher when patients lost to follow-up or dead from other causes were excluded.

F. J. Taussig (1943) reported the results of combined radiation therapy and iliac lymphadenectomy for cases of cervical cancer with involvement of the medial parametrium and upper third of the vagina; his operative mortality rate was 1.7% for 175 cases treated between 1930 and 1942. The 5-year survival rate was 38.6%, compared with 22.9% for 118 cases treated solely with radiation therapy. With the low primary mortality rate and the relatively high 5-year survival rate, Taussig was convinced of the value of this procedure.

J. C. Meigs (1944) reported a 5-year survival rate of 75% in patients with early invasive carcinoma treated surgically, and a reduced rate of complications that compared favourably to that of radiation therapy. He was a proponent of pelvic lymph node dissection, using the technique described by Taussig. In 1944 and 1951, Meigs reported the results of operations combining radical parametrial resection, hysterectomy and pelvic lymphadenectomy. In spite of the fact that a quarter of the women had stage II disease, 75% of them survived 5 years. He had no operative deaths in his last 100 patients. Metastases in lymph nodes were encountered in 22.4% of patients, which markedly decreased their survival (26.3%). Meigs' operative technique is that used currently by gynaecologic oncologists and differs from Wertheim's in the wider resection of the parametrial tissues and in the more thorough pelvic lymphadenectomy.

Brunschwig (1948) reported an ultra-radical operation for the treatment of advanced and recurrent cancer which he first performed in 1946. It consisted of an en bloc resection of the uterus, cervix, vagina and the adjacent pelvic organs with urinary and faecal diversion. Initially there was high mortality and morbidity and few survivors. In ensuing years, improvements in perioperative intensive care, diversionary procedures and methods of pelvic reconstruction have reduced operative mortality and increased survival rates. Pelvic exenteration has thus taken its place in the management of the patients who develop only central pelvic recurrence. Improved radiotherapeutic technique and equipment have reduced the need for this operation in recent years. High energy teletherapy equipment, introduced in the 1950s, has led to improved pelvic control of tumours with fewer complications.

Controversy between those who advocate radiation therapy and those who recommend radical pelvic surgery for primary treatment of early invasive carcinoma of the cervix has persisted through the years. However, a continuing process of advancement in new and existing techniques, coupled with a greater understanding of tumour biology, has led to a more individualised approach with the recognition that both techniques have a place in the treatment of this disease.

EPIDEMIOLOGICAL STUDIES

Rotkin (1973) reported that the first observations relating to the incidence, distribution and possible causative factors of carcinoma of the uterine cervix were made in 1842 by Rigoni-Stern, an Italian physician who examined the records of deaths in Verona from 1760 to 1839. He noted that the prevalence of uterine cancer was higher in married than in unmarried women, and that the rates increased steadily between the ages of 30 and 60 years. He also noted that uterine cancer was less common in unmarried women and extremely rare in nuns (a finding confirmed by reports published in the 1950s). In contrast, he noted that breast cancer was common in both of these groups of women.

Uterine cancer was one of the most prevalent neoplasms reported in Western Europe during the mid-19th century. It is thought that the cervix was the primary site in most of these cases. An increased risk was noted in the lower socio-economic classes, among multiparous women and in non-white women.

In 1919 Vineberg indicated that Jewish women had a less than average incidence of cervical cancer despite being a part of the lower socio-economic classes residing in New York City. From his case records between 1893 and 1906, Vineberg observed a 20-fold difference in the number of cases of cervical cancer in non-Jewish as opposed to Jewish women. Later studies on Jewish and non-Jewish populations conducted in the United States, Europe and Israel have also confirmed his findings. The inference that the circumcision status of the males in the population may be a contributing factor prompted the examination of other ethnic groups such as Moslems, who also practise circumcision. The results of these investigations suggest that the variation in incidence between the compared ethnic groups cannot be attributed solely to circumcision status but may be due to associated cultural differences or other factors.

In a World Health Organization publication (Waterhouse, 1976), the incidence of invasive cancer of the cervix was presented as a cumulative rate which was age standardised and which was expressed as a percentage lifetime risk from birth to age 74 (Fig. 1.1). Colombia had the highest and Spain had the lowest incidence rate. The variation between different areas within the countries is also demonstrated. A relatively high incidence is seen among those of Spanish origin in El Paso, Texas (USA) compared with other Caucasians in the same area. Black women residing in Detroit, Michigan (USA) have a higher rate of

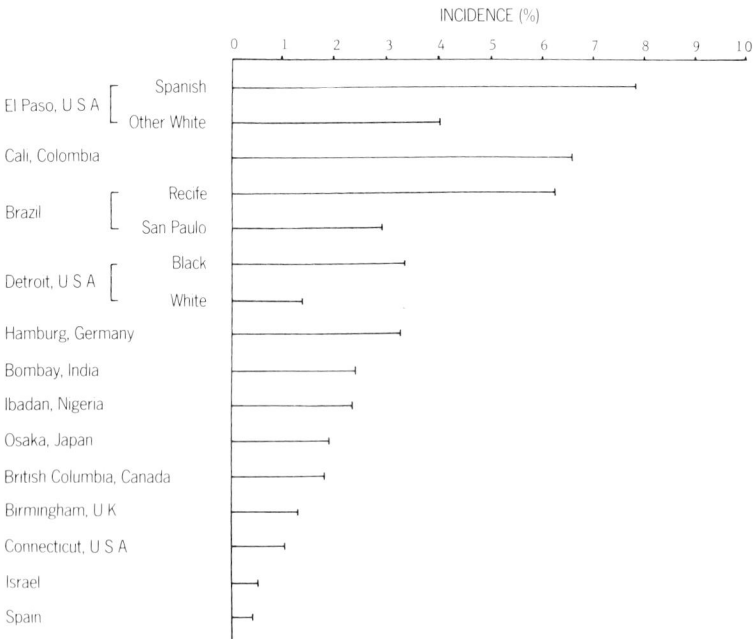

Fig. 1.1 Cumulative incidence rates for cancer of the cervix (birth to 74 years)

cervical cancer than Caucasians in the same area. A similar difference in incidence rates in two areas of Brazil also exists. The reasons for these varying rates are unclear, but speak for cultural or genetic factors, rather than locale.

In the United States, there is a significant difference in the incidence of cervical squamous cell carcinoma in black and white women. For example, in Birmingham, Alabama (USA) the incidence of squamous cell carcinoma was 20.7 per 100 000 in white women and 34.3 per 100 000 in black women. For the entire country, the average annual age adjusted incidence rate for squamous cell carcinoma was 13.7 per 100 000 for white women and 30.54 per 100 000 for black women. When age specific incidence rates for squamous cell carcinoma were considered, the rates for white women were seen to increase from the second to the fourth decade and to plateau thereafter whereas for black women the incidence rose steadily up to age 85 years. No reason is known for this difference. Henson (1977) also compared the age-adjusted and age-specific rates for the USA and England. The age-adjusted incidence rates were reported to be almost identical, whereas the age-specific rates increased at an earlier age in the USA when compared with England. (During the second decade of life, the incidence rate for cervix cancer per 100 000 was 12.12 in the United States and 1.9 in England). Henson suggested that these differences were probably a result of the screening programmes employed in the USA.

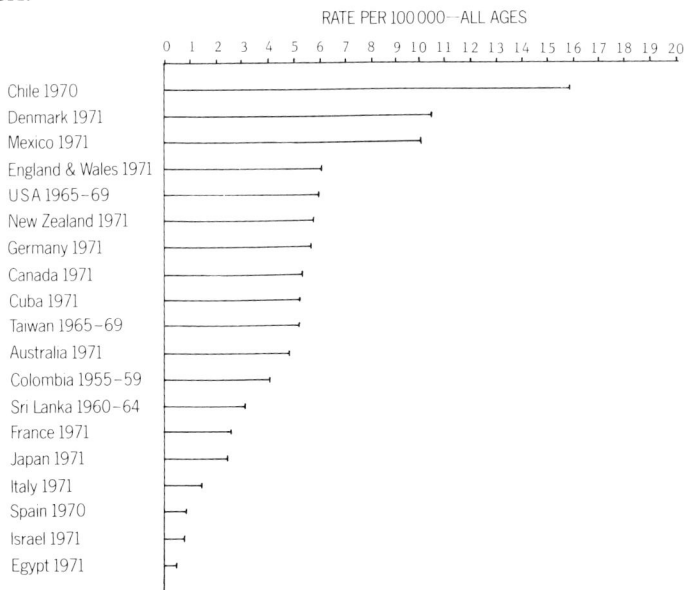

Fig. 1.2 Mortality rates for cancer of the cervix (age-standardised mortality rates per 100 000 women)

In another World Health Organization report (Hill 1975), the mortality rates for cancer of the cervix were published, using age-standardised figures (Fig. 1.2). Chile exhibits the highest mortality rate (15.7 per 100 000 women) while Egypt, Israel and Spain (0.3, 0.8 and 0.8 per 100 000 respectively) have low rates. Mortality rates presumably relate to stage of disease at time of treatment, as well as the availability and quality of treatment.

Cole, in an overview of cancer epidemiology (1978), reported the mortality rates in the United States. For cervical cancer, the mortality rate per 100 000 was 3.8 for whites and 11.5 for blacks. The US region with the highest mortality rate among whites only, based on figures from the 1950s and 1960s, was Appalachia. Figures published by Kessler in 1974, reviewing time trends for mortality and incidence in the USA between 1950 and 1969, suggest a decrease in the death rate from cervical cancer. This coincided with an increased incidence of carcinoma in situ, especially in women less than 50 years of age.

More specific epidemiological studies, in which the incidence of carcinoma of the cervix has been related to certain variable factors including race, communities and ethnic groups exhibiting cultural differences, socioeconomic status, pregnancy, sexual behaviour and

Table 1.1 Chronology of the diagnosis and treatment of cancer of the cervix

2000 BC	Gynaecologic medicine described in Egyptian papyrus
450 BC	Hippocrates referred to cancer of the uterus
600 AD	Aetius of Amida described cancer of the uterus
1575	Ambroise Paré recommended amputation of cancerous cervix
1652	Tulpius performed cervical amputation as treatment
1793	Baillie described invasion of bladder and rectum by cervical cancer
1813	Langenbeck performed vaginal hysterectomy for treatment
1895	Clark and Rumpf performed extended abdominal hysterectomy with removal of the pelvic nodes as treatment
	Roentgen discovered X-rays
1898	Wertheim devised an extended abdominal hysterectomy and node sampling as treatment
	Marie and Pierre Curie discovered radium
1899	Sjoegren and Stenbeck first used X-rays for treatment of cancer
1903	Danysz first used radium for treatment
1908	Schauta performed radical vaginal hysterectomy for treatment
1910	First Radium Hospital opened in Stockholm, Sweden
1925	Von Hinselmann introduced colposcopy for diagnosis
1935	Bonney reported improved results with radical surgical treatment
1943	Papanicolaou and Traut developed exfoliative cytology for diagnosis
1948	Alexander Brunschwig reported ultraradical surgical approach for advanced and recurrent cancer
1951	Meigs proved that a radical surgical approach for early stage cancer could equal radiation results with acceptable complications
1951	Cobalt 60 teletherapy introduced
1954	Linear accelerators introduced
1963	Suit introduced afterloading intracavitary applicator

venereal disease have been reported. In the USA a higher incidence of cervical cancer was observed in black populations, in urban populations, in low socioeconomic classes, in women with numerous pregnancies, in married women, in those with a history of venereal disease, in those with an early onset of sexual activity, and in those with numerous sexual partners. These factors have been examined for their possible aetiological significance and some of them are highly correlated. The most important covariable appears to be early onset of sexual activity. Thus Kessler (1974) concluded that 'several decades of clinical observations and epidemiological investigations have confirmed that squamous carcinoma of the cervix behaves as a venereal disease'.

BIBLIOGRAPHY

Anderson M C 1976 The aetiology and pathology of cancer of the cervix. Clinics in Obstetrics and Gynaecology 3: 317-337
Astruc 1762 A treatise on the diseases of women. (Translated from the French original and printed in London for J. Nocuse)
Bonney V 1935 The treatment of carcinoma of the cervix by Wertheim's operation. American Journal of Obstetrics and Gynecology 30: 815-830
Brunschwig A 1948 Complete excision of pelvic viscera for advanced carcinoma. Cancer 1: 177-
Castiglioni A 1941 In: Krumbhaar E B (ed) A history of medicine. Alfred A. Knopf, New York
Christenson A, Lange P, Nielsen E 1964 Surgery and radiotherapy for invasive cancer of the cervix. Acta obstetrica et gynecologica scandinavica 43: 59-87
Clark J G 1913 The radical abdominal operation for cancer of the uterus. Surgery, Gynecology and Obstetrics 16: 255-265
Cole P, Repetto F 1978 Cancer epidemiology. A summary of current information. Unit of Epidemiology and Biostatistics, International Agency for Research in Cancer, Lyon, France
Cullhed S 1978 Carcinoma cervicis uteri stages I and IA. Acta obstetrica et gynecologica scandinavica (supplement) 75: 1-28
Deeley T J, 1976 Cancer of the cervix uteri — an epidemiological survey. Clinical Radiology 27: 43-51
Donaldson R 1853 The practical application of the microscope to the diagnosis of cancer. American Journal of Medical Science 25: 43-70
Gellman D D 1976 Cervical cancer screening programs. I. Epidemiology and natural history of carcinoma of the cervix. Canadian Medical Association Journal 114: 1003-1012
Henson D, Tanone R 1977 An epidemiological study of cancer of the cervix, vagina and vulva based on the Third National Cancer Survey in the United States. American Journal of Obstetrics and Gynecology 129: 525-532
Hill G B 1975 Mortality from malignant neoplasms of the uterus since 1950. World Health Organization vol 28, no. 8, p 323-338
Holleb A I (ed) 1982 Ca — a cancer journal for clinicians. American Cancer Society, New York, vol 32
Jameson E (ed) 1936 Clio medica, gynecology and obstetrics. Paul B. Hoeber, New York
Kessler I I 1974 Cervical cancer epidemiology in historical perspective. Journal of Reproductive Medicine 12: 173-185

Kessler I I 1981 Histological concepts in cervical carcinogenesis. Gynecologic Oncology 12: S7–S24

Leonardo R 1944 History of gynecology. Froben Press, New York

Lerner H M, Jones H W, Hill C C 1980 Radical surgery for the treatment of early invasive cervical carcinoma (stage IB). Obstetrics and Gynecology 56: 413–418

Mann M 1887 A system of gynecology. Lea Bros, Pennsylvania

Masterson J G 1967 The role of surgery in the treatment of early carcinoma of the cervix. Clinical Obstetrics and Gynecology 10: 922–939

Mattingly R F 1977 Te Linde's operative gynecology. J B Lippincott, Philadelphia

Maughs G M B 1884 What the ancients knew concerning obstetrics and gynecology. Journal of the American Medical Association 2: 225–233

Meigs C D 1854 Carcinoma of the womb. In: Woman: her diseases and remedies. Blanchard and Lea, Pennsylvania, p 307–316

Meigs J C 1951 Radical hysterectomy with bilateral pelvic lymph node dissections. A report of one hundred patients operated on five or more years ago. American Journal of Obstetrics and Gynecology 63: 854–866

Mettler C 1947 History of medicine. Blakiston Company, Philadelphia

Papanicolaou G N, Traut H F 1943 Diagnosis of uterine cancer by the vaginal smear. Commonwealth Fund, New York

Ricci J V 1945 100 years of gynaecology. Blakiston Company, Philadelphia

Ricci J V 1950 The genealogy of gynaecology. Blakiston Company, Philadelphia

Rotkin I D 1973 A comparison review of key epidemiological studies in cervical cancer related to current searches for transmissible agents. Cancer Research 33: 1353–1367

Rowland B (translator) 1981 Medieval woman's guide to health. Croom Helm, London

Schmitz H G 1955 Lest we forget. American Journal of Obstetrics and Gynecology 69: 467–49

Suit H D, Moore E B, Fletcher G H et al 1963 Modification of Fletcher ovoid system for afterloading, using standard-sized radium tubes. Radiology 81: 126

Taussig F J 1943 Iliac lymphadenectomy for group II cancer of the cervix. American Journal of Obstetrics and Gynecology 45: 733–758

Terris M, Wilson F, Nelson J H Jr 1980 Comparative epidemiology of invasive carcinoma of the cervix, carcinoma in situ and cervical dysplasia. American Journal of Epidemiology 112: 253–257

Waterhouse, Muir, Correa, Powell (eds) 1976 Cancer incidence in 5 continents. World Health Organization vol III, no 15, IARC Scientific Publications

2

Pathological features

Surgical pathologists are key members of the group of physicians who diagnose and treat cervical cancer. Indeed, they may be considered the most important persons involved since any misinterpretation on their part is likely to be compounded by the clinicians. The pathologist is often confronted with and asked to make crucial decisions concerning presence or absence of invasive tumour, cell type and grade, evidence of tumour virulence, etc., and is expected to guide the clinicians in their decisions, which implies familiarity with all of the pertinent literature concerning treatment results as applied to cervical cancer. For all of these reasons, it is mandatory that surgical pathologist and oncologist work closely together in order that each may learn from the other and that clinical decisions are made in a careful, deliberate way so as to provide the greatest opportunity for a woman to survive the threat to her life from the neoplastic process.

PRECLINICAL CANCER

Preclinical or micro-invasive cancers, although constituting only a small part of cervical cancers, present a considerable problem of diagnosis for the pathologist and of treatment for the clinician. Creasman (1973) encountered only 98 examples of micro-invasion (depth of invasion of 5 mm or less) in a series of 2410 patients with invasive cervical cancer accumulated over a period of 26 years. These cases represented 4.1% of the invasive lesions in his series. Our experience is similar; using a 3 mm depth of invasion as the definition for micro-invasion, we have encountered 38 micro-invasive lesions in 1200 invasive cancer patients in 11 years (3.2%). Fennell (1978) reported a 3.8% incidence of micro-invasion in conisations performed for carcinoma in situ; we have encountered micro-invasion in 6.2% of 610 conisations performed as part of the evaluation of women with atypical cervical cytology.

The first responsibility of the pathologist is to determine the presence of any invasion in specimens submitted to him from patients with preclinical neoplasms. In former years, this was his only obligation, since patients with even focal invasion were treated by radiation or radical surgery. As time elapsed, it became apparent that many of the patients with the earliest forms of invasion did not have metastatic spread to lymph nodes, did not have recurrence and had survival rates approaching 100%. It seemed logical to separate out the early lesions that acted biologically like intra-epithelial neoplasia, in order to offer more conservative therapy. Unfortunately, the terminology used to describe stage IA cancer has not been uniform, and even the current (1976) FIGO staging for cancer of the cervix is not precise enough to guide the clinician in the treatment of the earliest forms of invasive cancer. FIGO stage IA is defined as 'micro-invasion (early stromal invasion)', terms which imply different things to different physicians. For the earliest form of invasion Lohe and associates (1978) recommended the term 'early stromal invasion', defined as stromal invasion to 1 mm by isolated projections arising from the base of neoplastic epithelium (Fig. 2.1). This entity is well documented and is only rarely associated with node metastasis (Table 2.1). Lohe concluded that the risk of dying from early stromal invasion, regardless of treatment, was very small since none of a collected series of 285 patients

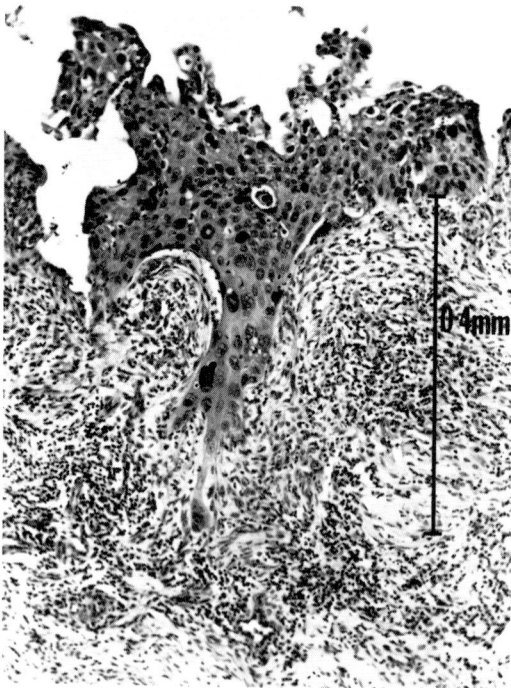

Fig. 2.1 Focal micro-invasion (early stromal invasion) occurring as an isolated tongue penetrating the stroma less than 1 mm. (H&E × 103)

Table 2.1 Positive nodes in focal micro-invasion (early stromal invasion)

Author	Year	No. of pts.	No. pos.	% pos.
Averette*	1976	162	0	0
Lohe*	1978	159	1	0.6
Hasumi	1980	61	1	1.6
Totals		382	2	0.5

*Collected series

from six gynaecology departments in Germany and only four of 895 collected from the literature died of cancer (0.34%). Wilkinson (1978) used the term 'borderline micro-invasion' for this lesion, describing it as invasion of 1 mm or less from the basement membrane of the epithelial surface immediately adjacent to the site of infiltration, without lymph-vascular space involvement. He observed 29 patients with this lesion treated by conservative hysterectomy, and none of them developed recurrent carcinoma. This entity comprised 4.8% of in situ carcinomas in his series and 27.1% of his cases of micro-invasion fell into this 'borderline' group.

The term 'microcarcinoma' was introduced by Mestwerdt in 1947. While early stromal invasion is not visible when the microscope slide is held up to the light, a microcarcinoma is a small visible lesion with both width and depth (Fig. 2.2). Burghardt (1979), using a three-dimensional volumetric technique, reported that microcarcinomas with a volume of

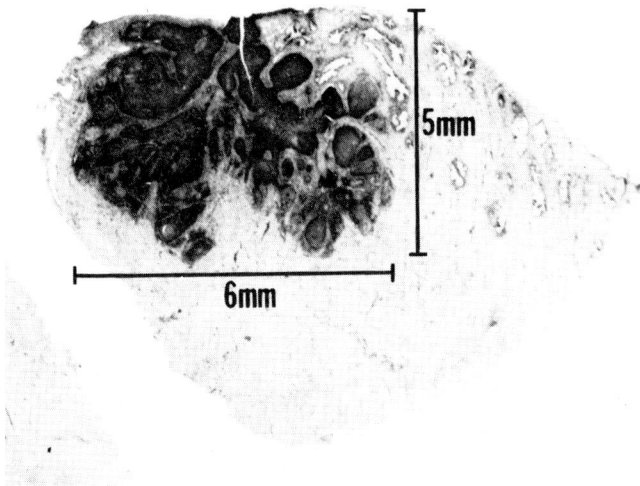

Fig. 2.2 A microcarcinoma consisting of coalescing masses of infiltrating tumour, often called a 'confluent' lesion. (H&E ×7.5)

Table 2.2 Positive nodes in microcarcinoma $\leqslant$ 5 mm depth

Author	Year	No. of pts.	No. pos.	% pos.
Foushee	1969	29	1	3.4
Mussey	1969	53	1	1.9
Sidhu	1970	41	2	5.0
Creasman	1973	19	1	5.3
Roche	1975	30	0	0
Leman	1976	47	0	0
Hasumi	1980	135	5	3.7
Boyce	1981	47	2	4.3
Totals		401	12	3.0

less than 400 mm³ do not metastasise to nodes. Lohe (1978) reported no positive nodes using a definition for microcarcinoma of width and length of up to 10 mm and a depth of penetration of 5 mm or less. Microcarcinoma expressed in only one measurement (depth of 5 mm or less) has a small, but appreciable risk of node metastases (Table 2.2). In spite of these precise definitions and the data on biological behaviour of these lesions, most authors fail to distinguish the two types of micro-invasion. Pathologists cannot routinely perform step sections that permit three-dimensional measurements; they rarely describe two dimensions, preferring a depth measurement only or using non-specific terms such as 'superficial', or 'confluent'. More pathologists are appreciating the importance of a width measurement as well as a depth measurement. Sedlis (1979), reporting the data from the Gynecologic Oncology Group (USA), stated that 43% of the patients with 'micro-invasion' had lesions wider than 4 mm and 22% of them had lesions wider than 8 mm. Even very superficial lesions may have a measurable width (Fig. 2.3).

The term 'confluence', meaning coalescence of invasion tongues, is widely used to describe micro-invasive lesions, although the term is misunderstood and is variously said to be significant or insignificant in regard to prognosis. Hasumi (1980) reported that lesions up to 3 mm in penetration were confluent in 25 out of 106 patients. In spite of this, he found no metastasis in pelvic nodes in any of the 25 patients with confluence and only one involved node in 106 patients with lesions invading to 3 mm. Ruch (1976) studied 115 cases of micro-invasive carcinoma and reported that lesions less than 2 mm in depth were confluent in only 4% of the cases. It would seem, therefore, that most of his patients had lesions that could be termed early stromal invasion. Lesions with 2 to 5 mm of invasion in Ruch's series had confluence in 39% of the cases and in those with 6 to 10 mm of invasion, 92% were confluent. Duncan (1982) found confluence in 8.9% of lesions up to 1

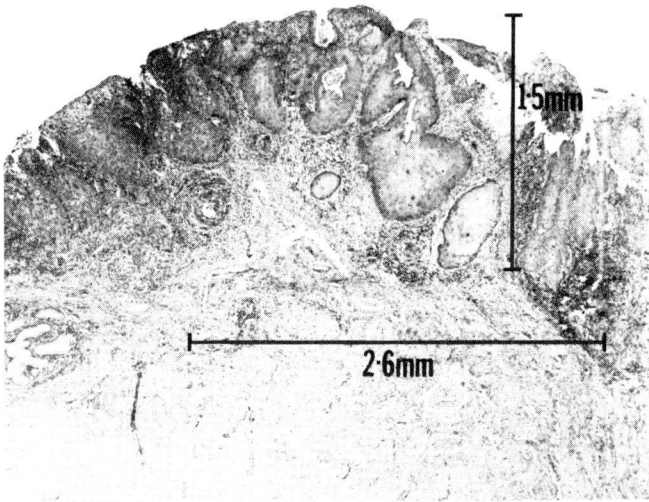

Fig. 2.3 A micro-invasive lesion measuring only 1.5 mm from surface to deepest penetration of the stroma with a measurable width of 2.6 mm. This illustrates the potential for lateral extension of very superficial lesions, and also illustrates the difficulty in measuring depth of invasion from the 'adjacent' basement membrane. (H&E ×25)

mm in depth, increasing to 14.3% of lesions invading 1 to 2 mm, and 75% in lesions 2 to 3 mm in depth. Sedlis (1979) reported confluence in 4% of lesions with invasion less than 1 mm, 32% in lesions 1 to 3 mm invasion, and 38% in lesions invading over 3 mm. Confluence per se does not imply that the tumour is more virulent, but indicates that the tumour volume is increasing. Currently, we use a width and a depth measurement and believe that references to tumour 'confluence' should be discontinued.

Much attention in recent years has been centred on whether radical treatment should be used when lesions invade to a depth beyond 1 mm, 3 mm, or 5 mm. Since there is a six-fold increase in positive nodes when comparing early stromal invasion to microcarcinoma (Tables 2.1, 2.2), the exact point at which one can neglect the lymph nodes and concentrate only on the primary lesion is of clinical importance. The Society of Gynecologic Oncologists (1974) adopted a definition of micro-invasion as invasion of the stroma in one or more places to a depth of 3 mm from the base of the epithelium without lymph-vascular space (LVS) involvement. Our practice for a number of years was to perform conservative hysterectomy as treatment for micro-invasion defined in this way, with one major exception: if confluence or tumour of measurable width was present, even in these superficial lesions, we performed an extended abdominal (modified radical) hysterectomy with lymphadenectomy. This is almost identical to the approach taken by

Yajima (1979) except that he did not perform lymphadenectomy in either group; he reported 5-year survival rates of almost 100% for both groups, which played down the importance of confluence in these superficial lesions. This work, the report by Hasumi (1980) and our own experience led to a change in management; we now ignore confluence and do not routinely perform a lymphadenectomy for lesions invading to a depth of 3 mm, unless obvious lymph-vascular space invasion is present. Hasumi reported a significant number of node metastases in lesions between 3 and 5 mm (13.8%). While this percentage is higher than we have encountered and that reported by others, we dissect pelvic nodes in lesions over 3 mm because of the increased risk of metastasis.

Much attention has focussed on the significance of lymph-vascular space (LVS) involvement in the preclinical lesions (Fig. 2.4). Duncan (1982) reported 5% LVS involvement in lesions invading to 1 mm and 27% LVS involvement in lesions invading between 1 and 3 mm. Leman (1976) found no LVS involvement in lesions invading to 1 mm but 26% invading from 1 to 3 mm and 43% invading between 3 and 5 mm. Roche (1975) observed that 57% of patients with lesions invading to 5 mm had LVS involvement if step sections were performed. While it can

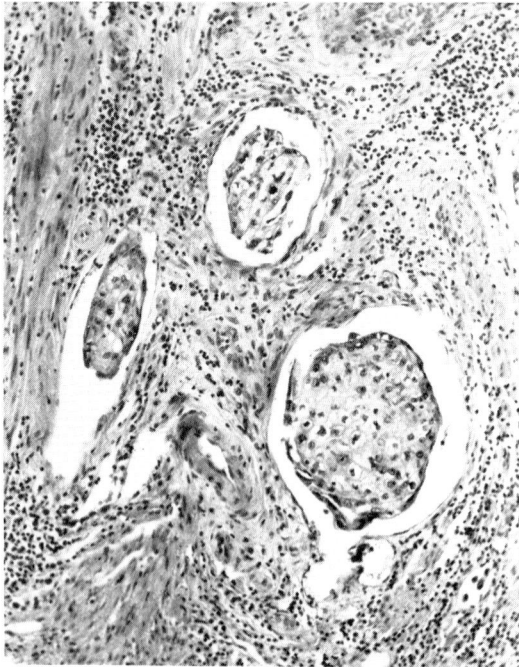

Fig. 2.4 Tumour present in endothelial lined spaces, presumably lymphatics. (H&E ×128)

be shown that tumour invasion into vascular spaces and blood vessels is associated with increased recurrence and death rates (Table 2.3), investigators such as Roche (1975) have tended to dismiss the significance of this finding in microscopic lesions invading to 5 mm. We feel that there is a considerable risk of recurrence or death even in these small lesions if LVS involvement is present and suggest that a modified hysterectomy and lymphadenectomy be performed on these patients. Lohe (1978) also recommended lymphadenectomy if LVS involvement was detected, although he stated that radical extirpation of the parametrial tissues was in no case indicated.

Table 2.3 Significance of lymph-vascular space involvement in microcarcinoma ≤ 5 mm depth

Author	Year	No. pts.	Recurrence	Deaths
Foushee	1969	7	1	1
Mussey	1969	19	2	1
Boyes	1970	12	1	1
Leman	1976	12	0	0
Burghardt	1979	53	2	1
Coppleson	1979	39	0	0
Iversen	1979	8	5	NS
Boyce	1981	10	3	1
Totals		160	14 (8.75%)	5 (3.1%)

Benson (1977) summarized the factors that affected the prevalence of positive nodes in reports about preclinical lesions. He stated that the rate of positive nodes was increased if all 'preclinical' lesions were included (rather than using strict microscopic criteria), if the diagnosis of micro-invasion was made by a small biopsy or an inadequate cone, i.e., if patients with more advanced tumours were included in the lymphadenectomy series. He pointed out that the prevalence of involved nodes is diminished if cases of 'questionable' invasion are included, if cases having LVS involvement are excluded, if patients with confluent growth patterns are excluded, and if external radiotherapy was given before lymphadenectomy. Benson emphasized the critical importance of reporting lesion size as defined by microscopic criteria. Since confusion exists in the literature, and inaccuracies of reporting data on this subject persist, a study group (Jordan 1982) met in October 1981 at the Royal College of Obstetricians and Gynaecologists and made the following observations and recommendations:

'Carcinoma of the cervix Stage Ia (micro-invasive carcinoma) is a histological diagnosis which should be made on a large biopsy which removes the whole lesion, preferably a cone biopsy.

Two groups should be recognised:
1. Early stromal invasion in which invasive buds are present either in continuity with an in situ lesion, or apparently separated cells not more than 1 mm from the nearest surface or crypt basement membrane.
2. Measurable lesions should be measured in two dimensions. The depth should be measured from the base of the epithelium from which it develops and should not exceed 5 mm, and the largest diameter should not exceed 10 mm on the section that shows the greatest extent.

When reporting Stage Ia lesions, the chosen depth and diameter for including the cases in the statistics should be given. Furthermore, the percentage of confluent lesions and of cases with involvement of endothelial lined spaces (vessels) should also be stated.'

Occult carcinomas are tumours originating within the endocervical canal, out of view of the clinician. They are ordinarily diagnosed by curettage performed because of abnormal bleeding or atypical Papanicolaou smears. Boronow (1977) demonstrated that the FIGO staging definition of stage IA used prior to 1976 was misleading about the incidence of positive nodes in stage IA because it grouped occult lesions with the microscopic lesions. Using this system, 9.4% of his stage IA patients had positive nodes. Using the modified FIGO system definition (1976) which separated occult lesions from the microscopic lesions, his stage IA patients (N = 35) had no positive nodes, while his IB occult group had 20.7% positive, similar to the rates usually quoted for clinical stage IB lesions.

CLINICAL INVASIVE CANCER

Henrikson (1960) in his classic study of the distribution of metastases in cancer of the cervix stated that 'cancer cells, regardless of the site of the primary lesion, the histologic grade, and the age and parity of the patient, can spread in any direction. The direction and the degree of spread are not predictable. The anterior and posterior spread is almost as frequent as the lateral extension. Thus, any attempt to remove all possible cancer-bearing tissue must include these areas.' Burghardt (1978), using large histological sections of radical hysterectomy specimens of 150 patients with cervical cancer, found medial parametrial involvement in 6.8% of patients in clinical stage IB and 23.1% and 19.3% involvement in clinical stage IIA and IIB respectively. In spite of this, he pointed out that the implication that tumour extends directly through the parametrium to the nodes is not true; parametrial involvement usually consists of spread to areas adjacent to the cervix, to parametrial vessels or to single parametrial nodes, none of which are palpable. Of 24 patients with histological parametrial involvement, only six had any direct extension from the cervical tumour, whereas the remainder had involved parametrial nodes, or tumour in parametrial blood vessels or lymphatics. Burghardt

Table 2.4 Stage IB, II: significance of lymph-vascular space involvement

Author	Year	No. of pts.	Stages	% Positive nodes		5-year survival	
				LVS involv.	No LVS involv.	LVS involv.	No LVS involv.
Gusberg**	1971	103	IB, IIA	44	4	–	–
Barber	1978	191	IB	–	–	59.4	90
Abdulhayoglu	1980	35	IB	60	20	–	–
Pagnini	1980	125	I–IV	–	–	47.2	83.3
Boyce	1981	139	IB	39	4	69	94
Baltzer**	1982	718	*	–	–	68.8	90.1
Burghardt	1982	–	IB	54.5	19.9	–	–

*Clinical stage not stated, but all observations were on extended hysterectomy specimens
**Lymphatic vessels only

Table 2.5 Most commonly involved node groups in stage I & II cancer of the cervix

Author	Year	Stage	No. of pts.	% Common iliac	% External iliac	% Obturator	% Hypogastric
Cherry	1953	I, II	213	14	47	20	7
Liu	1955	I, II	104	47	20.1	50	3.8
Plentl*	1971	*	744	13	23	19	17
Martimbeau	1982	IB	120	27	48	25	–
Totals			1181	17.9	29.6	22.5	13.7

*Collected series, stage not specified

believes that the palpable changes in the parametria that lead to the clinical designation of stage IIB are caused by shortening of the parametria brought about by the volume of cervical tumour or by inflammation simulating carcinomatous infiltration. When tumour involves the border zone between the cervix and the parametrium, the rate of pelvic node metastases increases from 15.7% to 47.8% and if there is further extension into the parametrium, the node involvement exceeds 80%. The size of the primary tumour was not found to correlate well with the number of lymph node groups involved.

Baltzer (1982) indicated that cervical squamous cell carcinoma expands as a closed, compact type of growth in most patients and observed that marked dissociation of tumour cells in the cervix of radical hysterectomy specimens is associated with a poorer survival rate.

Lymph-vascular space involvement

Lymph-vascular space involvement in the clinical stages of squamous cell carcinoma is associated with a significantly higher rate of pelvic node metastases and a significantly lower 5-year survival rate (Table 2.4). Baltzer (1982) found 50% LVS involvement in his series of 718 patients, and noted that such involvement has been reported in 25% to 50% of stage IB and II patients by other investigators. He found blood vessel invasion in 9.6% of specimens whereas other authors have reported blood vessels involved in up to 29% of patients. Whereas 31% of his patients with lymphatic vessel involvement died of cancer, 70% died if tumour was demonstrated in blood vessels.

The most commonly involved node groups in cancer of the cervix are the external iliac, the obturator, the common iliac, and the hypogastric nodes (Table 2.5, Fig. 2.5). The nodes are involved in sequence, i.e., the external iliac and internal iliacs, the common iliac, the aortic. In our experience, paracervical and presacral nodes are very rarely encountered. Cherry (1953) described two routes of lymphatic drainage from the cervix to the common iliac and para-aortic nodes, i.e., by the paracervical, external iliac and obturator groups and by the hypogastric node groups, and noted that the former mode of spread was more common. In studying 213 operative specimens, she concluded that rarely was the pattern of spread anomalous, i.e., the intermediate nodes negative and the higher nodes involved. We have not encountered such 'skip' metastases, although it has been reported in autopsy series.

Endometrial involvement

Cancer of the cervix extends into the lower uterine segment or into the endometrial cavity in 2–8.7% of patients, according to Perez (1977) and Spanos (1981). Both of these authors concluded that the prognosis was

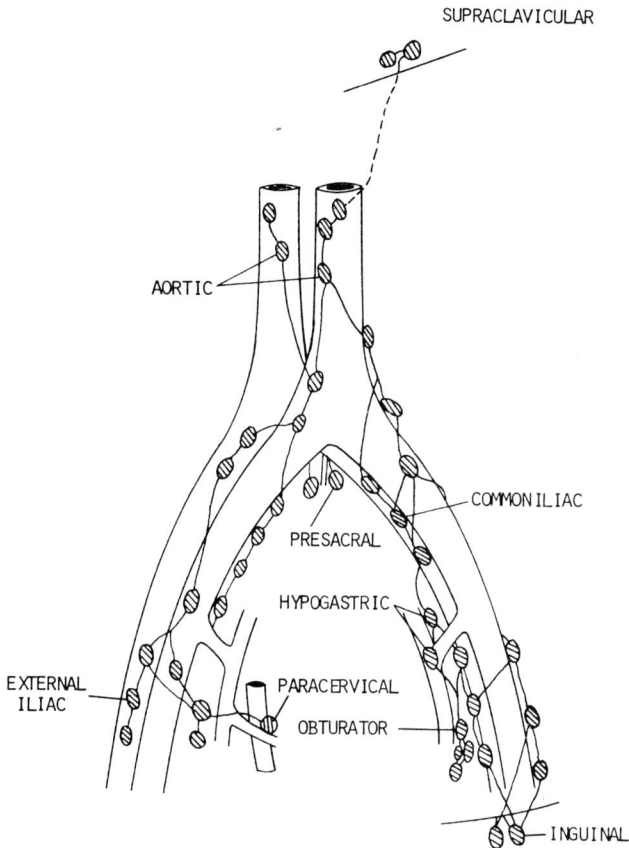

Fig. 2.5 Node groups potentially involved in patients with cervical carcinoma.

worse if endometrial extension was present. The problem of determining whether the endometrium is actually involved is an appreciable one, since the curette containing the specimen must be withdrawn through the tumour-filled cervix. Kotz (1979) suggested use of a suction curette since this would allow a cleaner, more accurate specimen.

Peritoneal involvement

The frequency of direct peritoneal involvement by carcinoma of the cervix has not been appreciated prior to the widespread use of surgical staging, yet is hardly surprising when one considers the anatomical relationship of the posterior cul-de-sac and tumour involving the posterior cervical lip and the posterior vaginal fornix. Welander (1981) reported finding direct peritoneal involvement by tumour in 12.6% of patients who underwent surgical staging procedures. Pelvic peritoneum was involved in 11 of 16 patients and extrapelvic peritoneum in five patients. We have encountered tumour breaking through the peritoneum in the cul-de-sac on a number of occasions. Our rate of malignant peritoneal cytology of 6.7% is less than that reported by Welander and by Hughes (1980), who reported 9.3% of 355 patients to have malignant peritoneal washings. Sotto (1960) found peritoneal involvement in 27 of 79 cervical cancer patients (34.1%) who underwent autopsies.

Metastatic cancer to the cervix
Although endometrial cancer not infrequently involves the cervix, metastatic carcinoma to the cervix from other organs is rare. Stanley Way (1980) observed only eight metastatic lesions to the cervix in 30 years; of these, three were from the liver, two from the stomach, one from the sigmoid colon, one from the breast and one from the fallopian tube. Yin-Chang (1982) reported six cases of metastatic disease from the gastro-intestinal tract to the cervix; five of these were from the stomach and one from the colon. A few cases of melanoma, leukaemia, breast cancer and ovarian cancer metastatic to the cervix have been reported.

SQUAMOUS CELL CARCINOMA: CELL TYPES

A histological staging classification introduced by Wentz and Reagan in 1959 has gained popularity and many investigators use this classification when reporting their data (Table 2.6). Large cell non-keratinizing tumours are most common (Fig. 2.6), followed by the large cell keratinizing type, an aberrant form of differentiation, since normal cervical squamous epithelium does not form keratin (Fig. 2.7). The small cell tumours are least common (Fig. 2.8). Mixtures of small cell and large types are also common (Fig. 2.9). Indeed, many tumours contain mixtures of cell types, although one type may predominate. Perhaps this explains the disagreement concerning the prognostic value of the Wentz-Reagan classification. In the keratinizing tumours, characteristic collections of keratin are present and pearls are formed. Non-keratinizing tumours are composed of large cells, some of which may contain keratin, but no pearls are present.

A number of authors have raised the question as to whether small cell tumours are epithelial in nature. Albores-Saavedra (1979) believes that most of them are carcinoids. These tumours are thought to originate from argyrophil cells of the endocervical epithelium and are part of tumours of the APUD (amine precursor uptake and decarboxylation) cell system. Cervical carcinoids may be malignant, with both local and distant metastases reported, but none has been reported to be associated

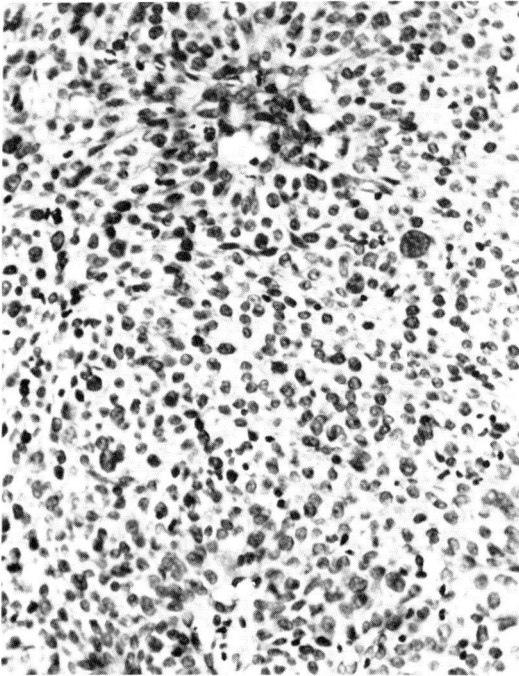

Fig. 2.6 Large cell non-keratinizing squamous cell carcinoma. Such tumours may have individual cell keratin, but do not form pearls. (H&E ×263)

with the carcinoid syndrome. Albores-Saavedra studied some of the tumours with the electron microscope and demonstrated tonofibrils in the cytoplasm; he postulated that this could represent squamous differentiation in a carcinoid and that it did not necessarily classify the tumour as squamous cell in type. Jones (1976) reporting a patient with Cushing's syndrome and a small cell cervical tumour, found that the tumour produced ACTH. Matsuyama (1979) reported another patient with Cushing's syndrome and a small cell tumour of the cervix. The metastatic lesions and the primary tumour in his patient contained high levels of ACTH as well as serotonin, histamine, amylase and beta MSH. Matsuyama reviewed all anaplastic cervical carcinomas at his institution and found that in about half of the cases argyrophil cells were identified. Those with such cells seemed to have a poorer prognosis than those without the cells. Habib (1979) also reported a patient said to have a primary carcinoid of the cervix because of demonstrable argyrophil granules. McKay (1979) performed electron microscopic studies on two small cell cervical tumours and concluded that they represented adult neuroblastomas.

The clinical behaviour of small cell tumours is also controversial. Van Nagell (1977) reported 41 patients with small cell carcinoma of the

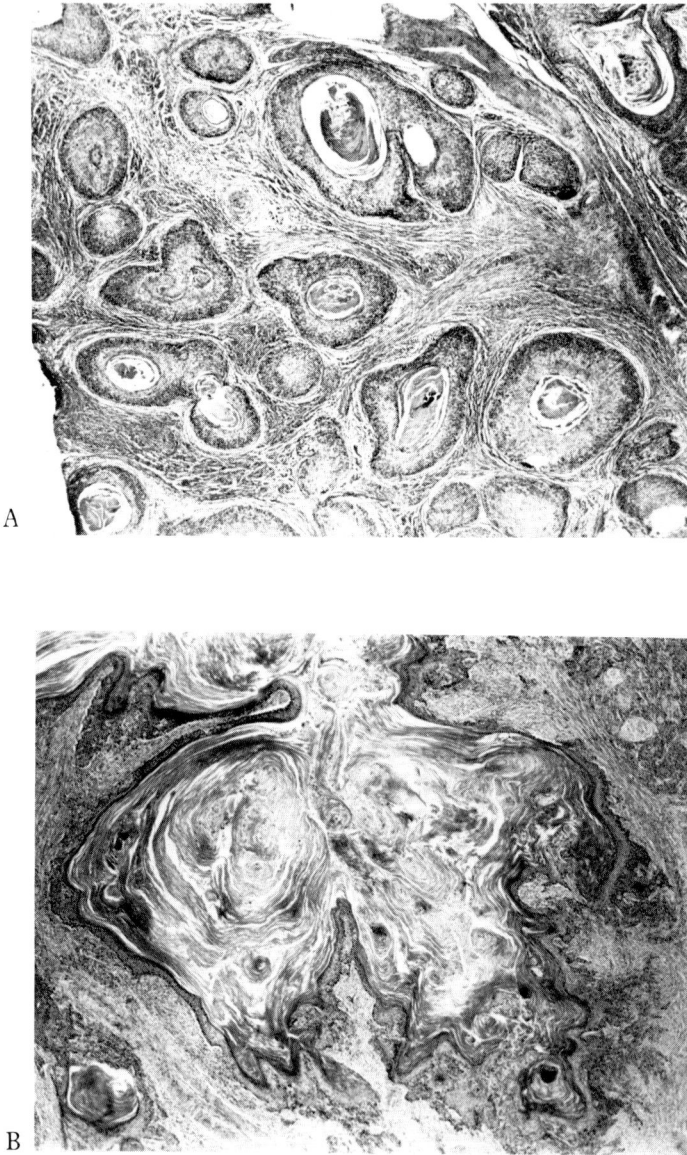

Fig. 2.7 Large cell non-keratinizing squamous cell carcinoma.
A. Keratin pearls are present in tumour nests. (H&E ×34)
B. A large collection of keratin within a tumour. (H&E ×25)

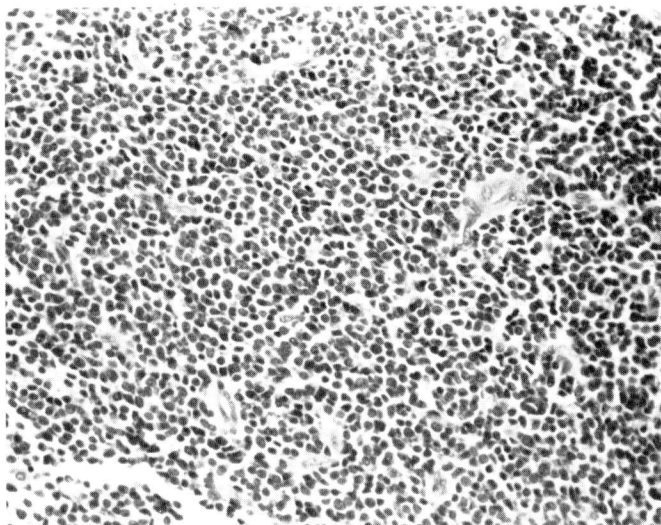

Fig. 2.8 A small cell tumour. The tissue type of these tumours is questioned (see text). (H&E ×263)

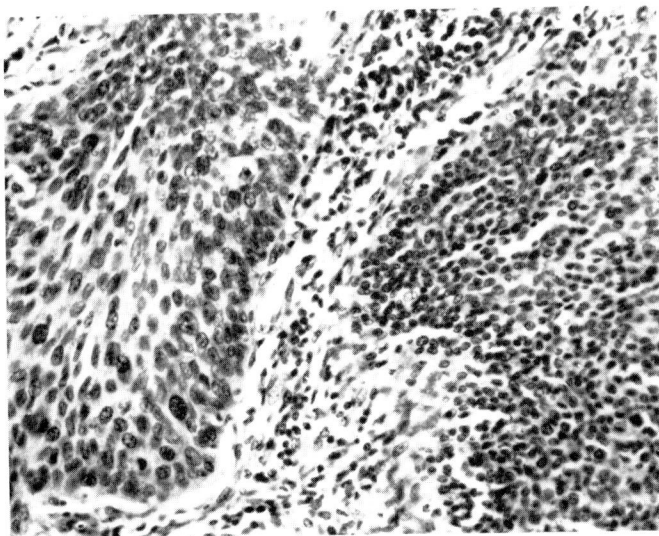

Fig. 2.9 Mixtures of the large cell type (left) and the small cell type (right) are not uncommon in cervical tumours. (H&E ×263)

cervix; 44% of these patients developed widespread metastases and died of recurrent cancer within 2 years. Van Nagell observed that the occurrence of LVS involvement in large cell keratinizing and non-keratinizing tumours was similar (20% and 24% respectively) but that 93% of patients with small cell tumours had LVS involvement, implying a special aggressiveness in small cell tumours. The increased LVS involvement and poor survival in small cell tumours has not been substantiated by other investigators. In fact, in surgical series, it is difficult to show any difference in 5-year survival for any of the cell types in the Wentz-Reagan classification (Table 2.7). Beecham (1978) could not show a difference in 2-year tumour-free rates, and Sidhu (1970) reported that the small cell lesions in the undifferentiated tumour group were more curable than the well-differentiated lesions.

SQUAMOUS CELL CARCINOMA: GRADE OR DIFFERENTIATION

Tumour grade (as contrasted to cell type) is said to have prognostic significance. Baltzer (1982), in a study encompassing 718 surgical specimens from patients with stage IB cervical cancer, found tumour differentiation in the invasive front of the tumour to correlate with survival more closely than differentiation in the centre of the tumour. Only 4% of patients died if their tumour was well differentiated in the invasive front whereas 27.7% died if it was poorly differentiated. Comparable mortality figures for the tumour centre were 14.4% (well differentiated) and 28.4% (poorly differentiated). Our mortality figures (387 stage IB patients) are 17% for well differentiated and 24% for poorly differentiated tumours, quite similar to the figures Baltzer quoted for the centre of the tumour.

Several investigators have studied the relationship of tumour differentiation and node metastasis. Lagasse (1979, 1980) reported no correlation of metastatic cancer in high (aortic or common iliac) nodes with tumour differentiation either in his own material or in that of the Gynecologic Oncology Group (USA). With the exception of the series reported by Chung (1981) there is no difference in the rate of positive pelvic nodes encountered in well differentiated and poorly differentiated tumours reported by several authors (Table 2.8). Since a tumour may vary in differentiation in different areas, small biopsy specimens may not be representative of the tumour, accounting for varying claims regarding the importance of tumour grading.

Since cell type and tumour grade considered alone do not invariably predict prognosis, a number of investigators have attempted to develop a scoring system, i.e., a method of judging the degree of malignancy of

Table 2.6 Squamous cell carcinoma incidence within Wentz-Reagan classification

Author	Year	No. of pts.	Large cell keratinizing % pos.	Large cell non-keratinizing % pos.	Small cell % pos.
Swan	1973	247	52.6	45.7	1.6
Johansson	1976	211	16.6	80.6	2.8
Beecham	1978	208	26.0	66.8	7.2
Ng	1979	1042	34.5	52.6	12.9
van Nagell	1979	482	36.7	53.5	9.8
Stendahl	1979	152	40.1	42.8	17.2
Pagnini	1980	125	45.6	32.8	21.6
Palma	1980	136	44.1	36.0	19.9
Stanhope	1980	194	31.9	53.9	9.3
Authors	1982	217	34.1	63.6	2.3
Totals		3014	35.5	54.2	10.3

Table 2.7 Stage IB squamous cell carcinoma treated by radical hysterectomy: survival by cell type

Author	Year	Large cell keratinizing 5-year survival		Large cell non-keratinizing 5-year survival		Small cell 5-year survival	
		No. of pts.	%	No. of pts.	%	No. of pts.	%
Sidhu	1970	13	77	63	90.5	38	85
Pagnini	1980	57	75	41	59	27	67
Authors	1982	50	80	82	82	3	33
Totals		120	77.5	186	79.6	69	75.4

Table 2.8 Positive pelvic nodes by differentiation of tumour

Author	Year	No. of pts.	WD % pos.	MWD % pos.	PD % pos.
Sidhu	1970	115	32.1	15.9	15.4
Underwood	1979	120	–	1.6	15.0
Chung	1981	142	–	8.2	50.0
Authors	1982	200	15.0	11.0	12.0
Totals		577	17.0	9.4	20.3

WD = Well differentiated, MWD = Moderately well differentiated, PD = Poorly differentiated

tumours using various or multiple histological criteria. Nodskov-Pederson (1971) did not think that nuclear size or DNA content was prognostic and could not correlate tumour morphology with degree of malignancy. Jakobsen (1979) studied nuclear DNA distribution in biopsy specimens from 46 patients with squamous cell carcinomas. He reported that poorly differentiated lesions contained hypertetraploid and aneuploid cell populations while highly differentiated tumours contained cells predominantly with hyperdiploid DNA content. Since he did not correct for stage of tumour, no conclusions can be drawn from his study. Stendahl (1979) developed a grading system based on numerous parameters including structure (solid, dissociated), differentiation, nuclear pleomorphism, number of mitoses, vascular invasion and stromal response. While he was able to establish that such a point system could correlate with survival, the classification appears too cumbersome for general use. Pagnini (1980) developed a similar scoring system, including histological type, vascular invasion, depth of invasion, mode of spread and presence or absence of necrosis in the tumour. He identified high and low malignancy groups with a highly significant difference in survival. Barber (1978) found no significant relationship of survival to cell type, histological or nuclear grades. Sidhu (1970), Gusberg (1971) and Baltzer (1982) pointed out the favourable influence on prognosis of dense lymphocytic infiltrate in the stroma around the tumour (Fig. 2.10); however, Barber (1978) found no relationship, and our experience is the same.

Van Nagell, studying pelvic lymph nodes from 80 patients with cancer of the cervix who had undergone radical hysterectomy and pelvic lymphadenectomy, observed that a lymphocyte predominant nodal pattern was associated with a statistically significant decrease in lymph node metastases and tumour recurrence. In contrast, patients with a lymphocyte depleted node pattern had a high incidence of metastasis and tumour recurrence, while those with germinal centre predominant

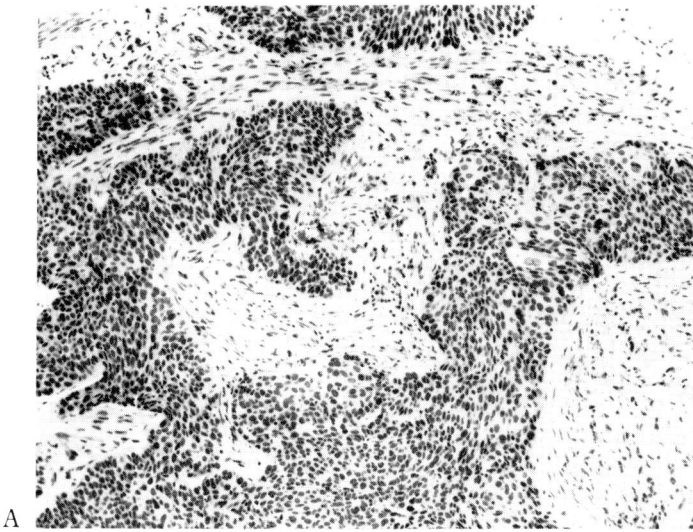

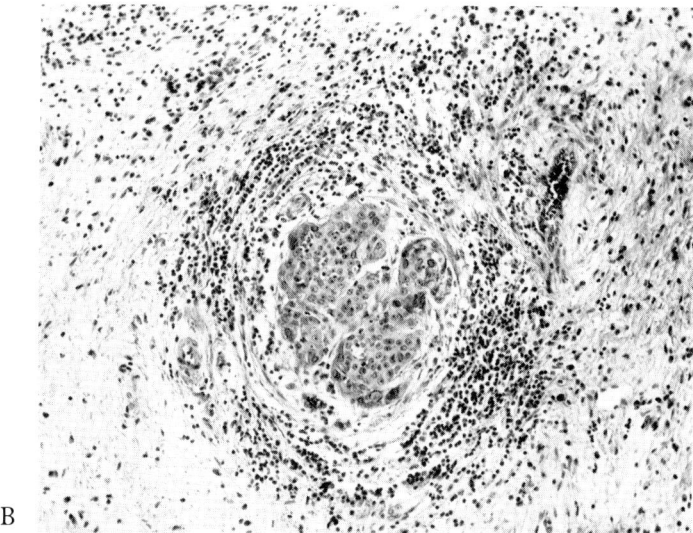

Fig. 2.10 Stromal reaction to tumour.
A. No stromal reaction is present. (H&E ×137)
B. A nest of tumour with adjacent round cell and leucocytic infiltration. (H&E ×171)

patterns had an intermediate incidence. He speculated, therefore, that regional lymph node morphology might be of prognostic significance; this observation bears further study and repetition.

ADENOCARCINOMA

Adenocarcinomas or mixed adenosquamous carcinomas range in incidence from 5% to 26% in recently reported series (Table 2.9). The overall percentage of approximately 10% is almost double the rate quoted in existing textbooks and raises the possibility that there is an increasing incidence of adenocarcinoma of the cervix. In our recent review of adenocarcinomas of the cervix, we concluded that the varied patterns (Fig. 2.11–2.17) had little prognostic significance and that tumour volume rather than histology correlated best with survival. In this study, which used matched squamous cell carcinoma controls, there was no difference in survival between adenocarcinomas and controls, and rates of positive pelvic nodes encountered in the two groups (stage IB) were identical.

We have not identified lesions that might be categorised as carcinoma in situ of the endocervix, although presumably atypical cells within the glands or clefts retaining their regular architectural pattern are diagnostic of this entity; certainly, it would seem reasonable that such a precursor lesion exists.

Significant numbers of patients have clearly recognisable elements of both epidermoid carcinoma and adenocarcinoma. A third of the patients in our series had such mixtures. Collision tumours are occasionally observed in which invasive squamous cell carcinoma abuts an invasive adenocarcinoma (Fig. 2.17). In most instances, however, admixtures of the tumour types can be demonstrated even at the ultrastructural level. We were not able to confirm the observations of Wheeless (1970) and Julian (1977) that, stage by stage, adenosquamous carcinomas of the cervix had a poorer 5-year survival.

Maier (1980) in reviewing 389 primary adenocarcinomas of the cervix at the Armed Forces Institute of Pathology (USA) reported a 43% association of cervical intra-epithelial neoplasia and cervical adenocarcinomas, especially in tumours with endometrioid and adenosquamous patterns. In our recent review, we found this association in 10% of the patients (Fig. 2.15).

Glassy cell carcinoma, first described by Glucksmann (1956) and said to occur in young, and especially in pregnant, women has been more recently studied by Littman (1976). The tumour, said to comprise 21% of mixed tumours (Glucksman), is characterized by cells with a moderate amount of cytoplasm having a 'ground glass' or finely

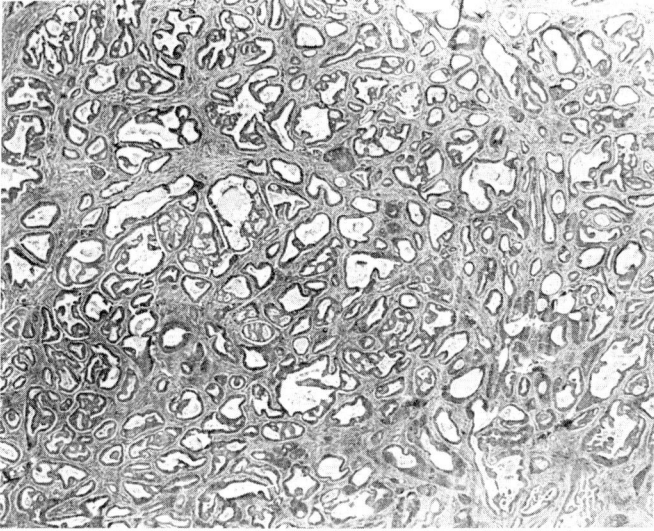

Fig. 2.11   Adenocarcinoma of the endocervical type. (H&E ×25)

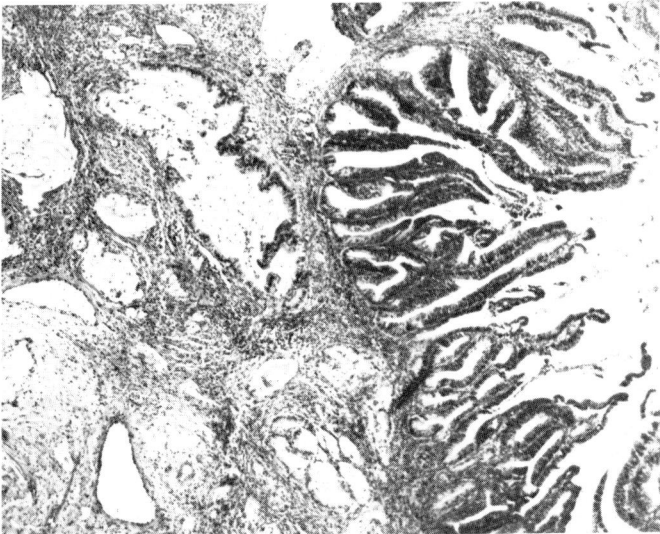

Fig. 2.12   Adenocarcinoma of mixed pattern. Mucin-containing area (left) is adjacent to a papillary area (right). (H&E ×49)

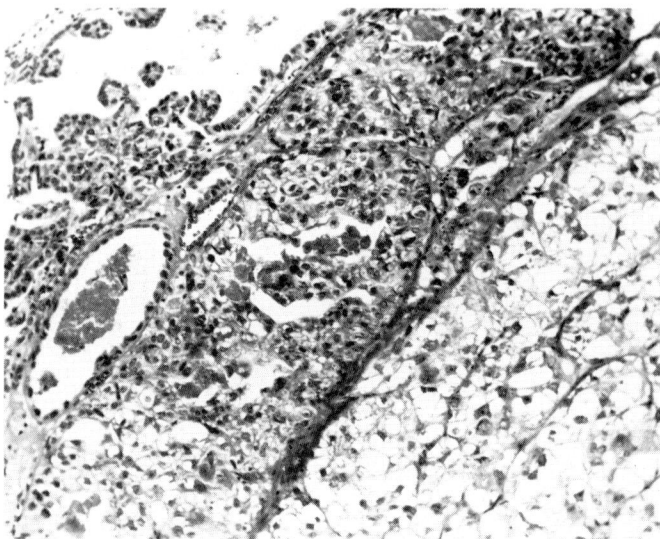

Fig. 2.13 Adenocarcinoma of mesometanephric pattern. Note hobnail cells (left) and clear cells with eccentric nuclei and vacuolated cytoplasm (lower right). (H&E ×103)

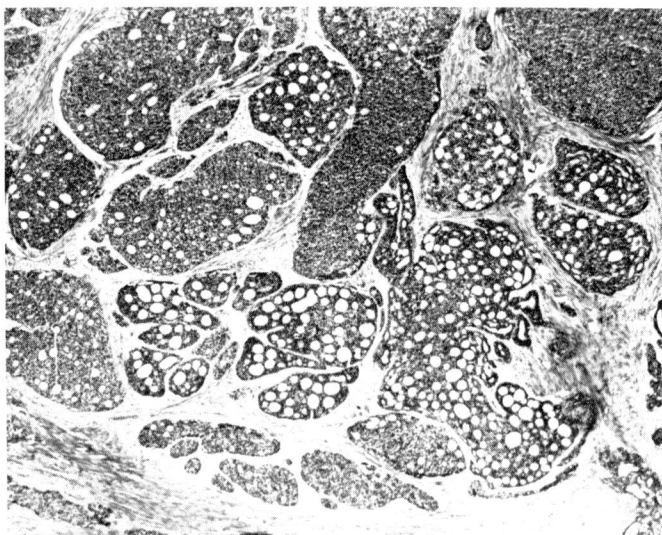

Fig. 2.14 Tumour with an adenoid cystic (microglandular pattern) basaloid type. (H&E ×25)

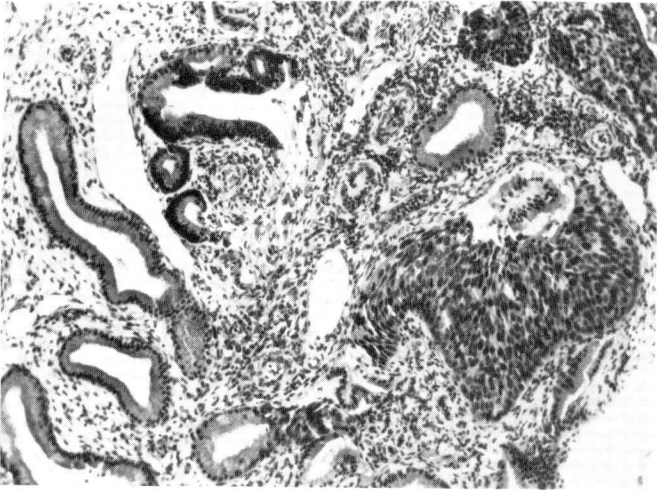

Fig. 2.15   Surface squamous carcinoma in situ (to right) overlying a well-differentiated carcinoma, endocervical pattern. (H&E ×103)

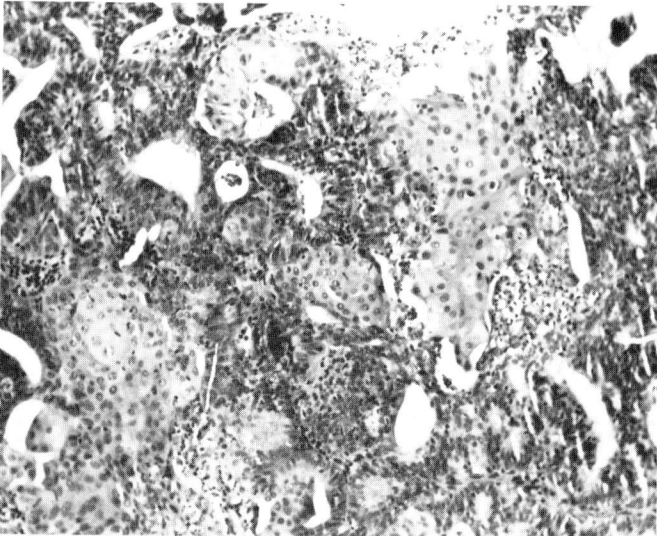

Fig. 2.16   An adenoacanthoma of the cervix. Benign metaplastic squamous cell nests are present in a well-differentiated adenocarcinoma.

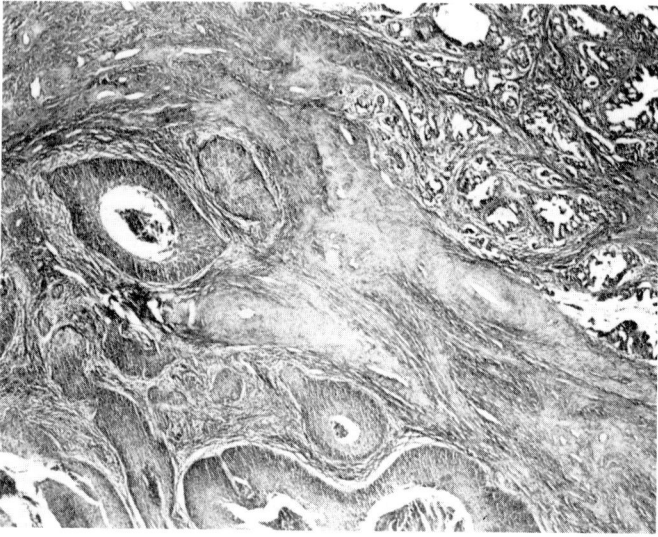

Fig. 2.17 An adenosquamous carcinoma. Squamous cell carcinoma adjoins a well-differentiated adenocarcinoma (upper right). In other areas admixtures are present leading to a designation of adenosquamous carcinoma. (H&E ×25)

granular appearance, a distinct cell wall that stains with eosin and PAS and enlarged nuclei with prominent nucleoli. It is thought to represent a variant of poorly differentiated mixed adenosquamous carcinoma. Littman found that it was associated with extrapelvic spread in half the cases and that results were poor with either surgery or radiation therapy. Using Glucksman's strict criteria for diagnosis that requires no significant differentiation to either a glandular or a squamous component, we have been able to make this diagnosis in only two or three instances. We are thus unable to say that 'glassy cell' tumours warrant a place in the classification of cancer of the cervix.

Table 2.9 Percentage of adenocarcinomas or mixed tumours

Author	Year	No. of patients	Total %
Swan	1973	308	10.4
Kjorstad	1977	2002	5.4
van Nagell	1977	82	8.5
Beecham	1978	245	15.0
Berkowitz	1979	27	26.0
Ng	1979	1236	13.4
Underwood	1979	178	15.1
van Nagell	1979	526	8.4
Benedet	1980	241	18.1
Volteranni	1980	417	9.1
Authors	1982	1390	9.9
Totals		6652	9.6

OTHER MALIGNANCIES

The term 'verrucous carcinoma' refers to well-differentiated squamous neoplasms which show evidence of maturation, extensive keratinization, but do not have sufficient atypia to merit a cytological diagnosis of malignancy. Crissman (1980) pointed out that biopsy confirmation of these lesions remains a difficult problem because, although they are often large bulky tumours (Fig. 2.17), superficial biopsies appear histologically benign and are easily confused with lesions such as condyloma accuminata. It is important, therefore, that the surgical pathologist be adequately briefed concerning the suspicious nature of the lesion. Partridge (1980), reporting our experience, noted that the tumours cause local destruction but rarely metastasise. Histologically, they are characterised by well-differentiated hyperplastic and hyperkeratotic squamous epithelium. Papillomatosis is marked and the line of demarcation between the tumour and the underlying stroma is characteristically sharp (Fig. 2.18). The treatment of choice is surgical, with wide local excision being sufficient in most cases. Radiotherapy is said to be ineffective in treating these lesions and is thought by Demian (1973) to result sometimes in anaplastic transformation of the tumour.

Abell (1973) reviewed the treatment of cervical sarcomas and carcinosarcomas. Regardless of treatment, leiomyosarcoma resulted in the death of six out of eight patients within 2 years. Six patients with carcinosarcoma all died within 15 months, and six of 12 patients with endocervical stromal sarcoma died within 2 years. Hysterectomy is indicated in patients with disease confined to the uterus, but the place of adjuvant therapy (radiation or chemotherapy) is unproven.

Tumours of adenoid cystic pattern are thought to be variants of adenocarcinoma or mixed adenosquamous carcinoma. Fowler (1978) indicated that such tumours are aggressive with lung metastases present in almost half of the patients in the 29 cases reported in the literature. Our experience leads us to conclude that the pattern is frequently present in cervical adenocarcinomas and mimics the adenoid cystic carcinomas of the head, neck and breast. However, it differs in several respects from those tumours, and the high metastasis rate is most likely because this pattern occurs in poorly differentiated adenosquamous carcinomas.

Lymphomas involving the female reproductive tract are very rare. We have only encountered one cervical lymphoma in a series exceeding 1500 invasive cervical cancer patients. Chorlton (1974) reported that lymphoma patients with FIGO stage I tumours have a 5-year survival of 60%.

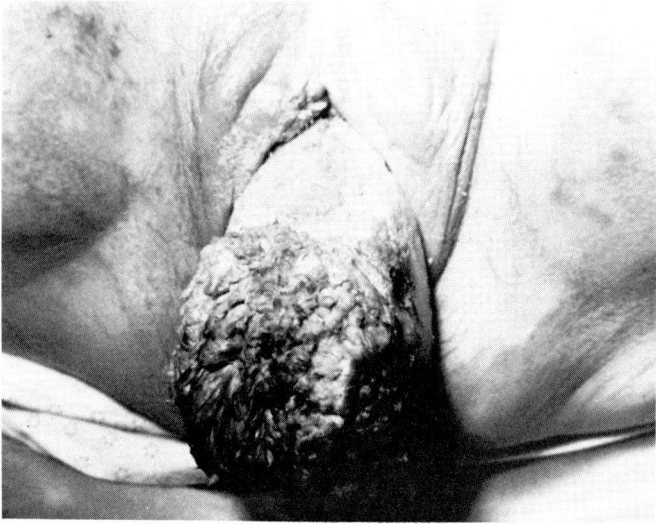

A

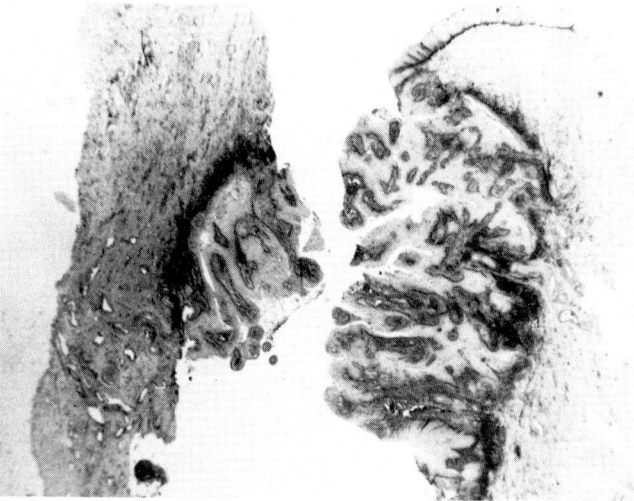

B

Fig. 2.18 Verrucous carcinoma of the cervix. A. A carcinoma occurring with uterine procidentia. B. Microscopic features include each of fibrovascular cover, lack of cytological atypia and an expanding, rather than an infiltrating tumour-stromal border. (H&E ×7)

POSTRADIATION DYSPLASIA

A small number of patients treated successfully by radiation therapy develop dysplastic epithelial changes in the vagina and cervix that lead to concern regarding possible recurrent disease. Such changes may be detected months or years following radiation and are not ordinarily associated with palpable findings suggesting recurrence. At one time, we made a practice of performing excision of the affected mucqsa by the vaginal route, both for diagnosis and treatment. Neither colposcopy nor Lugol's staining is always helpful in demarcating the lesions, since the atrophic and radiated mucosa may not have a normal appearance or usual staining reaction. Currently we are more conservative and follow these patients, unless invasion is suspected. We do not feel that the dysplastic changes are associated with recurrence and on follow-up they seem to have little tendency to progress.

BIBLIOGRAPHY

Abdulhayoglu G, Rich W M, Reynolds J, DiSaia P J 1980 Selective radiation therapy in stage IB uterine cervical carcinoma following radical pelvic surgery. Gynecologic Oncology 10: 84–92
Abell M R, Ramirez J A 1973 Sarcomas and carcinosarcomas of the uterine cervix. Cancer 31: 1176–1192
Averette H E, Sevin B-U 1979 Microinvasive (stage IA) carcinoma of the cervix. Obstetrical and Gynecological Survey 34: 833–834
Averette H E, Nelson J H Jr, Ng A B P, Hoskins W J, Boyce J G, Ford J H Jr 1976 Diagnosis and management of microinvasive (stage IA) carcinoma of the uterine cervix. Cancer 38: 414–425
Baltzer J, Lohe K J, Koepcke W, Zander J 1981 Formation of metastases in the ovaries in operated squamous cell carcinoma of the cervix uteri. Geburtshilfe und Frauenheilkunde 41: 672–673
Baltzer J, Lohe K J, Koepcke W, Zander J 1982 Histological criteria for the prognosis in patients with operated squamous cell carcinoma of the cervix. Gynecologic Oncology 13: 184–194
Barber H R K, Sommers S C, Rotterdam H, Kwon T 1978 Vascular invasion as a prognostic factor in stage IB cancer of the cervix. Obstetrics and Gynecology 52: 343–348
Beecham J B, Halvorsen T, Kolbenstvedt A 1978 Histologic classification, lymph node metastases and patient survival in stage IB cervical carcinoma. Gynecologic Oncology 6: 95–105
Benedet J L, Turko M, Boyes D A, Nickerson K G, Bienkowska B T 1980 Radical hysterectomy in the treatment of cervical cancer. American Journal of Obstetrics and Gynecology 137: 254–262
Benson W L, Norris H J 1977 A critical review of the frequency of lymph node metastasis and death from microinvasive carcinoma of the cervix. Obstetrics and Gynecology 49: 632–638
Berkowitz R S, Ehrmann R L, Lavizzo-Mourey R, Knapp R C 1979 Invasive cervical carcinoma in young women. Gynecologic Oncology 8:. 311–316
Bohm J W, Krupp P J, Lee F Y L, Batson H W K 1976 Lymph node metastasis in microinvasive epidermoid cancer of the cervix. Obstetrics and Gynecology 48: 65–67
Boronow R C, Hickman B T 1977 A comparison of two radiation therapy-treatment plans for carcinoma of the cervix. II. Complications and survival rates. American Journal of Obstetrics and Gynecology 128: 99–105
Boyce J, Fruchter R G, Nicastri A D, Ambinvagar P-C, Reinis M S, Nelson J H Jr 1981 Prognostic factors in stage I carcinoma of the cervix. Gynecologic Oncology 12: 154–165

Boyes D A, Worth A J, Fidler H K 1970 The results of treatment of 4389 cases of preclinical cervical squamous carcinoma. Journal of Obstetrics and Gynaecology of the British Commonwealth 77: 769—780

Brandt B, Lifshitz S 1981 Scalene node biopsy in advanced carcinoma of the cervix uteri. Cancer 47: 1920-1921

Buchsbaum H J 1979 Extrapelvic lymph node metastases in cervical carcinoma. American Journal of Obstetrics and Gynecology 133: 814-824

Burghardt E 1979 Microinvasive carcinoma. Obstetrical and Gynecological Survey 34: 836-838

Burghardt E 1982 Microinvasive and occult invasive carcinoma: pathology. In: Jordan J A, Sharp F, Singer A (eds) Pre-clinical neoplasia of the cervix. Royal College of Obstetricians and Gynaecologists, London

Burghardt E, Pickel H 1978 Local spread and lymph node involvement in cervical cancer. Obstetrics and Gynecology 52: 138-145

Cherry C P, Glucksmann A 1953 Observations on lymph node involvement in carcinoma of the cervix. Journal of Obstetrics and Gynaecology of the British Empire 60: 368-377

Chorlton I, Karnei R F, Norris H J 1974 Primary malignant reticuloendothelial disease involving the vagina, cervix and corpus uteri. Obstetrics and Gynecology 44: 735-748

Chung C K, Nahhas W A, Zaino R, Stryker J A, Mortel R 1981 Histologic grade and lymph node metastasis in squamous cell carcinoma of the cervix. Gynecologic Oncology 12: 348-354

Coppleson M 1979 Microinvasive cervical cancer. Obstetrical and Gynecological Survey 34: 840-841

Coppleson M 1982 Microinvasive and occult invasive carcinoma: colposcopic diagnosis and management. In: Jordan J A, Sharp F, Singer A (eds) Pre-clinical neoplasia of the cervix. Royal College of Obstetricians and Gynaecologists, London

Creasman W T, Parker R T 1973 Microinvasive carcinoma of the cervix. Clinical Obstetrics and Gynecology 16: 261-275

Crissman J, Flanagan R 1980 Verrucous carcinoma of the uterine cervix. Journal of Reproductive Medicine 25: 139-141

Demian S D E, Bushkin F L, Echevarria R A 1973 Perineal invasion and anaplastic transformation of verrucous carcinoma. Cancer 32: 395-401

Duncan I D 1982 Microinvasive and occult invasive carcinoma: the British 'experience' in the management of microinvasive carcinoma of the cervix. In: Jordan J A, Sharp F, Singer A (eds) Pre-clinical neoplasia of the cervix. Royal College of Obstetricians and Gynaecologists, London

Fennell R H Jr 1978 Microinvasive carcinoma of the uterine cervix. Obstetrical and Gynecological Survey 33: 406-411

Finck F M, Denk M 1970 Cervical carcinoma: relationship between histology and survival following radiation therapy. Obstetrics and Gynecology 35: 339-343

Foushee J H S, Greiss F C, Lock F R 1969 Stage IA squamous cell carcinoma of the uterine cervix. American Journal of Obstetrics and Gynecology 105: 46-58

Fowler W C Jr, Miles P A, Surwit E A, Edelman D A, Walton L A, Photopulos G J 1978 Adenoid cystic carcinoma of the cervix. Obstetrics and Gynecology 52: 337-342

Fuller A F, Elliott N, Kosloff C, Lewis J L Jr 1982 Lymph node metastases from carcinoma of the cervix, stages IB and IIA: implications for prognosis and treatment. Gynecologic Oncology 13: 165-174

Glucksmann A, Cherry C P 1956 Incidence, histology and response to radiation of mixed carcinomas (adenoacanthomas) of the uterine cervix. Cancer (Sept-Oct): 971-979

Gusberg S B, Yannopoulos K, Cohen C J 1971 Virulence indices and lymph nodes in cancer of the cervix. American Journal of Roentgenology, Radium Therapy and Nuclear Medicine 111: 273-277

Habib A, Kaneko M, Cohen C J, Walker G 1979 Carcinoid of the uterine cervix. Cancer 43: 535-538

Hasumi K, Sakamoto A, Sugano H 1980 Microinvasive carcinoma of the uterine cervix. Cancer 45: 928–931

Henriksen E 1960 Distribution of metastases in stage I carcinoma of the cervix. American Journal of Obstetrics and Gynecology 80: 919–932

Hughes R R, Brewington K C, Hanjani P, Photopulos G, Dick D, Votava C et al 1980 Extended field irradiation for cervical cancer based on surgical staging. Gynecologic Oncology 9: 153–161

Hurt W G, Silverberg S G, Frable W J, Belgrad R, Crooks L D Jr 1977 Adenocarcinoma of the cervix: histopathologic and clinical features. American Journal of Obstetrics and Gynecology 129: 304–315

Iversen T, Abeler V, Kjorstad K E 1979 Factors influencing the treatment of patients with stage IA carcinoma of the cervix. British Journal of Obstetrics and Gynaecology 86: 593–597

Jakobsen A, Bichel P, Sell A 1979 Correlation of DNA distribution and cytological differentiation of human cervical carcinomas. Virchows Archiv B Cell Pathology 31: 75–79

Jennings R H, Barclay D L 1972 Verrucous carcinoma of the cervix. Cancer 30: 430–434

Johansson O, Johnsson J E, Lindberg L G, Sydsjo A 1976 Prognosis, recurrences and metastases correlated to histologic cell type in carcinoma of the uterine cervix. Acta obstetrica et gynecologica scandinavica 55: 255–259

Jones H W III, Plymate S, Gluck F B, Miles P A, Greene J F Jr 1976 Small cell nonkeratinizing carcinoma of the cervix associated with ACTH production. Cancer 38: 1629–1635

Jordan J A, Sharp F, Singer A (eds) 1982 Preclinical neoplasia of the cervix. Proceedings of the Ninth Study Group of the Royal College of Obstetricians and Gynaecologists, October 1981, Appendix 1. Royal College of Obstetricians and Gynaecologists, London, p 301

Julian C G, Daikoku N H, Gillespie A 1977 Adenoepidermoid and adenosquamous carcinoma of the uterus. American Journal of Obstetrics and Gynecology 128: 106–116

Kjorstad J E 1977 Carcinoma of the cervix in the young patient. Obstetrics and Gynecology 50: 28–30

Kotz H L 1979 Endometrial extension of cervical tumor: a new technique for definitive detection. Maryland State Medical Journal (December): 61

Lagasse L D, Creasman W T, Shingleton H M, Ford J H, Blessing J A 1980 Results and complications of operative staging in cervical cancer: experience of the gynecologic oncology group. Gynecologic Oncology 9: 90–98

Lee R B, Weisbaum G S, Heller P B, Park R C 1981 Scalene node biopsy in primary and recurrent invasive carcinoma of the cervix. Gynecologic Oncology 11: 200–206 (abstract)

Leman M H, Benson W L, Kurman R J, Park R C 1976 Microinvasive carcinoma of the cervix. Obstetrics and Gynecology 48: 571–578

Littman P, Clement P B, Henriksen B, Wang C C, Robboy S J, Taft P D et al 1976 Glassy cell carcinoma of the cervix. Cancer 27: 2238–2246

Liu W, Meigs J V 1955 Radical hysterectomy and pelvic lymphadenectomy. American Journal of Obstetrics and Gynecology 69: 1–32

Lohe K J 1978 Early squamous cell carcinoma of the uterine cervix. I. Definition and histology. Gynecologic Oncology 6: 10–30

Mackay B, Osborne B M, Wharton J T 1979 Small cell tumor of cervix with neuroepithelial features. Cancer 43: 1138–1145

Maier R C, Norris H J 1980 Coexistence of cervical intraepithelial neoplasia with primary adenocarcinoma of the endocervix. Obstetrics and Gynecology 56: 361–364

Martimbeau P W, Kjorstad K E, Iversen T 1982 Stage IB carcinoma of the cervix, The Norwegian Radium Hospital. Results of treatment and major complications. II. Results when pelvic nodes are involved. Obstetrics and Gynecology, in press

Martzloff K H 1928 Epidermoid carcinoma of the cervix uteri. A histologic study to determine the resemblance between biopsy specimens and the parent tumor obtained by radical panhysterectomy. American Journal of Obstetrics and Gynecology 16: 578–594

Matsuyama M, Inoue T, Ariyoshi Y, Doi M, Suchi T, Sato T et al 1979 Argyrophil cell carcinoma of the uterine cervix with ectopic production of ACTH, β-MSH, serotonin, histamine and amylase. Cancer 44: 1813–1823

Morley G W, Seski J C 1976 Radical pelvic surgery versus radiation therapy for stage I carcinoma of the cervix (exclusive of microinvasion). American Journal of Obstetrics and Gynecology 126: 785–798

Mussey E, Soule E H, Welch J C 1969 Microinvasive carcinoma of the cervix. American Journal of Obstetrics and Gynecology 104: 738–742

van Nagell J R Jr, Donaldson E S, Parker J C, van Dyke A H, Wood E G 1977 The prognostic significance of pelvic lymph node morphology in carcinoma of the uterine cervix. Cancer 39: 2624–2632

van Nagell J R Jr, Rayburn W, Donaldson E S, Hanson M, Gay E C, Yoneda J et al 1979 Therapeutic implications of patterns of recurrence in cancer of the uterine cervix. Cancer 44: 2354–2361

Ng A B P 1979 Pathological factors significant in management and prognosis of cervical carcinoma. University of Miami Medical School, Miami, Florida

Nodskov-Pedersen S 1971 Degree of malignancy of cancer involving the cervix uteri, judged on the basis of clinical stage, histology, size of nuclei and content of DNA. Acta pathologica et microbiologica scandinavica section A 79: 617–628

Pagnini C A, Palma P D, DeLaurentiis G 1980 Malignancy grading in squamous carcinoma of uterine cervix treated by surgery. British Journal of Cancer 41: 415–421

Palma P D, Pagnini C A, DeLaurentiis G 1980 Prognostic significance of the cyto-histological classification of infiltrating cervical epidermoid carcinoma. Tumori 66: 183–190

Partridge E E, Murad T, Shingleton H M, Austin J M, Hatch K D 1980 Verrucous lesions of the female genitalia. II. Verrucous carcinoma. American Journal of Obstetrics and Gynecology 137: 412–424

Perez A C, Zivnuska F, Askin F, Camel H M, Ragan D, Powers W E 1977 Mechanisms of failure in patients with carcinoma of the uterine cervix extending into the endometrium. International Journal of Radiation Oncology, Biology and Physics 2: 651–659

Pilleron J P, Durand J C, Hamelin J P 1974a Location of lymph node invasion in cancer of the uterine cervix: study of 140 cases treated at the Curie Foundation. American Journal of Obstetrics and Gynecology 119: 453–457

Pilleron J P, Durand J C, Hamelin J P 1974b Prognostic value of node metastasis in cancer of the uterine cervix. American Journal of Obstetrics and Gynecology 119: 458–462

Plentl A A, Friedman E A 1971 Lymphatic system of the female genitalia. W B Saunders, Philadelphia

Powell J L, Burrell M O, Franklin E W III 1981 Radical hysterectomy and pelvic lymphadenectomy. Gynecologic Oncology 12: 23–32

Roche W D, Norris H G 1975 Microinvasive carcinoma of the cervix. Cancer 36: 180–186

Ruch R M, Pitcock J A, Ruch W A Jr 1976 Microinvasive carcinoma of the cervix. American Journal of Obstetrics and Gynecology 125: 87–92

Sedlis A, Sall S, Tsukada Y, Park R, Mangan C, Shingleton H M et al 1979 Microinvasive carcinoma of the uterine cervix: a clinical-pathologic study. American Journal of Obstetrics and Gynecology 133: 64–74

Shingleton H M, Lawrence W D, Gore H 1977 Cervical carcinoma with adenoid cystic pattern; a light and electron microscopic study. Cancer 40: 1112–1121

Shingleton H M, Gore H, Bradley D H, Soong S-J 1981 Adenocarcinoma of the cervix. I. Clinical evaluation and pathologic features. American Journal of Obstetrics and Gynecology 139: 799–814

Sidhu G S, Koss L G, Barber H R K 1970 Relation of histologic factors to the response of stage I epidermoid carcinoma of the cervix to surgical treatment. Obstetrics and Gynecology 35: 329–338

Sotto L S J, Graham J B, Pickren J W 1960 Postmortem findings in cancer of the cervix. American Journal of Obstetrics and Gynecology 80: 791–794

Spanos W J, Greer B E, Hamberger A D, Rutledge F N 1981 Prognosis of squamous cell carcinoma of the cervix with endometrial involvement. Gynecologic Oncology 11: 230–234

Stanhope C R, Smith J P, Wharton J T, Rutledge F N, Fletcher G H, Gallager H S 1980 Carcinoma of the cervix: the effect of age on survival. Gynecologic Oncology 10: 188–193

Stendahl U, Willen H, Willen R 1979 Classification and grading of invasive squamous cell carcinoma of the uterine cervix. Acta radiologica 18: 481–496

Swan D S, Roddick J W 1973 A clinical-pathological correlation of cell type classification for cervical cancer. American Journal of Obstetrics and Gynecology 116: 666–670

Underwood P B Jr, Wilson W C, Kreutner A, Miller M C III, Murphy E 1979 Radical hysterectomy: a critical review of twenty-two years' experience. American Journal of Obstetrics and Gynecology 134: 889–898

Volterrani F, Sigurta D, Gardani G, Milani A, Musumeci R 1980 Role of lymphography in cancer of the uterine cervix. Radiologia medica (Torino) 66: 611–614 (abstract)

Wallach J B, Edberg S 1959 Carcinoma metastatic to the uterine cervix. American Journal of Obstetrics and Gynecology 77: 990–995

Way S 1980 Carcinoma metastatic in the cervix. Gynecologic Oncology 9: 298–302

Welander C E, Pierce V K, Nori D, Hilaris B S, Kosloff C, Clark D G C et al 1981 Pretreatment laparotomy in carcinoma of the cervix. Gynecologic Oncology 12: 336–347

Wentz W B, Reagan J W 1959 Survival in cervical cancer with respect to cell type. Cancer 12: 384–388

Wheeless C R Jr, Graham R, Graham J B 1970 Prognosis and treatment of adeno-epidermoid carcinoma of the cervix. Obstetrics and Gynecology 35: 928–932

Wilkinson E J, Komorowski R A 1978 Borderline microinvasive carcinoma of the cervix. Obstetrics and Gynecology 51: 472–476

Yajima A, Noda K 1979 The results of treatment of microinvasive carcinoma (stage IA) of the uterine cervix by means of simple and extended hysterectomy. American Journal of Obstetrics and Gynecology 135: 685–688

Yin-Chang Z, Pei-Fan Z, Yung-He W 1982 Metastatic carcinoma of the cervix uteri from the gastrointestinal tract. Department of Oncology, China Medical College, in press

Zander J, Baltzer J, Lohe K J, Ober K G, Kaufmann C 1981 Carcinoma of the cervix: an attempt to individualize treatment; results of a 20-year cooperative study. American Journal of Obstetrics and Gynecology 139: 752–759

3

Diagnosis, staging and selection of treatment

DIAGNOSIS

The most common symptom in patients with cancer of the cervix is vaginal bleeding. This may occur as postcoital bleeding or as irregular bleeding, which may be mistaken by younger women as an abnormality of the menstrual cycle. Many patients with this disease, however, have postmenopausal bleeding as the primary symptom. Patients with advanced disease (large volume stage IIB or stage III) often have a malodorous or bloody vaginal discharge. Additionally, patients with advanced disease often are nutritionally depleted and have a low performance status.

During the past decade, 1197 patients with cervical cancer have been treated at the University of Alabama in Birmingham Medical Center. Approximately half of these patients were less than 50 years old. Our experience would suggest that invasive cancer occurs uncommonly before age 30, however it is quite common in patients between 30 and 70 years of age and beyond (Table 3.1).

Women fear the diagnosis of cancer and despite symptoms often delay in seeking a physician's opinion. In fact, Fruchter (1980) reported that a third of patients delayed seeing their physician for over 6 months after their initial symptoms. In a similar report, Flowers (1958) concluded that half of the patients theoretically could have had their disease diagnosed in a less advanced stage; this paper implicated both patient and physician delay. The latter was usually attributed to an inadequate initial physical examination or to inadequate evaluation and treatment of inconclusive cervical smears or biopsies.

The cytological diagnosis of invasive cancer of the uterine cervix is fraught with error, due to sampling problems and to misinterpretation by the cytopathologist. In general, atypical cervical smears in young women are predominantly associated with dysplasia. Cavanagh (1966) screened 18 160 women less than 30 years of age and of the 424 women (2.3%) with abnormal smears, he discovered 19 invasive cancers (4.5% of the abnormal smears). In older women, more invasive lesions will be

44

Table 3.1 Cancer of the cervix. No previous treatment 1970–1981. Age group by clinical stage.

Age Group	Clinical stage* I Pts	I %	II Pts	II %	III Pts	III %	IV Pts	IV %	Total Pts	Total %
10–19	1	50.0	1	50.0	0	0	0	0	2	0.2
20–29	68	90.7	5	6.7	2	2.7	0	0	75	6.3
30–39	177	76.7	39	16.9	11	4.8	4	1.7	231	19.3
40–49	137	56.2	65	26.7	31	12.7	11	4.5	244	20.4
50–59	117	45.2	99	38.2	35	13.5	8	3.1	259	21.6
60–69	74	35.2	92	43.8	25	11.9	19	9.1	210	17.5
70–79	37	28.9	61	47.7	21	16.4	9	7.0	128	10.7
80–89	10	22.7	15	34.1	13	29.6	6	13.6	44	3.7
90–99	0	0	2	50.0	1	25.0	1	25.0	4	0.3
Totals	651	51.9	379	31.7	139	11.6	58	4.9	1197	100.0

*Current data – University of Alabama, Birmingham. An additional 387 patients who had received previous treatment were also registered

found, but because of inflammation and necrosis, the cytological examination may be unsatisfactory and will result in an appreciable false-negative rate. After all, the cytological smear is only a screening method and histological confirmation or investigation is required either because of an atypical smear or a visible lesion on the cervix.

A particular problem of diagnosis occurs in younger women where the physicians' index of suspicion is low. Berkowitz (1979) reported a high false-negative smear rate when screening young women and recommended that all suspicious or symptomatic cervical lesions should be biopsied promptly, regardless of previous cytology. Visible or palpable cervical abnormalities during pregnancy or at the time of the postpartum examination should not be ignored simply because cytological smears are 'negative'. Adenocarcinomas which occur in young women are more commonly associated with negative cytology than are squamous cell carcinomas.

Colposcopic examination can aid in the diagnosis of micro-invasion and microcarcinoma (definition: see Ch. 2). At the time of colposcopic examination, adequate biopsies should be obtained from areas showing a mosaic pattern, punctation or atypical vessels. Sugamori (1979) indicated that the important colposcopic findings of micro-invasive carcinomas are an irregular mosaic pattern, papillary punctation or atypical vessels. Coppleson (1979) indicated, however, that with the exception of atypical vessels, the colposcopic findings of early invasion may be less impressive than those of carcinoma in situ. Atypical vessels (Fig. 3.1) should prompt the colposcopist to obtain ample biopsies in order to detect early invasive lesions. A punch biopsy diagnosis of micro-invasion is never sufficient; whenever there is a question as to the extent or depth of invasion on a biopsy, cervical conization is mandatory.

In addition to directed biopsies, we consider the endocervical curettage (Fig. 3.2) an important diagnostic tool since occasionally an occult lesion will be uncovered in the endocervical canal. This is especially true in postmenopausal women. Invasive cancer of the cervix usually involves the canal and the endocervical curettage will therefore contain malignant tissue fragments. It is a simple procedure that, together with the directed biopsies and smears, allows the clinician accurately to diagnose cervical precancer or cancer in an outpatient setting. Cold knife conization is an essential part of the evaluation in patients who have abnormal endocervical curettages or biopsies suggesting or demonstrating superficial invasion, since it will provide the pathologist with adequate material to establish the presence of and the extent of invasion.

Even if colposcopy is not available, the physician can often diagnose

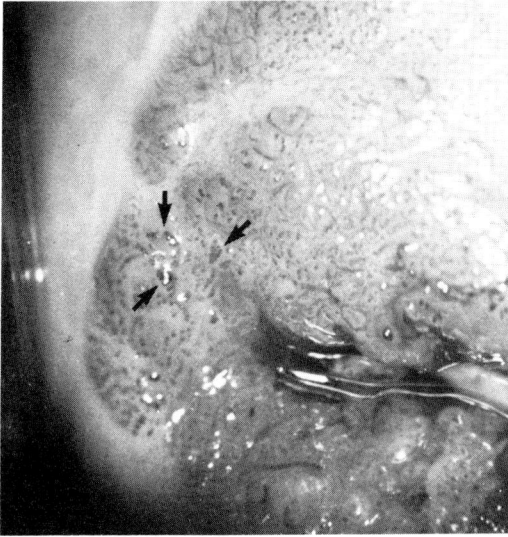

Fig. 3.1 Detail of atypical vessels (arrows) in a patient with micro-invasive carcinoma. (Colpophotograph courtesy of Dr Kenneth Hatch)

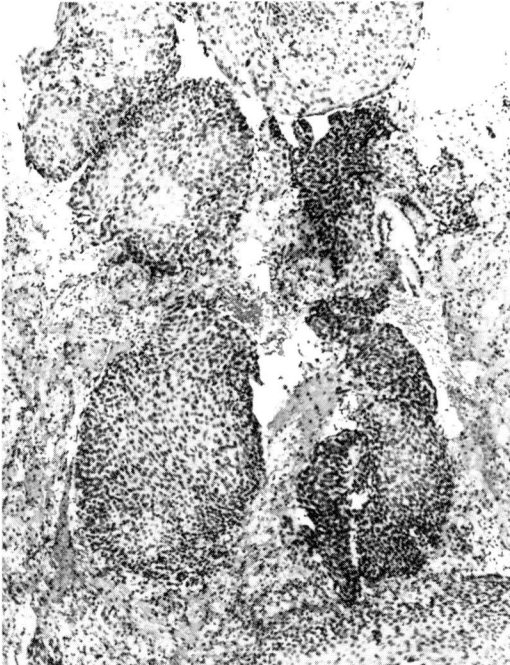

Fig. 3.2 Endocervical curettage specimen containing fragments of neoplastic squamous epithelium. A diagnosis of invasive carcinoma is not possible unless stromal invasion is demonstrated. Conisation of the cervix is necessary for a precise diagnosis. (H&E × 107)

early cancer of the cervix in his office; by staining with Lugol's iodine, multiple punch biopsies of non-staining areas and endocervical curettage, one can achieve an accuracy almost equal to that of colposcopy. The physician should biopsy any suspicious cervical lesion, regardless of the status of the cervical cytology. If conization is necessary, certain steps should be taken to ensure adequate histological evaluation. The pathologist should obtain a large number of tissue blocks (Fig. 3.3) in order that the entire specimen may be studied. If indicated, additional levels may be obtained from the blocks containing the most abnormal areas.

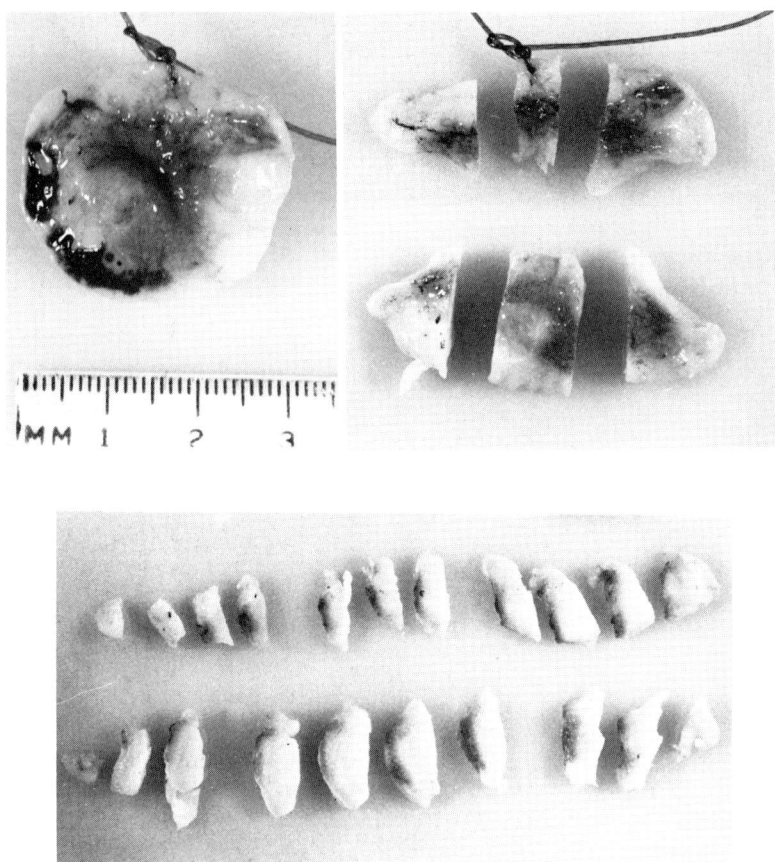

Fig. 3.3 Handling of a conisation specimen for optimal study. The tie indicates the 12 o'clock position. Cone is opened at 3 and 9 o'clock. The central segment from each lip is complete from endocervix to portio. Each of these segments is divided into blocks taking care to preserve the lines of surgical excision. The lateral segments are also divided into blocks, realising that only the portio (?vaginal) margin is a line of surgical excision. (Technique of Hazel Gore MB BS.)

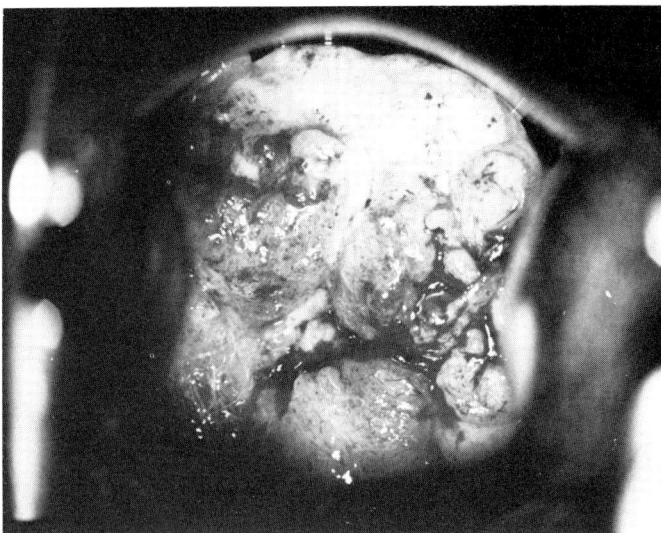

Fig. 3.4 An exophytic squamous cell carcinoma involving all quadrants of the cervix.

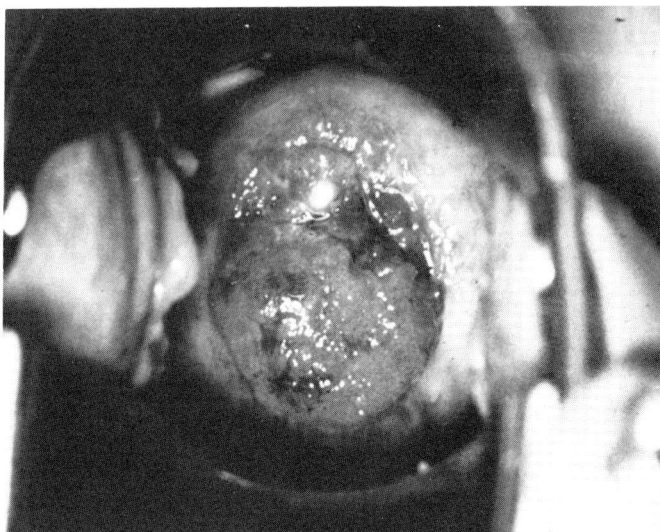

Fig. 3.5 An exophytic adenosquamous carcinoma.

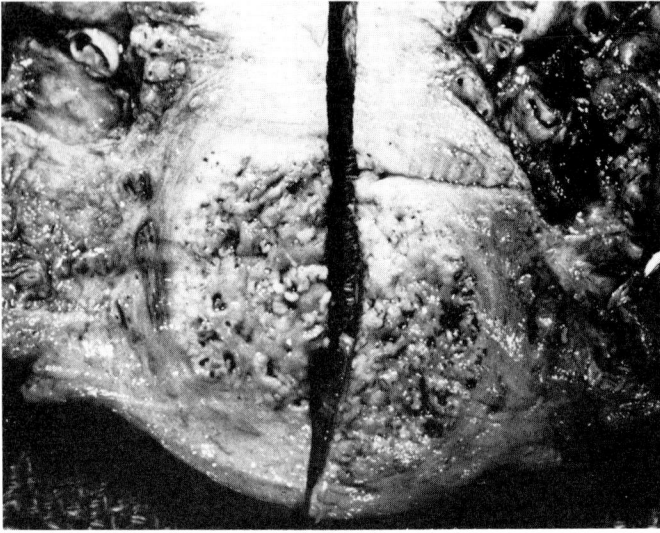

Fig. 3.6 A section of a radical hysterectomy specimen containing a squamous cell carcinoma confined to the endocervical canal. This tumour deeply invaded the stroma but was not apparent clinically.

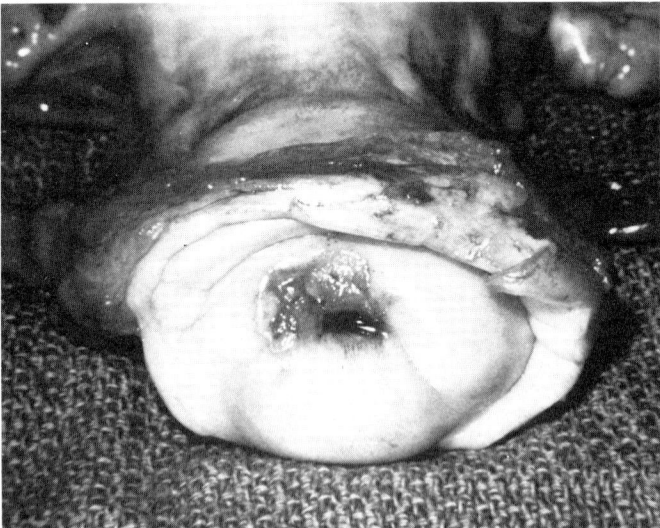

Fig. 3.7 A one-quadrant superficial ulcerative carcinoma. Maximum depth of invasion in this tumour was 8 mm.

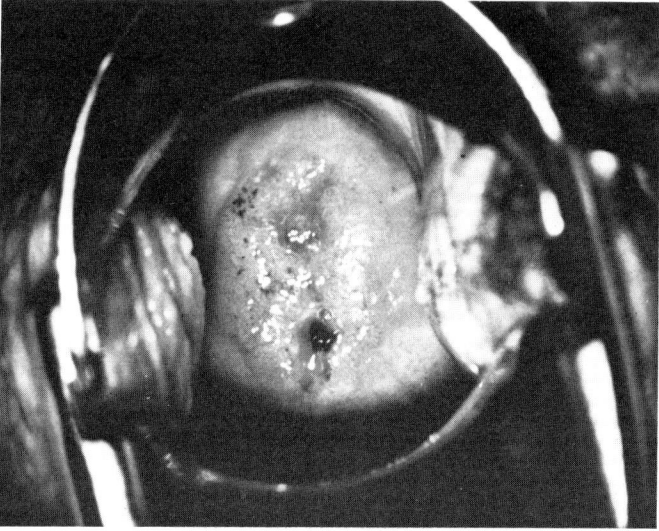

A

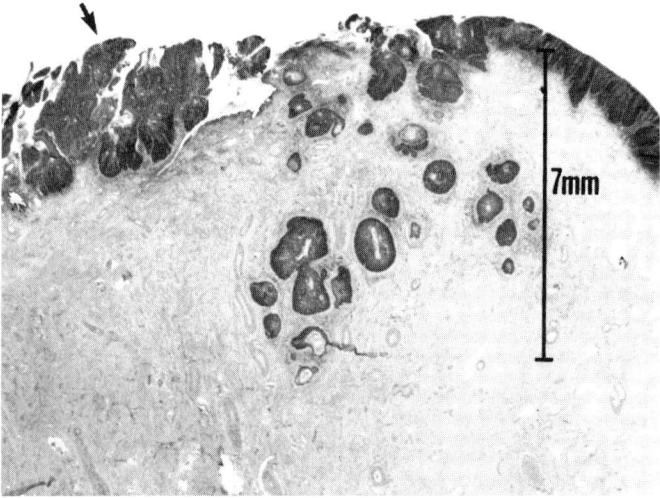

B

Fig. 3.8(A) A superficial papillary squamous cell carcinoma involving all four quadrants of the cervix. The histological features (B) include superficial invasion to 7 mm at one point; the papillary configuration is shown at the left (arrow). (H&E ×5)

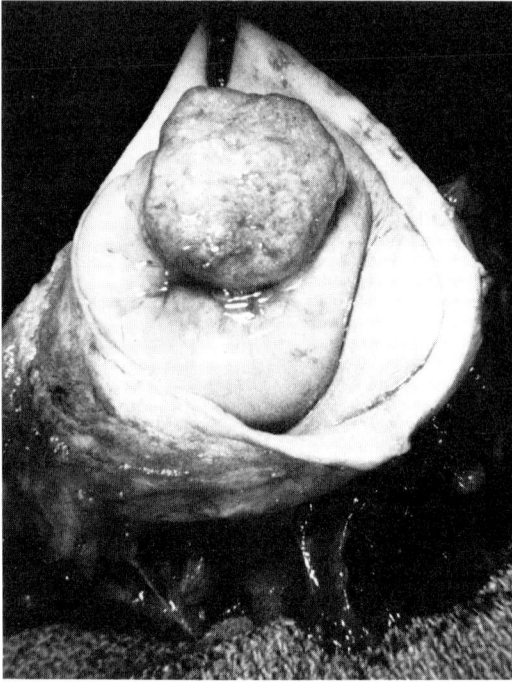

Fig. 3.9 A radical hysterectomy specimen in which a large polypoid adenosquamous carcinoma extends from the endocervical canal. (Photograph courtesy of Dr J. Max Austin, Jr)

Clinically, cervical cancers may appear as exophytic, endophytic, ulcerative, or polypoid lesions (Fig. 3.4–3.9). The exophytic configuration occurs slightly more often in squamous cell carcinomas than the ulcerative lesion (38% and 33% respectively). About 24% of lesions are endophytic in type while 5% are polypoid. Adenocarcinomas of the cervix are not markedly different in their clinical presentation (exophytic 40%, endophytic 32%, ulcerative 19%, polypoid 9%). It is interesting and perhaps surprising that the majority of adenocarcinomas are not endophytic in type, probably due to the eversion of the histological endocervix in women in the reproductive ages.

The nodular cervical carcinoma without a mucosal lesion is rarely encountered. The cervix that is unusually large or that is abnormal to palpation should be biopsied, just as all visible lesions require biopsy.

Occult carcinomas are small non-palpable endophytic lesions which have not expanded the endocervix. Unlike the micro-invasive group of lesions in which nodal metastases are rare (3% or less), occult lesions behave like larger, clinically apparent lesions. Boronow (1977) reported a high rate (20.7%) of pelvic nodal metastases in patients with IB occult tumours. Our experience is almost identical; occult lesions were commonly associated with bilaterally involved pelvic nodes (15%), and involved aortic nodes (8%). Presumably this is related to increased access to lymphatic vessels when the tumours invade the cervical stroma high in the endocervical canal.

Endometrial extension of cervical cancer has been reported by a number of authors to result in a poor prognosis. Perez (1978) reported that 9% of patients have extension of their cervical tumours to the lower uterine segment. Baltzer (1981) reported that three of four patients who were found to have ovarian metastases at the time of radical hysterectomy, had extension into the endometrium as well. It is difficult to determine the frequency of endometrial extension, since a large number of patients with cancer of the cervix do not have the uterus available for pathological study. Additionally, it is not easy to retrieve a specimen from the uterus that is not contaminated by the cervical tumour. In our patients undergoing radical hysterectomy, only a very few (2–4%) have had invasive tumour extension into the endometrial cavity. However, patients treated by radical hysterectomy have smaller tumours and cannot be compared to patients with larger volume lesions, which may involve the endometrial cavity more commonly. Because of uncertainty of the significance of this finding, the current FIGO staging system does not alter the stage for its presence (Table 3.2).

The large endophytic lesion that has distorted and expanded the endocervix to a barrel shape (Fig. 3.10) is associated with a poorer prognosis. Distortion of the lower uterine segment implies large tumour volume, and with the expansion, clinical staging becomes difficult. This configuration is associated with a high incidence of nodal metastases and a high failure rate, regardless of treatment modality.

With fewer indications for subtotal hysterectomy, carcinoma of the cervical stump is uncommonly seen in the United States. Staging considerations are the same; however,these lesions sometimes present problems in treatment because of distorted anatomy and adhesions of bowel to the upper part of the remaining cervix. Sala (1963) pointed out that although stump carcinomas have decreased in numbers, a more serious problem has emerged; i.e., postsurgical referral after hysterectomy, at which point the operative specimen was discovered to contain invasive cancer of the cervix. Green (1969) stated that 'simple hysterectomy had no place in the primary treatment of invasive cervical cancer.' He advocated early reoperation with radical surgical removal of the residual tumour-bearing area, as did Barber (1968). With this approach, Green achieved a 67% 5-year survival (21 patients) compared to a 30% 5-year survival for 30 patients treated by postoperative radiotherapy. Andras (1973) and Davy (1977) have reported excellent

Table 3.2 Staging classification for carcinoma of the cervix as adopted by the International Federation of Gynaecology and Obstetrics (1976)

Pre-invasive carcinoma

Stage 0   Carcinoma in situ, intra-epithelial carcinoma
Cases of stage 0 should not be included in any therapeutic statistics for invasive carcinoma

Invasive carcinoma

Stage I   Carcinoma strictly confined to the cervix (extension to the corpus should be disregarded)

     Stage Ia   Micro-invasive carcinoma (early stromal invasion)
     Stage Ib   All other cases of stage I. Occult cancer should be marked 'occ'

Stage II   The carcinoma extends beyond the cervix, but has not extended on to the pelvic wall
The carcinoma involves the vagina, but not the lower third

     Stage IIa   No obvious parametrial involvement
     Stage IIb   Obvious parametrial involvement

Stage III   The carcinoma has extended on to the pelvic wall. On rectal examination there is no cancer-free space between the tumour and the pelvic wall. The tumour involves the lower third of the vagina. All cases with a hydronephrosis or non-functioning kidney should be included, unless they are known to be due to another cause

     Stage IIIa   No extension on to the pelvic wall
     Stage IIIb   Extension on to the pelvic wall and/or hydronephrosis or non-functioning kidney

Stage IV   The carcinoma has extended beyond the true pelvis or has clinically involved the mucosa of the bladder or rectum. A bullous oedema as such does not permit a case to be alloted to stage IV

     Stage IVa   Spread of the growth to adjacent organs
     Stage IVb   Spread to distant organs

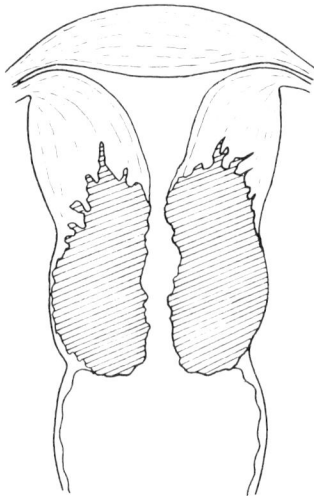

Fig. 3.10 Diagram of an infiltrating endocervical tumour causing expansion of the lower uterine segment, the so-called 'barrel-shaped' tumour (see text).

survival (over 80%) with high energy radiation treatment delivered promptly after discovery of the tumour. We have used both methods and favour reoperation in young patients. It is unacceptable to withhold additional potentially curative therapy after an inadequate operation, since nodal metastases and high recurrence rates increase with increasing tumour volume. The situation emphasises that cervical cytology is mandatory before a hysterectomy is performed for any indication.

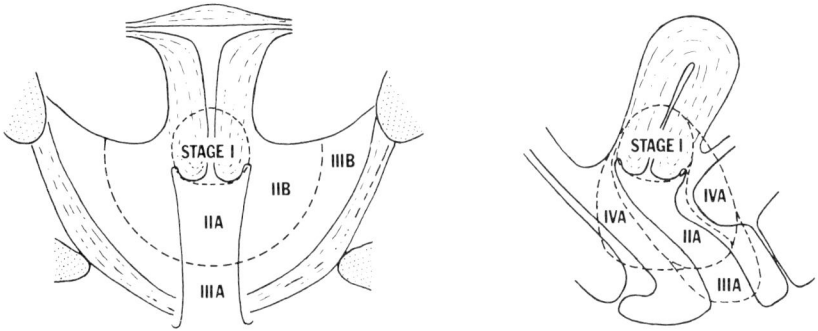

Fig. 3.11 Schematic representation of the clinical stages of cervical cancer. A. Anterior projection; B. Lateral projection.

STAGING

The current staging system of the International Federation of Gynaecology and Obstetrics is depicted in Table 3.2 and in Figure 3.11. Van Nagell (1971) compared this staging system to all previous staging systems, including that of the League of Nations and to the TNM (Tumour, Node, Metastasis) system and indicated that the FIGO staging system was as good as or superior to the others. In a recently collected series of 5810 patients (Table 3.3), about one-half of patients are FIGO stage I. This increasing rate of early stage lesions may be related to successful screening programmes. It coincides with the increasing numbers of patients diagnosed with pre-invasive lesions of

Table 3.3 Cancer of the cervix: percentage in various stages

Author	Year	No. of pts	I	II	III	IV
Kjorstad	1977	2002	47	37	11	5
Jiminez	1979	1227	31	55	12	2
Volterrani	1980	417	45	24	30	1
Zander	1981	980	77.7	22.5	0.3	–
Authors	1981	1184	52.4	31.1	11.7	4.8
Totals		5810	49.7	36.2	10.9	3.2

the cervix and the falling death rate from cancer of the cervix which has been noted in the United States and other countries in recent years.

Routine studies

In addition to a general physical and pelvic examination, the patient with cancer of the cervix requires other investigative studies to delineate the extent of disease and aid in selection of proper therapy (Table 3.4).

Table 3.4 Evaluation of cervical cancer patients

Category	Routine	Optional
Haematological Blood chemistry	Packed cell volume White cell count and differential Blood urea nitrogen, creatinine Liver enzymes Electrolytes	Coagulation studies Carcinoembryonic antigen (CEA) Nutritional screen (serum albumin, transferrin)
Radiographic Imaging	Chest X-rays Intravenous pyelography Barium enema	Computerized axial tomography (chest, abdomen, pelvis) Ultrasonography (abdomen, pelvis) Lymphangiography (pelvis) Radio-isotope scans (renal, liver, bone)
Endoscopic	Cystoscopy Proctosigmoidoscopy	Flexible colonoscopy Retrograde pyelography Bronchoscopy
Other	Nodal assessment (supraclavicular, inguinal) Abdominal palpation Pelvic assessment (bimanual, rectovaginal)	Delayed sensitivity skin testing Urodynamic testing Pulmonary function studies Electrocardiography Exam under anaesthesia

The importance of an examination under anaesthesia (EUA) was demonstrated by van Nagell (1971) with his report that it increased the accuracy of staging by 25%. The EUA allows a better inspection of the upper vagina and more precise palpation of the parametrial and lateral sidewall tissues than the routine office examination. Opportunities for an EUA occur either at the time of surgical treatment or at the time of intracavitary radio-isotope application. We rarely utilize such an examination other than in conjunction with the procedures mentioned above, unless primary therapy decisions cannot be made without clarification of the pelvic findings. In these circumstances, both the gynaecologic oncologist and the radiation therapist should be present for the EUA. At the time of examination or during other screening studies, abdominal or pelvic masses or enlarged lymph nodes (para-aortic, inguinal or pelvic sidewall) may be detected. Fine-needle aspiration may be performed under sonar or computerised tomography guidance (Table 3.5, Fig. 3.12); in experienced hands, the accuracy of

Table 3.5 Accuracy of fine-needle aspiration

Author	Year	No. of pts	Site	Accuracy (%)
Nordquist	1979	58	Abdominal/pelvic masses	95.0
Belinson	1981	90	Abdominal/pelvic masses	96.5
Shepherd	1981	50	Abdominal/pelvic masses	96.0
Dolan	1981	51	Retroperitoneal nodes	86.0
McDonald	1982	56	Retroperitoneal nodes	85.4
Totals		304		92.4

this technique is high and should be considered a part of modern management. Its use may obviate many laparotomies and eliminate other diagnostic studies.

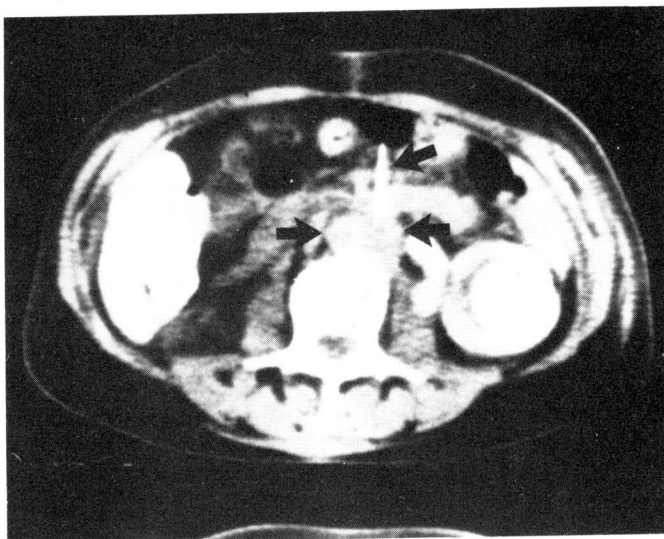

Fig. 3.12 Computerised axial tomography (CAT) scan demonstrating a needle (upper arrow) inserted into an enlarged para-aortic node (lower arrow). The path of the needle is only partially in the plane of the tomogram. (Photograph courtesy of Dr Peyton Taylor, University of Virginia, Charlottesville)

Radiographic studies including chest X-rays (Fig. 3.13) and intravenous pyelograms are essential. If either demonstrates extracervical disease, the treatment and prognosis are altered. Recognition that ureteral obstruction alters the prognosis is reflected in a recent change in the staging system. Currently, patients with this finding are assigned to stage III, whereas prior to 1971 other criteria (sidewall fixation or lower vaginal involvement) were required for assignment to this stage. Intravenous pyelograms rarely reveal obstruction in patients with palpable stages I and II disease; however, 33–42% of patients with palpable stage IIIB disease will have abnormal pyelograms (Shingleton 1971, van Nagell 1975).

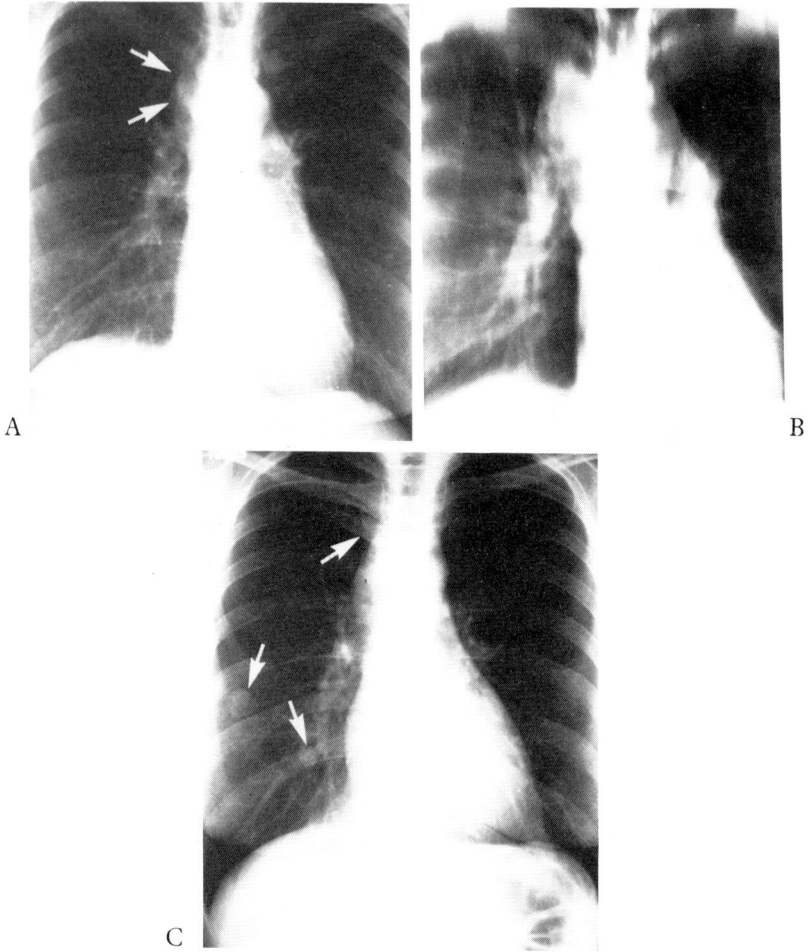

Fig. 3.13 Mediastinal and pulmonary metastases from cervical cancer. A. & B. Chest films demonstrating a mass in the right paratracheal and azygos region of a 39-year-old woman with squamous cell carcinoma. The whole lung tomography (B) delineates the mass, which consisted of enlarged malignant lymph nodes. C. Rounded opacities (arrows) in the right mid-lung field which represented metastatic disease in a 33-year-old woman with adenosquamous carcinoma.

The barium enema is especially important in older women as it may identify intrinsic colon disease, such as diverticulitis, ulcerative colitis, polyps or other conditions that may modify the treatment plan. Large bowel involvement by cervical cancer is almost always contiguous, i.e. a direct extension from the cervix to the rectum. This is better evaluated by proctoscopy than by barium enema.

Cystoscopy and proctoscopy are important studies if the lesion is bulky and especially if it involves the anterior or posterior vagina. If positive biopsies are obtained, the patient is relegated to stage IVA and has a poorer prognosis. The presence of bullous oedema in the base of the bladder is an ominous finding since it indicates tumour invasion of the bladder muscularis and is associated with a poor prognosis, even though it does not change the stage of the patient.

Screening blood chemistries are important as they may predict or confirm other abnormal findings, i.e., elevated serum blood urea nitrogen and creatinine are associated with ureteral obstruction as demonstrated by the intravenous pyelogram. Abnormal liver enzymes may accompany advanced metastatic disease but are more likely to identify patients with non-malignant liver disease. Elevated serum calcium values secondary to bone metastases or ectopic parathormone production may accompany advanced disease.

The usefulness of carcinoembryonic antigen (CEA) testing has been studied in squamous cell carcinoma of the cervix. Van Nagell (1979) performed immunoperoxidase staining of tumour tissues and found CEA to be present in 63% of 241 patients with squamous cell carcinoma. The recurrence rate of patients with the CEA-producing tumours was slightly higher than that of those with non-CEA-producing tumours; however, the difference was not statistically significant. He concluded that patients whose tumours stain for CEA could benefit from serial plasma CEA determinations, since rising plasma levels correlate directly with recurrent cancer in over 80% of such patients. At the present time, this technique is investigational and is not applicable to the routine follow-up of patients with squamous cell carcinoma.

Wahlstrom (1979), also using immunoperoxidase tissue staining, demonstrated the presence of CEA in 80% of cervical biopsies from patients with adenocarcinoma of the endocervix (exception: mesonephric tumours). He concluded that the technique may be helpful in distinguishing endocervical tumours from endometrial tumours, which contain CEA in only 8% of patients.

Ultrasonography and computerised axial tomography are helpful in the diagnosis and measurement of enlarged retroperitoneal nodes, abdomino-pelvic masses and abscesses (Figs. 3.14–3.16), but are not mandatory in the evaluation of cervical cancer patients. The studies are accurate in delineation of liver metastases and are capable of detecting ureteral obstruction. It has been suggested that CAT scans might replace intravenous pyelograms as part of the metastatic work-up; however the cost of the intravenous pyelogram is much less and it serves as an important part of the post-treatment surveillance. The limitations of the CAT scan in the pelvis were indicated by Grumbine (1981) who indicated that only 58% of scans accurately predicted parametrial

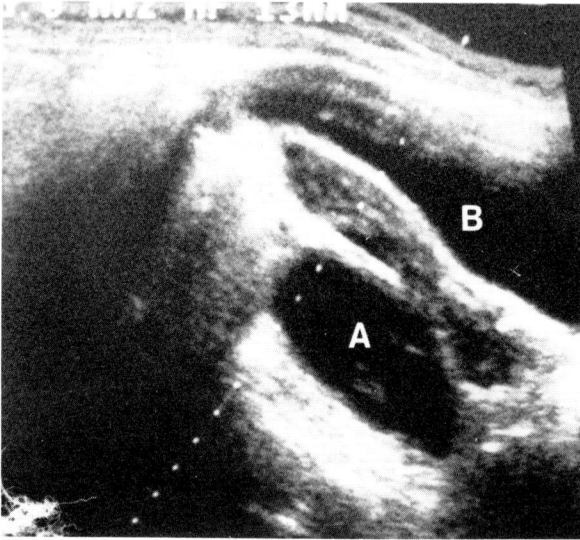

Fig. 3.14 A longitudinal midline ultrasound scan which reveals a large abscess in the cul-de-sac in a patient with squamous cell carcinoma of the cervix. A = abscess; B = bladder.

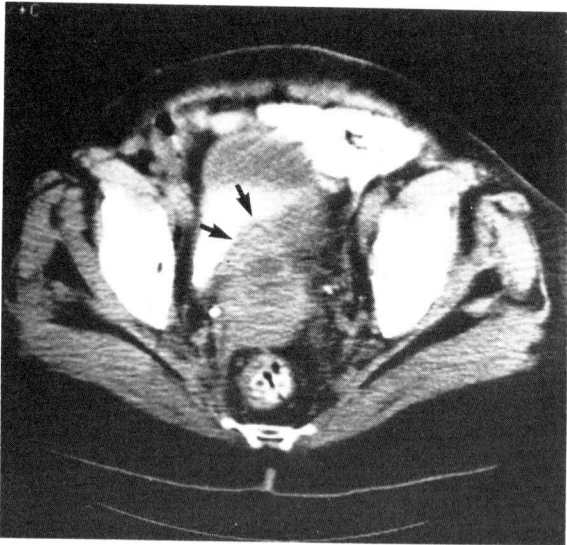

Fig. 3.15 A pelvic computerised axial tomography (CAT) scan in which a pelvic mass elevates the bladder base. The interface between the mass and the bladder is irregular (arrows), secondary to invasion of the bladder wall by carcinoma.

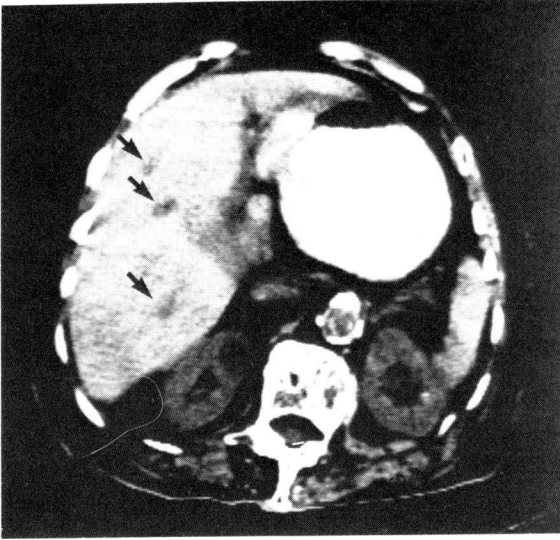

Fig. 3.16 A computerised axial tomography (CAT) scan through the liver of a 46-year-old woman with squamous cell carcinoma. Several metastatic areas are demonstrated (arrows). Enlarged para-aortic lymph nodes, presumably due to metastatic disease, were present though not demonstrated in this section.

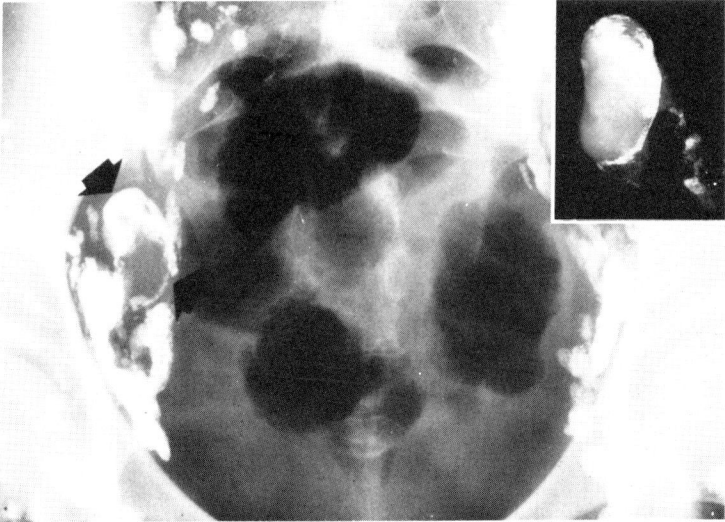

Fig. 3.17 Details of a lymphangiographic study of pelvic lymph nodes. A large right pelvic node (arrows) has a filling defect secondary to invasion by squamous cell carcinoma. The inset shows the same node after removal. (Films courtesy of Dr Peyton Taylor, University of Virginia, Charlottesville)

extension. Experience with both ultrasonography and CAT scanning has demonstrated the inherent difficulty of interpretation of these images unless radiologists and surgeons jointly view the films before and after each laparotomy. The main value of these techniques is in identifying enlarged retroperitoneal nodes, especially in the para-aortic area, and in giving additional information about abdomino-pelvic masses.

Lymphangiography (Fig. 3.17) has been advocated by many authors for evaluation of pelvic and aortic nodes. There are significant false-positive and false-negative rates, especially in regard to the evaluation of aortic nodes (Tables 3.6, 3.7). For these reasons and because in contrast to CAT scans and ultrasound, it is invasive and morbid, we seldom use the technique at this institution. It also shares with CAT scans and ultrasonography the problem of interpretation; all of these studies should be interpreted with caution.

Renal scans using ^{131}I-labelled hippuran provide superior information on renal function and are complementary to intravenous pyelograms, which primarily demonstrate renal anatomical changes. Patricio (1968) indicated that over half the patients with stages III and IV disease had abnormal renographic studies and about a third of these changes improved after irradiation. While scans are not recommended routinely, they can be of value in determining the degree of function of a poorly visualised collecting system demonstrated with intravenous pyelography.

Radionucleotide scans of the liver are seldom helpful and have been replaced by the more accurate ultrasound or CAT scans. It provides, however, an alternate method of evaluation of patients whose blood chemistries reveal abnormal liver function. Nuclear isotope bone scans are rarely indicated unless the patient has bone pain and should be preceded by skeletal films of the affected area. Routine long bone X-ray studies are not indicated, since they are rarely positive in the absence of bone pain. The routine chest films and pyelograms offer an opportunity to survey the vertebral column, ribs and pelvic bones (Figs. 3.18, 3.19).

Surgical staging

In recent years a number of studies regarding the value of surgical staging for cancer of the cervix have been completed. It is apparent, based on these studies, that clinical staging is highly inaccurate (Table 3.8). Overall errors range from 25% of patients with clinical stage I to 50% or more of patients with stage III disease. These inaccuracies have prompted many institutions to utilise surgical staging to better localise tumour spread. The main benefit of surgical staging is the diagnosis of extrapelvic disease which markedly alters treatment. It is noted,

Table 3.6 Accuracy of lymphangiography: pelvic nodes

Author	Year	No. of pts	False +	False −	Overall accuracy
Piver	1971	103	2.4	19.7	76.9
Averette	1972	70	–	–	79.0
Leman	1975	60	42.9	5.9	51.2
Lagasse	1979	95	–	–	67.0
Pellier	1979	200	12.5	8.8	78.7
Volteranni	1980	145	–	–	82.8
Dolan	1981	50	–	–	38.0
Totals		723			75.4

Table 3.7 Accuracy of lymphangiography: aortic nodes

Author	Year	No. of pts	False +	False −	Overall accuracy
Averette	1972	70	–	–	50.0
Piver	1973	26	–	–	95.8
Brown	1979	21	62.5	12.5	25.0
Totals		117			55.6

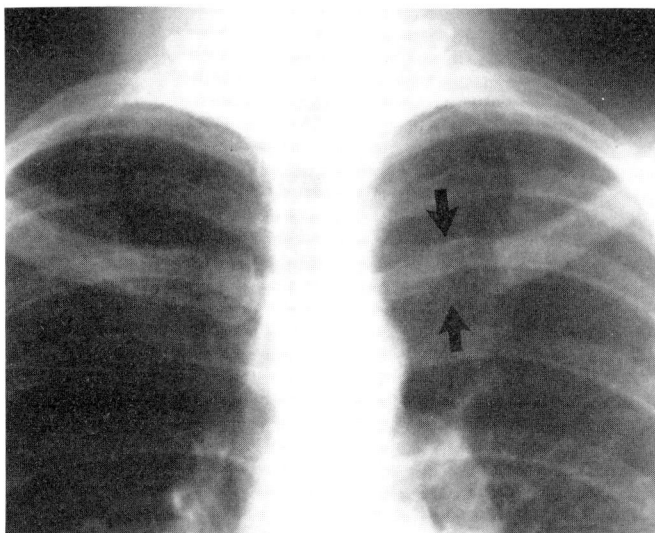

Fig. 3.18 Bony metastasis in a 27-year-old woman with squamous cell carcinoma. The medial portion of the left clavicle has been destroyed by tumour (arrows).

Table 3.8 Differences in clinical and surgical staging

Author	Year	No. of pts	Stage I inaccuracy %	Stage II inaccuracy %	Stage III inaccuracy %	Stage IV inaccuracy %	Overall inaccuracy %
van Nagell	1971	125	–	–	–	–	33.0
Averette	1972	82	–	–	–	–	38.6
Sudarsanam	1978	220	28.0	48.8	89.5	0	36.8
Lagasse	1979	95	–	–	–	–	33.6
Lagasse*	1980	290	24.4	50.0	44.4	50.0	38.3
Chung	1981	159	17.3	21.9	42.9	66.7	21.4
Totals		971	24.1	42.9	58.9	37.5	34.2

*Gynecologic Oncology Group data

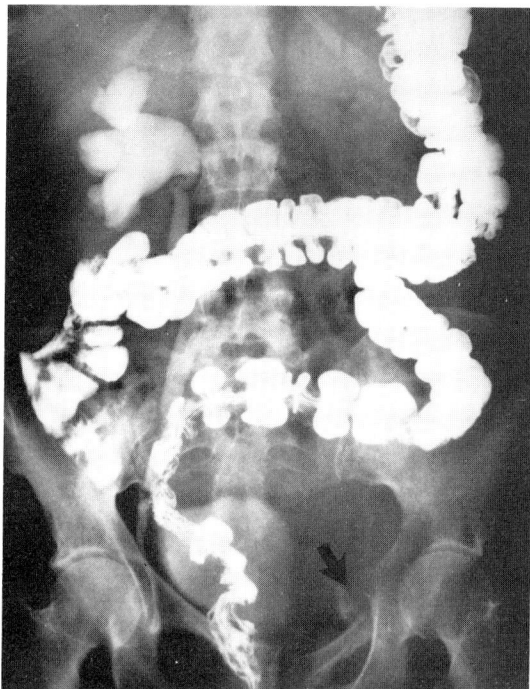

Fig. 3.19 Radiographic findings in a 44-year-old woman with advanced squamous cell cancer. The left kidney is non-visualising; there is right hydronephrosis and hydro-ureter of a marked degree. A pelvic mass displaces the bladder and rectosigmoid to the right. In addition, bony invasion has occurred in the right pelvis (arrow). (Film courtesy of Dr Larry Kilgore)

however (Table 3.9), that the transperitoneal surgical staging procedures are associated with appreciable major complications and occasional deaths, which may outweigh the benefits. The more extensive the nodal dissection the more serious the complications, as demonstrated by Wharton (1977) who reported 120 patients who had

Table 3.9 Complications of transperitoneal surgical staging procedures

Author	Year	No. of pts	Complications (%)	Deaths(%)
Piver*	1973	24	4.1	0
Berman	1977	31	43.0	0
Nelson*	1977	104	18.3	1.9
Buchbaum	1979	150	12.0	0.7
Bonanno*	1980	150	12.6	0
Lagasse	1980	245	15.5	0
Welander	1981	127	1.6	0
Totals		831	13.2	0.4

*Aortic dissection/biopsy

undergone extensive periaortic dissections. Thirteen of the patients (10.8%) experienced major complications and four patients (3.3%) died as a result of the procedure itself.

Alternate methods of exploration have been offered by Schellhas and Berman. Berman (1977) noted significantly fewer complications utilising an extraperitoneal approach through a lower abdominal J-shaped incision. This incision allows dissection of the pelvic nodes as well as the low aortic and common iliac nodes. The pelvic nodes are already in the treatment field and removal of nodal metastases offers little benefit; however, patients with occult disease at the time of periaortic dissection are potentially curable with extended radiation fields. Schellhas (1975) described a vertical abdominal incision for an extraperitoneal approach which allows sampling of the aortic and pelvic nodes and pointed out that his procedure is associated with very few complications and fatalities. In our modification of Schellhas' operation, a small incision (Fig. 3.20) is made above the pelvic radiation field. We have utilised this technique even in quite obese patients with very little morbidity and usually no delay in initiation of radiation therapy. Whereas we had experienced a number of serious small bowel complications associated with transperitoneal aortic node sampling followed by periaortic irradiation, we have not observed this using the modified Schellhas surgical staging procedure. When using the latter technique, we make a window in the peritoneum and obtain cul-de-sac washings, since free tumour cells in the peritoneal cavity are associated with a poor prognosis.

Certain authors have reported the ability to perform ancillary procedures including salpingo-oöphorectomy, ovarian biopsies, liver biopsies, resection of bowel lesions, or peritoneal biopsies at the time of transperitoneal exploratory laparotomy for surgical staging. The more recent shift to extraperitoneal techniques which avoid entering the pelvis preclude these procedures in most instances, however.

Surgical staging has provided new information concerning nodal metastases (Tables 3.10 and 3.11). The risk of metastases in pelvic nodes ranges from 15.9% in stage IB to 55% in stage IVA. The incidence of involved para-aortic nodes ranges from 6.5% in stage IB to 40.3% in stage IV. It is apparent that previously a large number of patients with extrapelvic disease have been treated with pelvic ports only. Since it appears that some patients with microscopic metastatic disease in the aortic nodes can be salvaged by extended field irradiation, it seems important to surgically stage those patients who are at high risk for affected aortic nodes, especially young patients.

Before beginning radiotherapy to the para-aortic nodes it is important to prove that there is no spread beyond this treatment field; it appears

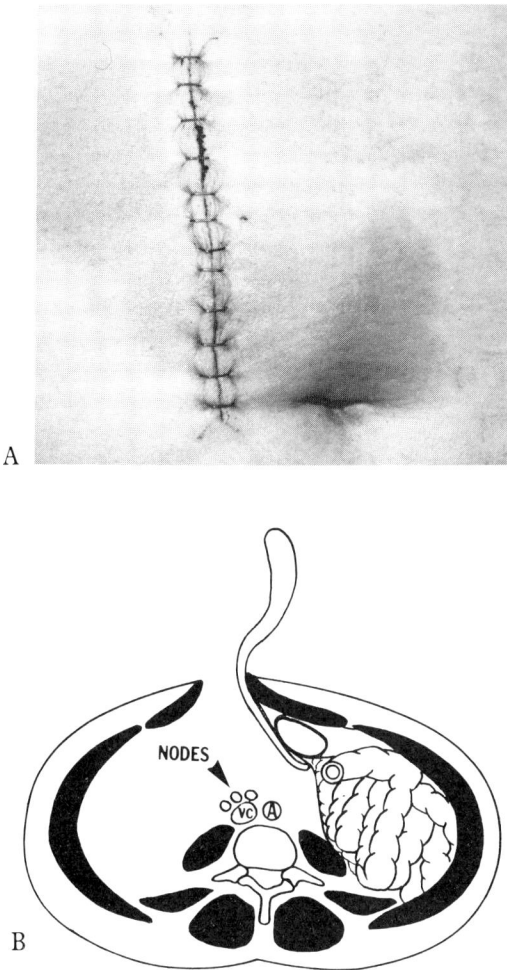

Fig. 3.20 An extraperitoneal approach to the para-aortic node area for surgical staging. A. The incision is above the umbilicus and out of the pelvic radiation field; B. Schematic representation of the abdominal contents in the peritoneal envelope displaced to the patient's left, allowing dissection of nodes between the renal vessels and the bifurcation of the iliac vessels. vc = vena cava; a = aorta

that approximately a third of patients with metastases to para-aortic nodes will have involved scalene nodes (Table 3.12). Currently our practice is to perform left supraclavicular fat-pad biopsy under the same anaesthetic when metastatic disease is found in para-aortic nodes.

Table 3.10 Incidence of pelvic node metastases by stage

Author	Year	IB		IIA		IIB		III		IVA	
		Pts	% Pos.	Pts	% Pos.	Pts	% Pos.	Pts	% Pos.	Pts	% Pos.
Navratil	1954	383	11.2	–	–	–	–	232	43.5	–	–
Sidhu	1970	115	16.5	–	–	–	–	–	–	–	–
Hsu	1972	670	12.4	–	–	–	–	32	50.0	16	56.3
Berman	1977	12	16.7	8	50.0	26	19.2	22	40.9	–	–
Boronow	1977	73	26.0	–	–	–	–	–	–	–	–
Burghardt	1978	44	15.9	13	33.3	93	36.5	106	35.8	–	–
Langley	1980	152	21.0	–	–	–	–	–	–	–	–
Ballon	1981	22	27.0	16	38.0	32	16.0	24	37.5	1	0
Chung	1981	110	12.7	15	20.0	17	17.6	14	50.0	3	66.6
Martimbeau	1981	562	21.3	–	–	–	–	–	–	–	–
Authors	1982	200	14.0	–	–	–	–	–	–	–	–
Totals		2343	15.9	52	32.7	168	28.0	234	43.8	20	55.0

Table 3.11 Incidence of para-aortic node metastases by stage

Author	Year	IB		IIA		IIB		III		IV	
		Pts	% Pos.	Pts	% Pos.	Pts	% Pos.	Pts	% Pos.	Pts	% Pos.
Nelson	1977	–	–	16	12.5	47	14.9	39	38.0	–	–
Wharton	1977	21	0	10	0	47	21.2	34*	32.3	8**	37.5
Sudarsanam	1978	153	7.0	21	14.0	22	18.0	19	26.3	–	–
Buchsbaum	1979	16	25.0	4	0	15	6.7	104	32.7	10	40.0
Bonanno	1980	–	–	23	4.0	73	12.0	52	31.0	3	33.0
Hughes	1980	140	4.3	35	8.5	45	24.4	96	23.9	23	43.5
Lagasse	1980	143	5.6	22	18.2	58	32.8	63	30.2	3	33.0
Ballon	1981	22	23.0	16	19.0	32	19.0	24	16.7	–	–
Chung	1981	110	4.5	15	6.7	17	17.6	14	42.9	3	66.6
Welander	1981	14	28.6	22	22.7	41	19.5	38	25.3	12	33.3
Authors	1982	187	4.8	–	–	–	–	–	–	–	–
Totals		806	6.5	184	11.9	397	19.6	483	29.6	62	40.3

Table 3.12 Scalene node metastases in untreated patients with para-aortic node metastases

Author	Year	No. of pts	% pos.
Buchsbaum	1979	23	35
Brandt	1981	25	28
Lee	1981	10	30
Totals		58	31

SELECTION OF THERAPY

Several factors are important in the selection of treatment: preservation of sexual function, the age of the patient, tumour volume, and demonstrated extrapelvic disease. All therapy for cancer of the cervix will alter or potentially alter sexual function. If the patient has stage IB disease and surgery can be used, the vagina, although shortened, is not otherwise changed. Too often the physician, adhering to the concept that older women should have no interest in sexual activity, ignores this important feature of treatment planning. Abitbol (1974) reported that radiation therapy markedly alters the vagina, and is associated with sexual dysfunction in 78% of patients, making intercourse impossible or less pleasurable. In contrast, only 6% of his surgically treated patients experienced sexual dysfunction. Our experience is similar to Abitbol's, although with the use of vaginal dilatation in the immediate postradiation period, stricturing of the vagina can perhaps be reduced from the levels he reported. The treatment of the great majority of patients with cancer of the cervix must be with radiation and every effort should be made (by vaginal dilations, local oestrogens, local antibacterial agents) to minimise the damage to the vagina in order that the patient can resume a normal sexual life after the therapy.

Whether young patients have a lower survival rate than older patients with the same stage cancer of the cervix is still controversial. Kjorstad (1977), studying a group of over 2000 patients, reported that young patients had a more favourable stage distribution and a better prognosis than older ones. Our patients with stage IB cancer of the cervix have no significant difference in survival rates in younger and older groups, using an age cut-off of either 40 years or 30 years. Stanhope (1980) reported a significantly lower 5-year survival in women under age 35. Cullhed (1978) quoted a 9% poorer survival rate for women under age 30. It is difficult to resolve this question in view of the fact that the current FIGO staging system allows great variation in tumour volume within a given stage, and accurate assessment of tumour volume and extent is impossible except in the surgically treated or surgically staged patients.

While some authors have stated that radical hysterectomy can be performed on women of almost any age, we have used primary surgical treatment in women over age 60 only when the patient is an excellent operative candidate. O'Leary (1966) considered age not to be a deterrent to radical hysterectomy and felt that the presence of cardiovascular or renal impairment was the most important consideration in selecting therapy.

Tumour volume is the single most important factor in predicting survival in patients with cancer of the cervix. It is also apparent that the clinical FIGO staging system is not an accurate measure of tumour volume and in many instances surgical staging procedures may improve the physician's ability to treat all of the disease. Bulky tumours, especially those involving the endocervical canal, may lead to consideration of a combination of irradiation and surgery, based on the observations of some authors that central pelvic failure is often seen following radiation treatment of bulky lesions of the endocervix. However, it has not been shown conclusively that increased survival is associated with combined treatment. It is our experience that most recurrences following irradiation treatment of bulky central pelvic disease are other than in the central pelvis, suggesting that routine adjunctive conservative hysterectomy does not alter survival rates.

Demonstration of extrapelvic tumour in the pretreatment evaluation usually alters treatment. Microscopic disease in the aortic nodes, in the absence of demonstrated spread to the scalene nodes, allows modification of the irradiation port to include the aortic nodes. Distant disease otherwise requires consideration of a chemotherapeutic approach with or without palliative radiation.

BIBLIOGRAPHY

Abitbol M M, Davenport J H 1974 The irradiated vagina. Obstetrics and Gynecology 44: 249–256
Andras E J, Fletcher G H, Rutledge F 1973 Radiotherapy of carcinoma of the cervix following simple hysterectomy. American Journal of Obstetrics and Gynecology 115: 647–655
Averette H E, Dudan R C, Ford J H Jr 1972 Exploratory celiotomy for surgical staging of cervical cancer. American Journal of Obstetrics and Gynecology 113: 1090–1096
Baltzer J, Koepcke W 1979 Tumor size and lymph node metastases in squamous cell carcinoma of the uterine cervix. Archives of Gynecology 227: 271–278
Baltzer J, Lohe K J, Kopcke W, Zander J 1981 Formation of metastases in the ovaries in operated squamous cell carcinoma of the cervix uteri. Geburtshilfe und Frauenheilkunde 41: 672–673
Baltzer J, Lohe K J, Kopcke W, Zander J 1982 Histological criteria for the prognosis in patients with operated squamous cell carcinoma of the cervix. Gynecologic Oncology 13: 184–194

Barber H R K, Pece G V, Brunschwig A 1968 Operative management of patients previously operated upon for a benign lesion with cervical cancer as a surprise finding. American Journal of Obstetrics and Gynecology 101: 959–965

Beecham J B, Halvorsen T, Kolbenstvedt A 1978 Histologic classification, lymph node metastases, and patient survival in stage IB cervical carcinoma. Gynecologic Oncology 6: 95–105

Belinson J L, Lynn J M, Papillo J L, Lee K, Korson R 1981 Fine-needle aspiration cytology in the management of gynecologic cancer. American Journal of Obstetrics and Gynecology 139: 148–153

Benedet J L, Turko M, Boyes D A, Nickerson K G, Bienkowska B T 1980 Radical hysterectomy in the treatment of cervical cancer. American Journal of Obstetrics and Gynecology 137: 254–262

Berkowitz R S, Ehrmann R L, Lavizzo-Mourey R, Knapp R C 1979 Invasive cervical carcinoma in young women. Gynecologic Oncology 8: 311–316

Berman M L, Lagasse L D, Watring W G, Ballon S C, Schlesinger R E, Moore J G et al 1977 The operative evaluation of patients with cervical carcinoma by an extraperitoneal approach. Obstetrics and Gynecology 50: 658–664

Bonanno J P, Boyce J, Fruchter R, Khulpateea N, Macasaet M, Remy J C 1980 Involvement of para-aortic lymph nodes in carcinoma of the cervix. Journal of American Osteopathic Association 79: 567–571

Boronow R C 1977 Stage I cervix cancer and pelvic node metastasis. Special reference to the implications of the new and the recently replaced FIGO classifications on stage Ia. American Journal of Obstetrics and Gynecology 127: 135–137

Brandt B, Lifshitz S 1981 Scalene node biopsy in advanced carcinoma of the cervix uteri. Cancer 47: 1920–1921

Brascho D J, Diagnostic and staging work-up (including ultrasound) in treatment planning. Course 116A, Department of Radiation Oncology, UAB School of Medicine, Alabama

Brown R C, Buchsbaum H J, Tewfik H H, Platz C E 1979 Accuracy of lymphangiography in the diagnosis of para-aortic lymph node metastases from carcinoma of the cervix. Obstetrics and Gynecology 54: 571–575

Buchsbaum H J 1979 Extrapelvic lymph node metastases in cervical carcinoma. American Journal of Obstetrics and Gynecology 133: 814–824

Buchsbaum H J, Lifshitz S 1976 The role of scalene lymph node biopsy in advanced carcinoma of the cervix uteri. Surgery, Gynecology and Obstetrics 143: 246–248

Buchsbaum H J, Rice A C 1972 Cerebral metastasis in cervical carcinoma. American Journal of Obstetrics and Gynecology 114: 276–278

Bueschen A J, Witten D M 1979 Radionuclide evaluation of renal function. Division of Urology, University of Alabama Medical School Symposium on Advances in Imaging Techniques. Urologic Clinics of North America 6: 307–320

Burghardt E 1982 Microinvasive and occult invasive carcinoma: pathology. In: Jordan J A, Sharp F, Singer A (eds) Pre-clinical neoplasia of the cervix. Royal College of Obstetricians and Gynaecologists, London

Cavanagh D, McLeod A G W, Ferguson J H 1966 Carcinoma of the cervix among women in their twenties. Journal of the American Medical Association 195 (10): 146–148

Chen S S, Kumari S, Lee L 1980 Contribution of abdominal computed tomography (CT) in the management of gynecologic cancer: correlated study of CT image and gross surgical pathology. Gynecologic Oncology 10: 162–172

Chung C K, Nahhas W A, Stryker J A, Curry S L, Abt A B, Mortel R 1980 Analysis of factors contributing to treatment failures in stages IB and IIA carcinoma of the cervix. American Journal of Obstetrics and Gynecology 138: 550–556

Coppleson M 1979 Microinvasive cervical cancer. Obstetrics and Gynecology Survey 34: 840–841

Cullhed S 1978 Carcinoma cervicis uteri stages I and IIA. Acta obstetrica et gynecologica scandinavica (supplement) 75: 1–28

Davy M, Bentzen H, Jahren R 1977 Simple hysterectomy in the presence of invasive cervical cancer. Acta obstetrica et gynecologica scandinavica 56: 105–108

Deale C J C, Du Toit M P 1980 Routine investigations in the clinical staging of invasive carcinoma of the cervix. South African Medical Journal 29: 895–898

Delgado G 1978 Stage IB squamous cancer of the cervix: the choice of treatment. Obstetrical and Gynecological Survey 33: 174–183

Dolan T E, McIntosh P K 1981 Percutaneous retroperitoneal lymph node biopsy: an appraisal for a substitute to laparotomy in far advanced metastatic carcinoma. Gynecologic Oncology 11: 364–370

Fisher M S 1980 Lumbar spine metastasis in cervical carcinoma: a characteristic pattern. Radiology 134: 631–634

Fletcher G H 1979 Predominant parameters in the planning of radiation therapy of carcinoma of the cervix. Bulletin of Cancer 66: 561–572

Flowers C E Jr, Ross R A, Pritchett N L 1958 Delay by physician and patient in the diagnosis and treatment of pelvic cancer. Southern Medical Journal 51: 1497–1504

Freiman D B, Ring E J, Oleaga J A, Carpiniello V C, Wein A J 1978 Thin needle biopsy in the diagnosis of ureteral obstruction with malignancy. Cancer 42: 714–716

Fruchter R G, Boyce J, Hunt M, Sillman F, Medhat I 1980 Invasive cancer of cervix: failures in prevention. II. Delays in diagnosis. New York State Journal of Medicine (May): 913–917

Fuller A F, Elliott N, Kosloff C, Lewis J L Jr 1982 Lymph node metastases from carcinoma of the cervix, stages IB and IIA: implications for prognosis and treatment. Gynecologic Oncology 13: 165–174

Ginaldi S, Wallace S, Jing B-S, Bernardino M E 1981 Carcinoma of the cervix: lymphangiography and computed tomography. American Journal of Roentgenology 136: 1087–1091

Gore H, Shingleton H M, Austin J M Jr 1976 A classification of endocervical curettings. Gynecologic Oncology 4: 53–65

Green T H, Morse W J Jr 1969 Management of invasive cervical cancer following inadvertent simple hysterectomy. Obstetrics and Gynecology 33: 763–769

Grumbine F C, Rosenshein N B, Zerhouni E A, Siegelman S S 1981 Abdominopelvic computed tomography in the preoperative evaluation of early cervical cancer. Gynecologic Oncology 12: 286–290

Hughes R R, Brewington K C, Hanjani P, Photopulos G, Dick D, Votava C et al 1980 Extended field irradiation for cervical cancer based on surgical staging. Gynecologic Oncology 9: 153–161

Jiminez J, Alert J, Beldarrain L, Montalvo J, Roca C 1979 Carcinoma of the uterine cervix. Acta radiologica: Oncology, Radiation, Physics, Biology 18: 465–469

Ketcham A S, Chretien P B, Hoye R C, Harrah J D, Deckers P J, Sugarbaker E V et al 1973 Occult metastases to the scalene lymph nodes in patients with clinically operable carcinoma of the cervix. Cancer 31: 180–183

Kjorstad J E 1977 Carcinoma of the cervix in the young patient. Obstetrics and Gynecology 50: 28–30

Kolstad 1982 Colposcopy services: discussion. In: Jordan J A, Sharp F, Singer A (eds) Pre-clinical neoplasia of the cervix. Royal College of Obstetricians and Gynaecologists, London

Kotz H L 1979 Endometrial extension of cervical tumor: a new technique for definitive detection. Maryland State Medical Journal (Dec.): 61

Lagasse L D, Ballon S C, Berman M L, Watring W G 1979 Pretreatment lymphangiography and operative evaluation in carcinoma of the cervix. American Journal of Obstetrics and Gynecology 134: 219–224

Lagasse L D, Creasman W T, Shingleton H M, Ford J H, Blessing J A 1980 Results and complications of operative staging in cervical cancer: experience of the gynecologic oncology group. Gynecologic Oncology 9: 90–98

Lang E K 1980 Angiography in the diagnosis and staging of pelvic neoplasms. Radiology 134: 353–358

Lee R B, Park R C 1981 Bladder dysfunction following radical abdominal hysterectomy. Gynecologic Oncology 11: 304–308

Lee R B, Weisbaum G S, Heller P B, Park R C 1981 Scalene node biopsy in primary and recurrent invasive carcinoma of the cervix. Gynecologic Oncology 11: 200–206

Lee K F, Greening R, Kramer S, Hahn G A, Kuroda K, Lin S-R et al 1971 The value of pelvic venography and lymphography in the clinical staging of carcinoma of the uterine cervix. American Journal of Roentgenology 3: 284–296

Leman M H, Park R C, Barham E D, Chism S E, Petty W M, Patow W E 1975 Pretreatment lymphangiography in carcinoma of the uterine cervix. Gynecologic Oncology 3: 354–360

McDonald T W, Morley G W, Choo Y C, Shields J J, Cordoba R B, Naylor B 1982 Fine needle aspiration of intra-abdominal lymph nodes showing lymphangiographic abnormalities in patients with gynecologic neoplasms. Obstetrics and Gynecology, in press

Maier R C, Norris H G 1980 Coexistence of cervical intraepithelial neoplasia with primary adenocarcinoma of the endocervix. Obstetrics and Gynecology 56: 361–364

Mann W J Jr, Jander H P, Orr J W Jr, Taylor P T, Hatch K D, Shingleton H M 1980 The use of percutaneous nephrostomy in gynecologic oncology. Gynecologic Oncology 10: 343–349

van Nagell J R Jr, Roddick J W Jr, Lowin D M 1971 The staging of cervical cancer: inevitable discrepancies between clinical staging and pathologic findings. American Journal of Obstetrics and Gynecology 110: 973–978

van Nagell J R, Sprague A D, Roddick J W Jr 1975 The effect of intravenous pyelography and cystoscopy on the staging of cervical cancer. Gynecologic Oncology 3: 87–91

van Nagell J R, Donaldson E S, Parker J C, van Dyke A H, Wood E G 1977 The prognostic significance of cell type and lesion size in patients with cervical cancer treated by radical surgery. Gynecologic Oncology 5: 142–151

van Nagell J R Jr, Rayburn W, Donaldson E S, Hanson M, Gay E C, Yoneda J et al 1979 Therapeutic implications of patterns of recurrence in cancer of the uterine cervix. Cancer 44: 2354–2361

Nelson J H Jr, Boyce J, Macasaet M, Lu T, Bohorquez J F, Nicastri A D et al 1977 Incidence, significance and follow-up of para-aortic lymph node metastases in late invasive carcinoma of the cervix. American Journal of Obstetrics and Gynecology 128: 336–340

Nordqvist S R B, Sevin B-U, Nadji M, Greening S E, Ng A B P 1979 Fine-needle aspiration cytology in gynecologic oncology. I. Diagnostic accuracy. Obstetrics and Gynecology 54: 719–724

O'Leary J A, Symmonds R E 1966 Radical pelvic operations in the geriatric patient: a 15-year review of 133 cases. Obstetrics and Gynecology 28: 745–753

Pagnini C A, Palma P D, DeLaurentiis G 1980 Malignancy grading in squamous carcinoma of uterine cervix treated by surgery. British Journal of Cancer 41: 415–421

Patricio M B, Baptista A M 1968 Renographic analyses in radiation therapy for carcinoma of the uterus. Acta radiologica: Therapy, Physics, Biology 7: 97–107

Pellier D, Chavanne G, Thu N T 1979 Lymphographic evaluation of cervico-uterine carcinoma. Bulletin of Cancer (Paris) 66: 515–518

Perez C A, Zivnuska F, Askin F, Camel H M, Ragan D, Powers W E 1977 Mechanisms of failure in patients with carcinoma of the uterine cervix extending into the endometrium. International Journal of Radiation Oncology, Biology, Physics 2: 651–659

Perez-Mesa C, Spratt J S Jr 1976 Scalene node biopsy in the pretreatment staging of carcinoma of the cervix uteri. American Journal of Obstetrics and Gynecology 125: 93–95

Pierson R L, Figge P K, Buchsbaum H J 1975 Surgery for gynecologic malignancy in the aged. Obstetrics and Gynecology 46: 523–527

Piver M S, Barlow J J 1973 Para-aortic lymphadenectomy, aortic node biopsy, and aortic lymphangiography in staging patients with advanced cervical cancer. Cancer 32: 367–370

Piver M S, Wallace S, Castro J R 1971 The accuracy of lymphangiography in carcinoma of the uterine cervix. American Journal of Roentgenology 111: 278–283

Rousseau J, Fenton J, Debertrand P, Mathieu G 1972 Carcinoma of the cervix. Radiology 103: 413–418

Rutledge F N, Galakatos A E, Wharton J T, Smith J P 1975 Adenocarcinoma of the uterine cervix. American Journal of Obstetrics and Gynecology 122: 236–245

Sakkas J L, Androulakis J, Pisidis A 1979 Ureteral obstruction due to carcinoma of the cervix uteri: a study by means of intravenous pyelography and lymphography of the cervix. American Surgery (Sept.): 569–574

Sala J M, deLeon A D 1963 Treatment of carcinoma of the cervical stump. Radiology 81: 300–306

Schellhas H F 1975 Extraperitoneal para-aortic node dissection through an upper abdominal incision. Obstetrics and Gynecology 46: 444–447

Selim M A, Kurohara S S, Webster J H 1971 Surgical or radiation therapy for cancer of the cervix stage I. Obstetrics and Gynecology 38: 251–255

Shepherd J H, Cavanagh D, Ruffolo E, Praphat H 1981 The value of needle biopsy in the diagnosis of gynecologic cancer. Gynecologic Oncology 11: 309–320

Shingleton H M, Fowler W C, Koch G G 1971 Pretreatment evaluation in cervical cancer. American Journal of Obstetrics and Gynecology 110: 385–389

Shingleton H M, Gore H, Bradley D H, Soong S-J 1981 Adenocarcinoma of the cervix. I. Clinical evaluation and pathologic features. American Journal of Obstetrics and Gynecology 139: 799–814

Spanos W J, Greer B E, Hamberger A D, Rutledge F N 1981 Prognosis of squamous cell carcinoma of the cervix with endometrial involvement (Abstract). Gynecologic Oncology 11: 230–234

Stanhope C R, Smith J P, Wharton J T, Rutledge F N, Fletcher G H, Gallager H S 1980 Carcinoma of the cervix: the effect of age on survival. Gynecologic Oncology 10: 188–193

Sudersanam A, Charyulu K, Belinson J, Averett H, Goldberg M, Hintz B et al 1978 Influence of exploratory celiotomy on the management of carcinoma of the cervix. Cancer 41: 1049–1053

Sugimori H, Matsuyama T, Kashimura M, Kashimura Y, Tsukamoto N, Taki I 1979 Colposcopic findings in microinvasive carcinoma of the uterine cervix. Obstetrical and Gynecological Survey 34: 804–807

Tao L C, Pearson F G, Delarue N C, Langer B, Sanders D E 1980 Percutaneous fine-needle aspiration biopsy. I. Its value to clinical practice. Cancer 45: 1480–1485

Volterrani F, Sigurta D, Gardani G, Milani A, Musumeci R 1980 Role of lymphography in cancer of the uterine cervix (Abstract). Radiologia medica (Torino) 66: 611–614

Wahlstrom T, Lindgren J, Korhonen M, Seppala M 1979 Distinction between endocervical and endometrial adenocarcinoma with immunoperoxidase staining of carcinoembryonic antigen in routine histological tissue specimens. Lancet 2: 1159–1160

Wallace S, Jing B-S, Zornoza J, Hammond J A, Hamberger A, Herson J et al 1979 Is lymphangiography worthwhile? Radiation Oncology, Biology, Physics 5: 1873–1876

Walsh J W, Rosenfield A T, Jaffe C C, Schwartz P E, Simeone J, Dembner A G et al 1978 Prospective comparison of ultrasound and computed tomography in the evaluation of gynecologic pelvic masses. American Journal of Roentgenology 131: 955–960

Welander C E, Pierce V K, Nori D, Hilaris B S, Kosloff C, Clark D G C et al 1981 Pretreatment laparotomy in carcinoma of the cervix. Gynecologic Oncology 12: 336–347

Wentz W B, Lewis G C 1965 Correlation of histologic morphology and survival in cervical cancer following radiation therapy. Obstetrics and Gynecology 26: 228–232

Wharton J T, Jones H W III, Day T G Jr, Rutledge F N, Fletcher G H 1977
Preirradiation celiotomy and extended field irradiation for invasive carcinoma of
the cervix. Obstetrics and Gynecology 49: 333–338

Wheeless C R Jr, Graham R, Graham J B 1970 Prognosis and treatment of adenoepidermoid carcinoma of the cervix. Obstetrics and Gynecology 35: 928–932

Yin-Chang Z, Pei-Fan Z, Yung-H W 1982 Metastatic carcinoma of the cervix uteri
from the gastrointestinal tract. (In press)

Zander J, Baltzer J, Lohe K J, Ober K G, Kaufmann C 1981 Carcinoma of the
cervix: an attempt to individualize treatment; results of a 20-year cooperative
study. American Journal of Obstetrics and Gynecology 139: 752–759

4

Primary surgical and combined treatment

SURGERY OR RADIATION?

When one compares cure rates between surgical and radiation treatment for stage IB cancer of the cervix, the survival rates are almost identical. Delgado (1978), in a collected series, reported 83.4% 5-year survival following radical surgery (2600 patients) and 85.5% 5-year survival following radiotherapy (1995 patients). But apart from survival, there are other advantages of surgical treatment for patients with small volume stages I and IIA (Table 4.1). Although radiation can be used in all patients, the bladder and bowel damage incurred in 2% to 6% of patients may present chronic problems for the patient and her physician. Radiation cystitis or proctitis may occur months or years following treatment and persist for long periods of time. Bladder and rectal fistulae following radiation treatment are difficult to correct surgically, since the endarteritis associated with radiation treatment reduces blood supply to the pelvic tissues and impedes healing. Abitbol (1974), comparing sexual dysfunction between surgery and radiation treated patients, found that compared to surgically treated patients, a

Table 4.1 Selection of treatment for stage IB cancer of the cervix

	Advantages	Disadvantages
Radiation	Can apply to all patients	Serious bladder or bowel damage 2–6%
	Survival rates equal to surgery	Vaginal stenosis
		Sexual dysfunction
		Complications are delayed, difficult to correct
Surgery	Ovarian conservation	Urological complications: fistulae/strictures 1–2%
	Establishes exact extent of tumour	Other operative complications
	More functional vagina	Must select patients
	Complications early, correctable	Postoperative radiation required in a few patients
	Psychological advantage	

large percentage of those treated with radiation experienced vaginal shortening that interfered with sexual function. He pointed out that while the rectal and bladder complications following radiation have been emphasised in the literature, the vaginal complications and sexual problems associated with cervical cancer treatment have been ignored.

One reason for selecting surgery is ovarian conservation. Metastases to the ovaries are quite rare with small volume cervical tumours. We have encountered only one ovarian metastasis in 258 consecutive primary radical operations for stage IB cancer of the cervix (0.4%), an almost identical rate to that reported by Baltzer (1981). Reoperation for cystic degeneration of the remaining ovary (or ovaries) was required in only three patients of our 258 (1.2%). Webb (1975) reported a reoperation rate of 7.6% for cysts or torsion of ovaries. If they appear normal, our current practice is to conserve both ovaries in women 40 years or younger and to remove them after that age.

With the surgical approach, the extent of tumour can be established (Tables 3.8, 3.10, 3.11, Ch. 3). The vagina will be slightly shortened but otherwise normal, and removal of the tumour appears to offer a psychological advantage to the patient. The complications of surgical treatment occur early and are usually correctable; for instance, the urological fistula rate is 2% or less in centres where this operation is performed routinely. Operative deaths very rarely occur (Table 4.2).

Table 4.2 Urinary fistulae and operative deaths in non-irradiated patients treated by radical hysterectomy

Author	Year	No. of pts.	Ureteral fistulae (%)	Vesical fistulae (%)	Operative deaths (%)
Käser	1973	717	3.3	0.6	NS
Park	1973	156	0	0	0.64
Hoskins	1976	224	1.3	0.45	0.89
Morley	1976	208	4.8	0.5	1.4
Sall	1979	349	2.0	0.8	0
Webb	1979	423	1.4	0.7	0.3
Benedet	1980	241	1.2	0.4	0.4
Langley	1980	284	5.6	1.4	0
Lerner	1980	108	0.9	0	0
Bostofte*	1981	479	3.8	1.4	0.2
Powell	1981	135	1.5	0	0.74
Zander	1981	1092	1.4	0.3	1.0
Authors	1982	300	1.3	0	0.3
Totals		4716	2.3	0.57	0.55

*Okabayashi techinique

We have favoured a radical surgical approach in women under 60 with small stage IB lesions because of the short treatment time and the other previously stated advantages. It seems very appropriate to consider this form of therapy for patients under 60, since it eliminates the risk of long-term complications secondary to arteritis and the potential carcinogenic effects of radiation in women who are likely to live several decades.

Nordqvist (1979), in summarizing the selection criteria for surgical treatment at the University of Miami, stated that age above 70 years, obesity, cardiovascular disease, diabetes and serious pulmonary disease constituted contra-indications to surgery. Between 1967 and 1976, 75.4% of 337 patients with stages IB or IIA were treated primarily by radical hysterectomy and node dissection. By comparison, the operability rate at the University of Alabama in Birmingham for stage I disease has been 51% (314 of 615 stage I patients).

The requirement that one must select the younger, healthier patients is one disadvantage of surgery as primary treatment. The obese, the diabetic, the patient with cardiac problems will be treated with primary radiation. Critics of radical surgery have emphasized that postoperative radiation therapy is still given to 15% or more of patients.

Rutledge (1979) stated that the issue is not how many radical surgical procedures should be employed, but how best to select patients for a surgical approach. Certainly, primary surgical treatment should not be attempted when the lesion is so large that it precludes tumour-free margins. The majority of patients with surgical margins less than 1 cm recur within 12–18 months of the operation and the salvage rate is not impressive even if postoperative pelvic radiation is administered. The likelihood of adequate resection, therefore, is a prime consideration before embarking on extended operations as primary treatment. While it is true that one can deliver postoperative irradiation therapy to these patients, the normal anatomy is altered and adhesions may diminish mobility of the small bowel in the lower abdomen, resulting in increased numbers of complications. The prudent surgeon should consider these risks, just as the radiotherapist should consider a primary surgical approach for young women with small cervical lesions, when a qualified pelvic surgeon is available.

SELECTION OF OPERATION

The appropriate operative procedures for cervical neoplasia diagnosed by conisation are determined by the size of the lesion (Table 4.3). In focal micro-invasion (early stromal invasion), total abdominal or vaginal hysterectomy (type I — Piver 1974) is sufficient, since this lesion is associated with recurrence and death in less than 1% of patients. Burghardt (1982) indicated that in unusual circumstances, i.e., young

Table 4.3 Choice of operative procedure for cervical neoplasms diagnosed by
conization

Histological findings	Terminology	Recommended procedure
Stromal invasion: to 1 mm as isolated projections arising at base of CIS or dysplasia	Focal Micro-invasion (Early stromal invasion)	Total hysterectomy (abdominal or vaginal) Therapeutic conization*
Stromal invasion: to 3 mm Width: to 10 mm	Micro-invasion**	Abdominal hysterectomy Node assessment
Stromal invasion: 3–5 mm Width: to 10 mm	Microcarcinoma	Extended abdominal (modified radical) hysterectomy Pelvic node dissection
Stromal invasion: over 5 mm or Width: over 10 mm	Invasive carcinoma	Pelvic node dissection Aortic node assessment Radical hysterectomy

* See text
** If lymph-vascular spaces are involved, treat as microcarcinoma

women who desire to retain their childbearing capabilities, a
therapeutic conisation of the cervix can be considered.

In micro-invasive lesions (stromal invasion up to 3 mm depth and a
width not greater than 10 mm) abdominal hysterectomy seems prudent
in order that nodal assessment may be carried out at the same time.
Clinically, non-suspicious pelvic and para-aortic nodes are left
undisturbed, while suspicious nodes may be selectively removed and
examined by frozen section. This recognises the slight risk of node
spread in lesions of this size, yet does not subject the patient to either an
extended hysterectomy or to a full lymphadenectomy.

Yajima (1979) treated 188 patients with micro-invasive lesions (up to
3 mm depth of invasion) by either conservative abdominal or vaginal
hysterectomy (69 patients) or modified type II radical hysterectomy
without lymphadenectomy (119 patients). Those with neither
confluence nor lymph-vascular space invasion were treated by the
conservative method while those with either confluence or lymph-
vascular involvement were treated by the more radical method. He
achieved a 99% 5-year survival in both groups, which seems to justify
his selection of therapy. It is important to note that the depth of
invasion used for selection of patients was 3 mm or less, and thus not
comparable to the figures quoted (Table 2.3, Ch. 2) for lesions up to 5
mm depth of invasion.

A microcarcinoma is defined as stromal invasion between 3 and 5 mm
with a width not exceeding 10 mm. Patients with this lesion are treated

at our institution by extended abdominal (modified radical) hysterectomy and pelvic node dissection (Fig. 4.1). We perform the lymphadenectomy because of the 2.7% incidence of positive nodes in this group of patients and because we do not feel that the node dissection adds appreciably to the operative morbidity. The excision of only the medial third of the cardinal ligament (type II operation — Fig. 4.1) and a 2 or 3 cm vaginal cuff guarantees adequate local resection yet avoids some of the bladder denervation associated with more radical resection of the cardinal ligaments. It also recognizes the fact that microcarcinoma virtually never involves the paracervical-parametrial tissues directly.

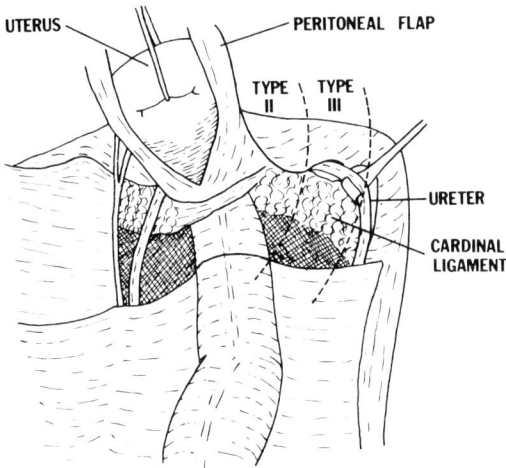

Fig. 4.1 Types of hysterectomy for invasive cancer of the cervix. In the type II operation, the ureter is partially dissected and pulled aside in order to allow resection of the medial portion of the cardinal ligament. In the type III operation, more extensive mobilisation of the ureter and ureterovesical junction is required in order to sever the cardinal ligaments at the pelvic sidewall.

Tumours that invade the stroma over 5 mm or that have a width of over 10 mm are classified as invasive carcinomas. These and adenocarcinomas are treated surgically by aortic node assessment, pelvic lymphadenectomy and radical hysterectomy with excision of the paracervical tissues at the pelvic sidewall (type III operation — Fig. 4.1).

When lymph-vascular spaces (LVS) are involved in the biopsy or conization specimen, the risks of recurrence and death increase appreciably (Table 2.3, Ch. 2). If such involvement is present, the patients are treated by abdominal (type II or III) radical hysterectomy and lymphadenectomy.

Selection of operation in special circumstances

Cancers of the cervical stump may be treated surgically. Selection of therapy involves the same consideration as does carcinoma in the intact uterus, i.e., estimation of tumour volume and of the likelihood of adequate margins. The operations are little different, other than the fact that bowel adhesions are often present and the bladder will ordinarily extend over the cervical stump as part of the peritonealisation. After mobilising the bladder, the stump can be grasped with a clamp for traction and the operation (type II or III) can proceed routinely. If the lesion is in the focal micro-invasion category, a trachelectomy from the vaginal approach will suffice.

Patients in whom invasive carcinoma has been found in a conventional vaginal or abdominal hysterectomy specimen may be treated by re-operation in order to complete therapy. This is considered in younger patients in whom ovarian conservation and vaginal preservation are important. The distorted anatomical relationships in the mid-pelvis require particular attention, but once the bladder and rectum are dissected away from the vaginal cuff, it can be grasped for traction and the parametrial tissues and upper vagina can be excised without undue difficulty. Care in dissecting the ureter and the ureterovesical junctions free from the vaginal cuff angles is important, since dense fibrous adhesions are to be expected secondary to the previous surgery.

Sarcomas of the cervix may be treated surgically but because sarcomas often recur distally, this should dampen enthusiasm for radical surgical procedures for this tissue type. A conservative hysterectomy or pelvic radiation may be used to treat the primary tumour. Chemotherapy has not been shown to be effective.

Patients with verrucous carcinoma of the cervix should be treated with type I or II hysterectomy depending on the size of the lesion. This ensures wide local excision of the tumour. Lymphadenectomy is not recommended (it is a local tumour and rarely metastasizes) and radiation is thought to be detrimental.

Consideration is given occasionally to primary pelvic exenteration for patients with advanced (stage IVA) disease in which the pelvic sidewalls are not involved. Involvement of the bladder or rectal walls by tumour leads one to expect that irradiation therapy would inevitably lead to fistula formation. However, Million (1973) reported that only two of 53 patients with stage IVA developed bladder fistulae during radiation treatment. For this reason, we do not employ exenterative surgery initially.

TOTAL HYSTERECTOMY

Many of the patients who are to be treated by conservative total hysterectomy will have had a recent conization of the cervix. Unlike patients treated by the type III hysterectomy, which includes radical excision of the paracervical tissues, those who undergo conservative total hysterectomy are at increased risk from pelvic infection if the hysterectomy is performed after 48 h but before 4 to 6 weeks following the conization. Following conization, it has been our practice to either proceed with total hysterectomy within 48 h or to delay hysterectomy 6 weeks. Orr (1982), reviewing the material at the University of Alabama Medical Center, and Webb (1979), reviewing the material from the Mayo Clinic, both indicated that the conization-radical hysterectomy interval was not an important factor in relation to postoperative morbidity. With this information, we feel that it is safe to proceed with a radical hysterectomy at any interval following conization.

When performing a vaginal hysterectomy for focal micro-invasion, the colposcope and Lugol's staining of the upper vagina and cervix should be performed to assure adequate margins. If necessary, a generous vaginal cuff can be developed prior to clamping the uterosacral and cardinal ligaments. In fact, we prefer the vaginal hysterectomy in these instances because the abdominal approach allows less predictable surgical margins.

Preoperative preparation for abdominal operations

Cruse (1980) indicated several important ways that the incidence of wound infections could be kept at a minimum. His recommendations included keeping the preoperative stay short, use of preoperative hexachlorophane showers, minimising the amount of shaving, avoiding use of drains in the wound, good surgical technique and minimising operative time. These can ordinarily be carried out with minimal difficulty.

While prophylactic antibiotics significantly decrease infectious morbidity in premenopausal women undergoing conservative hysterectomy, it is not clear that perioperative antibiotics are effective in reducing febrile morbidity in patients undergoing radical hysterectomy. We have not been able to demonstrate a significant difference in overall infectious morbidity when using perioperative antibiotics in radical hysterectomy patients, although we believe that there is a decreased risk of pelvic cellulitis and abscesses in patients receiving perioperative antibiotics.

Perioperative mini-dose heparin administration decreases the risk of subclinical venous thrombosis but there is little evidence that it prevents fatal pulmonary thromboembolism in radical gynaecological surgery. We presently administer mini-dose heparin only to patients at high risk, i.e., obese or with previous history of phlebitis. We no longer use it routinely, because of the significant increase (approximately 25%) in blood loss associated with its use.

Pneumatic calf compression by an externally applied device may be effective in prophylaxis against venous thrombosis. This has not gained popularity because the devices are expensive and cumbersome. The results with intravenous Dextran use for prophylaxis against thromboses are equivocal in radical gynaecologic surgery, although it has been shown to be effective in general surgical patients.

At the present time, we have no strong preference for the type of incision to be used for a radical hysterectomy and pelvic lymphadenectomy. If a transverse incision is selected, we prefer the Maylard muscle-cutting incision. In this, all layers are opened transversely which allows superior exposure for the pelvic node dissections.

Description of radical hysterectomy

After entering the abdomen, a careful exploration of all quadrants is carried out with particular attention paid to the pelvic, common iliac and aortic nodes. Clinical assessment has some error: Welander (1981) reported that if the nodes were negative to palpation, the surgeon would be correct 94% of the time. If the nodes were clinically suspicious, the accuracy of the assessment was only 59%.

If aortic nodes are found to contain metastatic tumour by frozen section, the procedure should be abandoned, since the drastically reduced survival rate in this situation does not justify the morbidity of the operation. Martimbeau (1982), reporting the experience at the Norwegian Radium Hospital, stated that positive common iliac nodes are an ominous finding, associated with a 23% 5-year survival; however, positive nodes below the common iliacs were associated with a 60% cure rate. A decision to abandon the procedure because of isolated metastases to external iliac or obturator nodes is more difficult. Because of the high recurrence rates with positive pelvic nodes, we have usually abandoned the radical operation if nodes above the bifurcation of the iliacs are involved with cancer, if more than one pelvic node is involved, if a cancerous node was stuck to a major vessel, or if bilaterally involved pelvic nodes are encountered. One might question this practice, however, in view of Heller's (1981) finding of a 71% 5-year survival in positive node patients whose lymphadenectomies and hysterectomies were followed by 5000 rad pelvic radiation, compared to 34% 5-year survival in those who had node sampling only, followed by radiation or chemotherapy.

Upon entering the abdomen, washings from each paracolic gutter and the cul-de-sac are taken for prognostic purposes. Welander (1981) reported peritoneal spread in 12.6% of patients and Hughes (1980) reported 9.3% of such involvement in cervical cancer. All 20 of Hughes' patients who received no additional treatment for this finding died within 2 years. Only two of 13 (15.4%) treated by whole abdominal radiation survived 5 years. The incidence of malignant cells in washings in our operative material is 5%. A rapid cytological evaluation technique would be helpful; if microscopic peritoneal involvement could be proven intraoperatively, it would constitute another reason for abandoning the procedure.

The comprehensiveness of the lymphadenectomy may not significantly alter survival, yet it may increase complications. One can increase the percentage of positive nodes encountered with pelvic node dissection by performing the node dissection under lymphangiographic control, as reported by Kolbenstvedt (1976), who increased the incidence of positive nodes by 10% using this method. Pilleron (1974) noted no significant difference in 5-year survival in patients having a limited versus extensive en bloc dissection of nodes (45% versus 50%). He stated that lymphocysts and lower extremity oedema were associated with the more extensive dissection. Martimbeau (1982) reported lower extremity oedema as a consequence of the en bloc dissection technique.

Pilleron (1974) stated that lymph nodes lateral to the external iliac arteries are never involved with tumour and recommended that, to avoid oedema, they should not be dissected. He also noted that the common iliac nodes are not involved in an isolated fashion. It has been our practice to dissect all visible nodes adjacent to the common iliac, the external iliac, the hypogastric vessels, and those in the obturator fossa. We do not routinely mobilise or dissect behind the vessels (with the exception of the external iliac vessels), nor do we use lymphangiography to increase the completeness of the dissection. In spite of this, 5-year survival of our patients with positive nodes is 60% (equal to that reported by Martimbeau for the more extensive dissection) and leg oedema has been quite rare (2% or less).

Dissection of the ureter and the bladder is the key to performing a wider parametrectomy-upper vaginectomy which distinguishes the type II and III operations (Fig. 4.1) from the conventional abdominal hysterectomy. The ureter is picked up on the medial peritoneal flap after opening the broad ligament. It is tunnelled bluntly through the cardinal ligament and after partial mobilisation of the bladder from the cervix, the vesico-uterine ligament anterior to the ureter is incised, 'unroofing' the ureter. Further dissection to free the ureter circumferentially from its attachments to the cardinal ligament is necessary to mobilise the uretero-vesical junction from the vagina; only in this way is one able to sufficiently isolate the cardinal ligaments to perform the type III radical operation. For the type II modified radical operation, the posterior attachments of the ureter can be left in place and the uretero-vesical junction can be pushed aside to perform the medial parametrial excision.

The ovaries are removed in women who are aged 40 years or older. If the ovary/ovaries is/are conserved, the fallopian tube is ordinarily taken with the specimen. Hodel (1982) suggested that the ovaries might be transposed and fastened to the gutter peritoneum in order that they are out of the (potential) pelvic radiation field. We have occasionally employed this method when intraoperative findings in younger patients make postoperative pelvic radiation necessary; however, the majority of patients who undergo this operation will not receive adjunctive radiation, making routine transposition unnecessary.

The mean operative time for the type III radical hysterectomy at the University of Alabama in Birmingham is 3.7 h and the mean blood loss is 1900 ml. These figures are quite similar to those reported by Hoskins (1976) from the University of Miami. The portion of the procedure associated with the greatest blood loss is the dissection of the bladder and uretero-vesical junction, where bleeding occurs from large veins in the vicinity of the vesico-uterine ligament. We do not routinely ligate the hypogastric arteries, nor do we sacrifice the superior vesical arteries.

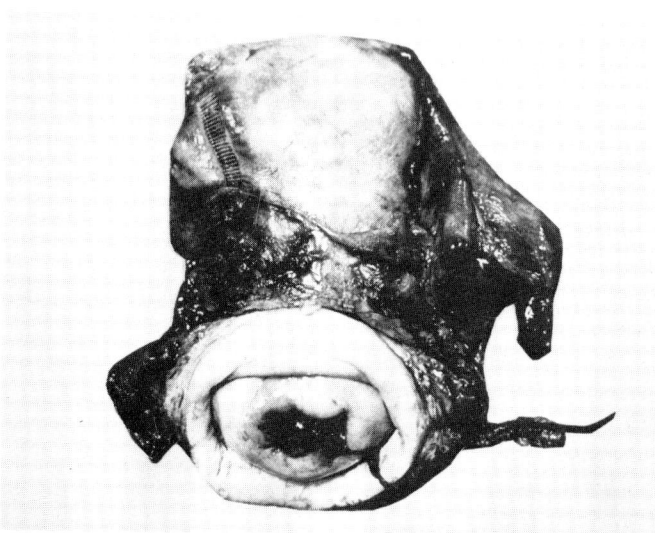

Fig. 4.2 A type III radical hysterectomy specimen. In this instance, both ovaries were conserved, although the fallopian tubes are contained in the specimen. The cardinal ligaments and paravaginal tissues were severed at the pelvic sidewall, and the upper third of the vagina was removed.

The specimen (Fig. 4.2), including the wide vaginal segment and the attached parametrial and paracervical tissues, is excised. After a haemostatic suture is placed around the cut vaginal edges, the peritoneum of the pelvis is closed in order to prevent small bowel adhesions to the vaginal cuff and denuded pelvic vessels. If the ovaries have been retained, they must be stabilised in the peritoneal closure to minimise chances of torsion. We usually place extraperitoneal Penrose drains in the obturator fossa, brought out through the open vaginal cuff. We only occasionally use suction drains in the pelvis. Our pelvic closure and pelvic drainage technique differs from that of Hoskins (1976) and van Nagell (1976), who have suggested that their low ureteral fistula rates were due at least in part to use of suction drains. We do not suspend the ureter from the iliac vessels, another technique suggested to reduce ureteral fistulae.

For several years, we have employed suprapubic catheters (16 French Foley catheter) placed directly in the dome of the bladder at the time of the abdominal closure.

At the end of the procedure, the surgical specimen is carefully inspected and in some instances the surgical pathologist is called to the operating room in order that he and the surgeon can have the opportunity to discuss areas of special concern (margins). This provides information that is necessary to allow the surgical pathologist to properly evaluate the excised tissues.

Postoperative care and complications

The mean postoperative stay of patients undergoing radical hysterectomy on our service is 9.7 d, with a range of 5 to 45 d. About one-third of the patients experienced febrile morbidity which prolonged the hospital stay. By comparison, Hoskins (1976) reported a mean hospital stay of 16 d (range 7 to 108 d). Early ambulation is practised. The patient is encouraged to be out of bed on the first postoperative day, and barring complications, is placed on a regular diet and is freely ambulatory within a week. The Penrose drain is removed on the second postoperative day. The suprapubic catheter is connected to straight drainage during the hospitalisation and no trial of voiding is attempted. The patient is discharged with the suprapubic catheter in place. A cystometrogram is performed 21–28 d postoperatively; if at that time the patient has bladder sensation, and a reasonable bladder capacity, she is asked to void. If this can be accomplished with a low residual urine (under 100 ml), the suprapubic catheter is removed. During the time the catheter is in place in the postoperative period, antibacterial agents such as nitrofurantoin or sulfisoxazole are administered. Using this regimen, we have experienced very few long-term bladder complications. A simple cystometrogram performed as a baseline study before surgery and repeated at intervals following surgery has been helpful in the management of our patients, allowing decision about catheter removal based on data such as sensation of filling and bladder capacity. Bladder care should emphasise prevention of overdistension, since it can further damage the bladder. Suprapubic tubes have an advantage over transurethral catheters because the patient can open and close the catheter herself and thus can attempt voiding without the necessity of removal or replacement of the catheter, or the danger of overdistension. We have very rarely prescribed intermittent self-catheterisation for patients, although it is an acceptable technique and is preferable to long-term indwelling catheter use.

Langley (1980) defined an atonic bladder (after radical hysterectomy) as a residual urine of over 100 ml 3 months postoperatively. Although he used suprapubic drainage postoperatively, 3.5% of his patients had bladder atony, treated by intermittent self-catheterisation. Thomas Green (1969) reported a 3% incidence of atonic bladders in an earlier series and recommended that prolonged Foley catheter drainage (6 weeks) might reduce the ureteral and bladder complications, by allowing time for healing. While episodes of overdistension (usually associated with voiding trials and with blocked catheters) may compound the injury to the partially denervated bladder, the remarkable consistency of the percentage of patients with long-term atonic bladders in Langley's, Green's and our series suggests that this is the incidence of atony due to bladder denervation and not to the method of postoperative bladder drainage.

The exact nature of the bladder damage associated with radical hysterectomy is under investigation. It has been the subject of recent studies by Forney (1980), Lowe (1981), Carenza (1982) and others. Forney observed different degrees and types of damage with incomplete or complete transection of the cardinal ligaments. He noted that stress urinary incontinence occurred more frequently in those who had complete transections. He felt that sympathetic denervation was responsible for most of the alteration, as did Lowe (1981) who noted a reduction in bladder compliance, elevated baseline bladder pressures and hyperreflexia in the immediate postoperative period. He also reported a significant decrease in the urethral pressure profile after surgery. Additional studies are needed to elucidate this complex problem.

Ureteral fistulae, formerly the most dreaded complication of this operation, are now relatively uncommon (Table 4.2). The urological injuries have decreased markedly from the rates encountered in series dating back 20 to 40 years, such as those reported by Liu (1955) and

Green (1969). No immediate explanation is apparent; however, advances in anaesthesia, use of perioperative antibiotics, more meticulous dissection, improved pelvic and bladder drainage, and other differences in postoperative care may be responsible in some way.

Intravenous pyelograms (IVP) are obtained prior to discharge of the patient from the hospital. Almost all patients will have transient ureteral dilatation above the pelvic brim, with associated dilatation of the renal pelvis: these changes return to normal within 3–6 weeks. The postoperative IVP is obtained to establish that there is no major obstruction or alteration of ureter or bladder attributable to the surgical procedure, to a lymphocyst or to a pelvic haematoma. It also serves as a baseline study for subsequent pyelograms.

Febrile morbidity is reported to occur in 25% to 50% of patients following radical hysterectomy, depending on the definitions used by the individual authors. In a recent report on 311 patients followed at this institution, febrile morbidity occurred in 33%. The major causes of febrile morbidity following radical hysterectomy are pulmonary atelectasis, urinary tract infections, wound infections or haematoma, pelvic cellulitis, pelvic or deep vein phlebitis, and pelvic abscess. Pulmonary morbidity is usually secondary to atelectasis; this is usually minor and responds well to conservative measures. Pneumonia following this procedure is extremely rare.

Morbidity of pelvic aetiology due to pelvic cellulitis or abscess occurred in 10% of patients in our series. These complications are thought to be potentially more serious as they may predispose patients to development of a later urinary fistula. Many authors indicate that because of this risk, the vaginal cuff should be closed, as an open vaginal cuff allows for ascending infection. Our experience is different and we have had few problems with open vaginal drainage. Interestingly, patients undergoing conization do not apparently have an increased risk of these complications, regardless of the interval between conization and radical hysterectomy.

Urinary tract infections following radical hysterectomy are seen in 5% to 10% of patients, even if perioperative antibiotics are used, and may be secondary to prolonged urethral or suprapubic drainage. We prefer to maintain patients on constant urinary prophylaxis during the period of bladder catheterisation. Other causes of febrile morbidity, such as wound infection or haematoma, are relatively rare and may be prevented by careful attention to surgical technique.

Pelvic lymphocysts following radical hysterectomy are usually asymptomatic. Other than the high rate (29%) quoted by Dodd (1970), most investigators have reported a low incidence of lymphocysts (Table 4.4). The cause of lymphocysts is not readily apparent. Pilleron felt that

Table 4.4   Incidence of pelvic lymphocytes following radical abdominal hysterectomy and pelvic lymphadenectomy

Author	Year	No. of pts.	% Lymphocysts
Dodd	1970	453	29
Käser	1973	717	1
Lagasse	1974	118	9
Sall	1979	349	2
Webb	1979	610	3
Benedet	1980	241	2
Authors	1982	350	1

they were more common in patients who had had extensive lymph node dissections. Others have observed that incomplete dissections cause the collections of lymph in the retroperitoneal space that results in lymphocysts; because of this, some surgeons have advocated ligating the afferent lymphatics. Others feel that proper drainage of the retroperitoneal area may prevent lymphocyst formation. Although we have never practised routine ligation of the lymphatics and have provided only short-term retroperitoneal drainage using Penrose drains, we have only rarely seen the condition, which is most often diagnosed on a routine postoperative intravenous pyelogram (Fig. 4.3).

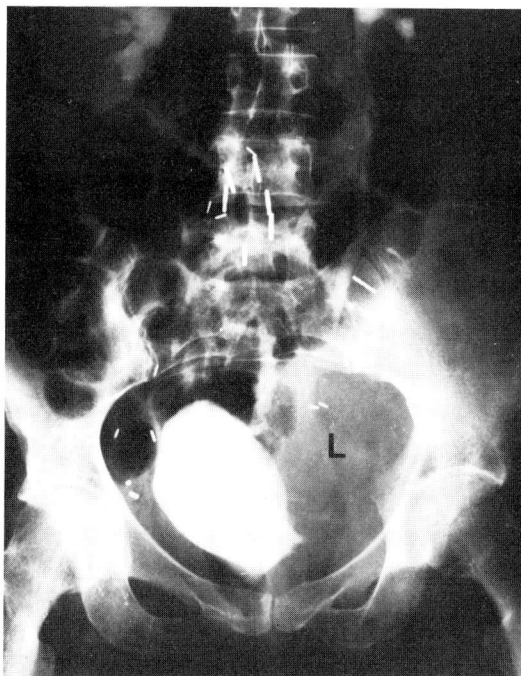

Fig. 4.3   A postoperative lymphocyst following radical hysterectomy. The lymphocyst (L) displaces the bladder and the left ureter medially.

Symptomatic lymphocysts require treatment. Simple aspiration with a needle is not curative but percutaneous catheters might be used to chronically drain the area and allow healing. Others advocate operative management, with transperitoneal marsupialisation of the lymphocyst for drainage.

Nerve injuries may occur during the course of the radical hysterectomy operation. The obturator nerve is the most likely to be damaged; however, the femoral or the peroneal nerves can be injured in the course of the surgery. The obturator nerve may be severed during the obturator fossa node dissection. It can be resutured and may regenerate, but other than possible weakness in adduction of the thigh, the patients experience no major disability. Femoral neuropathies may result from pressure by the blades of self-retaining retractors and care should be exercised that they do not rest on the psoas muscle. Peroneal nerve damage may occur as a result of pressure on the popliteal fossa when the patient is placed in stirrups. Careful attention to leg placement and padding of the stirrups decreases the risk of this type of nerve injury.

Vena caval lacerations or lacerations of the external iliac, the hypogastric or obturator veins may occur in the course of the node dissections. Such large vein injuries may be difficult to control and may result in major blood losses. Obturator fossa venous bleeding may respond best to packing of the fossa while vena caval and iliac vein injuries require suturing of the vessels.

Factors affecting survival after surgery

The survival of patients following radical hysterectomy is largely dependent upon an adequate surgical specimen, i.e., wide margins around the tumour. Most patients with margins of less than 1 cm will recur, and this rate is only slightly reduced by administration of postoperative pelvic radiation. With proper selection of therapy, this situation should arise rarely.

A number of investigators have related survival to lesion size for stage IB cervical cancer (Table 4.5). We have achieved a 5-year survival rate of 91.4% and encountered a node metastasis rate of 12% for lesions 2 cm or less in size, whereas with lesions above 2 cm in size, the node metastasis rate was 35.9% and the survival rate was 63.9%. Similar data have been obtained by others, using 3 cm size as the dividing point.

The depth measurement of cervical stromal invasion appears to be an important prognostic indicator. The deeper the tumour invades the stroma, the more likely it will invade lymphatics and embolise to the lymph nodes (Fig. 4.4). Deep invasion is in a sense another measure of

Table 4.5 Stage IB cancer of the cervix. Positive nodes and survival related to lesion size

Author	Year	No. of pts.	Size	Pos. node (%)	Surv.	%	Size	Pos. node (%)	Surv.	%
Piver	1977	157	≤3 cm	21.3	5 yrs	88.5	>3 cm	36.5	5 yrs	65.4
van Nagell	1977	82	<2 cm	9.0	1–10 yrs	94.0	≥2 cm	31.0	1–10 yrs	40.0
Chung	1980	85	<4 cm	16.0	2 yrs	92.0	≥4 cm	80.0	2 yrs	47.0
Authors	1982	200	≤2 cm	12.0	5 yrs	91.4	>2 cm	35.9	5 yrs	63.9

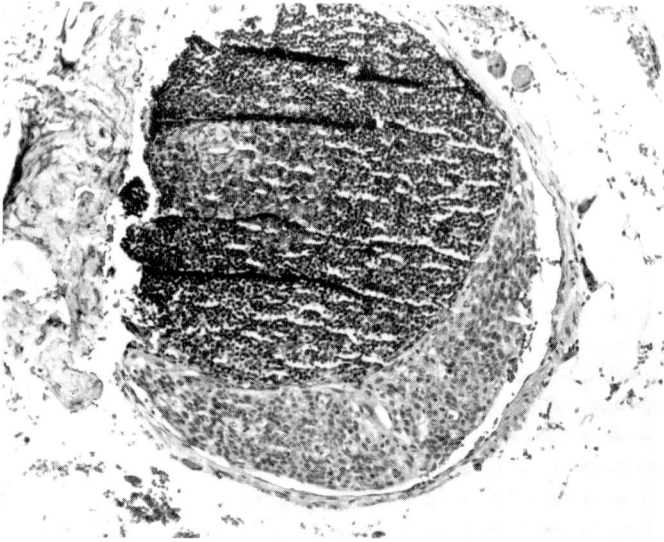

A

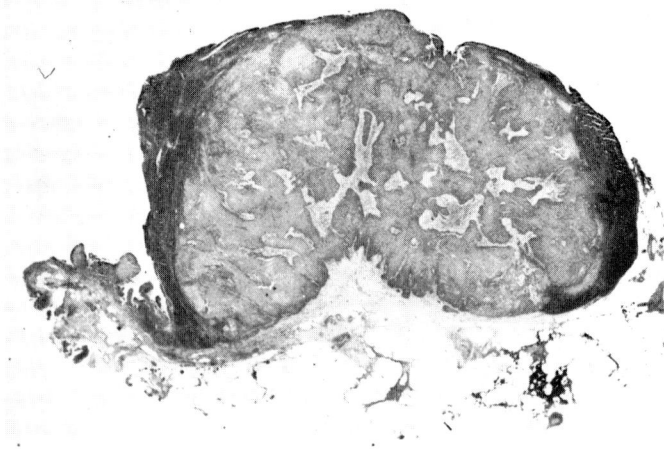

B

Fig. 4.4 A. Metastatic tumour involving the periphery of a small lymph node. (H&E ×103)
B. Almost complete replacement of a lymph node by metastatic squamous cell carcinoma. (H&E ×8)

total volume of tumour. Moreover, it is obvious that volume can only be of prognostic value in surgically treated patients.

Patients with negative nodes at the time of radical hysterectomy have about a 10% recurrence rate. Certain high-risk factors are apparent in these patients. If tumour is present in vascular spaces, if the endometrial cavity, the deep endocervical stroma or the paracervical (cardinal liagment) tissues are invaded; if the tumour is undifferentiated or 3 cm (or larger) in size, one may predict high recurrence rates. In these situations, adjunctive radiation may be of some benefit in a few patients; however, 80% of the recurrences will be in sites other than the central pelvis. For this reason, chemotherapy has been advocated to improve survival in this high-risk group. We have not employed adjunctive chemotherapy to date.

Metastases in pelvic nodes affect survival adversely and a number of authors agree that the number of involved pelvic nodes and their location (unilateral or bilateral) affect survival rates. Hsu (1972) reporting how many stage IB patients were treated surgically, reported a 48.5% 5-year survival with one to four positive pelvic nodes and 19% survival with five or more positive pelvic nodes. Boronow (1980) reported the results of a panel discussion at the Society of Gynecologic Oncologists. The collected material from several centres demonstrated a marked difference in survival if more than three pelvic nodes were involved by tumour, i.e., the 5-year survival fell from 70% (one to three nodes) to 35% (more than three nodes).

Pilleron (1974) reported 59% 5-year survival for unilaterally positive pelvic nodes, compared with 22% 5-year survival for bilaterally positive nodes. Hsu (1979) reported 57.1% survival with unilaterally positive and 34.9% with bilaterally positive pelvic nodes. These figures are contrasted to his 88% 5-year survival in patients with negative pelvic nodes. The figures in our patients are 70% for unilateral and 40% for bilateral node involvement. Webb (1979) and Martimbeau (1982), in contrast, ascribed no significance to bilaterality of pelvic node metastases.

Tumour in capillary-like spaces is an ominous finding even in the absence of demonstrated pelvic node metastasis. We have usually given postoperative pelvic radiation to these patients but many still recur. Positive peritoneal washings are also associated with poor survival rates. Radioactive chromic phosphate (^{32}P) might be considered in these circumstances, but its value to date is unproven.

COMBINED RADIOTHERAPY AND SURGERY

The role of combined radiotherapy and surgery in the treatment of cervical carcinoma remains controversial. There has been much speculation regarding the value of preoperative radiation in early stage tumours. Some have postulated that the rapidly dividing cancer cells can be destroyed by irradiation, thus lessening the risk of spread of cancer cells during the subsequent operation. The two major areas where combined radiation and surgery are advocated are in the treatment of barrel-shaped endocervical lesions (Fig. 3.10, Ch. 3) and in the preoperative use of intracavitary radiation prior to a radical abdominal hysterectomy.

Concerns about central pelvic recurrence due to the large volume of the barrel-shaped lesions has prompted some authors to advocate radiation followed by an extrafascial hysterectomy; whole-pelvis teletherapy (4000–5000 rad) followed by a single intracavitary application is recommended before the conservative hysterectomy. In advocating this approach, Fletcher (1979) achieved decreased rates of central pelvic recurrence, although a significant improvement in patient survival was not demonstrated. Nelson (1975) indicated that recurrences following combined radiation and extrafascial hysterectomy were much more likely in distant sites, not within the radiation field. Theoretically, since 6000 rad are required to destroy a 2 cm tumour nodule, and 5000 rad to destroy tumour less than 2 cm (Table 5.1, Ch. 5), one should be concerned about a dosage of only 4000 rad to the lateral pelvic walls in these patients because the expanded endocervix and large tumour volume is associated with a high rate of lymphatic metastases. Although many authors advocate combined radiation and hysterectomy in barrel-shaped lesions, in most instances their series contain too few patients to make a statement based on the data presented. We have only rarely used this approach but concede that in selected patients it may be advantageous. We prefer to carefully gauge radiation response and to make a decision concerning the adjunctive hysterectomy after the patient has received 4000 rad whole-pelvic teletherapy. If the response is excellent, the therapy is completed along conventional lines without surgical intervention.

The risk of complications in patients treated by irradiation and adjunctive hysterectomy is increased over that of patients treated by radiation alone. O'Quinn (1980) indicated a combined fistula rate of 11.6% and felt that the rate could be decreased by avoiding blunt dissection and excessive vaginal apex radiation dosages. She noted that the risk of fistulae was increased in patients who were found to have pelvic inflammatory changes prior to therapy.

The other form of combined therapy that has been widely advocated is intracavitary radiation followed at some interval by extended abdominal hysterectomy and pelvic lymph node dissection. Almost none of the series reporting this combination have randomised controls nor do they relate survival to lesion size. Perez (1980), who reported a randomised study of patients with stage IB and IIA carcinoma of the cervix, indicated that there was no survival advantage to patients treated by combined intracavitary radiation-radical hysterectomy compared to patients treated by conventional radiation alone. Some have stated that an advantage of the combined approach is that ureteral and paracervical dissection need not be so wide; this implies that such patients would not have recurrence often in the central pelvis and that one is therefore justified in reducing the radicality of the operation. Of Perez's patients treated by the combination therapy, however, 7.3% failed in the central pelvis. Although Einhorn (1980) concluded that survival was increased in patients treated with combined therapy compared with those receiving radiation therapy alone, she did not stratify patients according to volume of tumour and the two groups may not be comparable. Hansen (1981) reported superiority of radical surgery over combined radiation-surgery in stages IB and IIA.

We do not believe that in early stage disease, combined therapy improves survival rates when compared to full course radiation or radical surgery alone and know from considerable personal experience (Talbert 1965, Shingleton 1968) that urological complications are appreciably higher in those patients subjected to preoperative intracavitary radiation before extended hysterectomy. In changing our management in recent years to either radical surgery or radiation alone, we have maintained excellent survival rates, lowered the rate of complications, and have also eliminated the risk of an additional anaesthetic for the patient.

BIBLIOGRAPHY

Abdulhayoglu G, Rich W M, Reynolds J, DiSaia P J 1980 Selective radiation therapy in stage IB uterine cervical carcinoma following radical pelvic surgery. Gynecologic Oncology 10: 84–92

Abell M R, Ramirez J A 1973 Sarcomas and carcinosarcomas of the uterine cervix. Cancer 31: 1176–1192

Abitbol M M, Davenport J H 1974 Sexual dysfunction after therapy for cervical carcinoma. American Journal of Obstetrics and Gynecology 119: 181–189

Adcock L L 1979 Radical hysterectomy preceded by pelvic irradiation. Gynecologic Oncology 8: 152–163

Baltzer J, Lohe K J, Koepcke W, Zander J 1981 Formation of metastases in the ovaries in operated squamous cell carcinoma of the cervix uteri. Geburtshilfe und Frauenheilkunde 41: 672–673

Baltzer J, Lohe K J, Koepcke W, Zander J 1982 Histologic criteria for the prognosis in patients with operated squamous cell carcinoma of the cervix. Gynecologic Oncology 13: 184–194

Benedet J L, Turko M, Boyes D A, Nickerson K G, Bienkowska B T 1980 Radical hysterectomy in the treatment of cervical cancer. American Journal of Obstetrics and Gynecology 137: 254–262

Bonar L D 1980 Results of radical surgical procedures after radiation for treatment of invasive carcinoma of the uterine cervix in a private practice. American Journal of Obstetrics and Gynecology 136: 1006–1008

Bostofte E, Serup J 1981 Urological complications of Okabayashi's operation for cervical cancer. Acta obstetrica et gynecologica scandinavica 60: 39–42

Boyce J, Fruchter R G, Nicastri A D, Ambinvagar P-C, Reinis M S, Nelson J H Jr 1981 Prognostic factors in stage I carcinoma of the cervix. Gynecologic Oncology 12: 154–165

Burghardt E 1982 Microinvasive and occult invasive carcinoma: pathology. In: Jordan
    J A, Sharp F, Singer A (eds) Pre-clinical neoplasia of the cervix. Royal College of
    Obstetricians and Gynaecologists, London
Carenza L, Nobili F, Giacobini S 1982 Voiding disorders after radical hysterectomy.
    Gynecologic Oncology 13: 213–219
Chung C K, Nahhas W A, Stryker J A, Curry S L, Abt A B, Mortel R 1980 Analysis
    of factors contributing to treatment failures in stages IB and IIA carcinoma of the
    cervix. American Journal of Obstetrics and Gynecology 138: 550–556
Churches C K, Kurrle G R, Johnson B 1974 Treatment of carcinoma of the cervix by
    combination of irradiation and operation. American Journal of Obstetrics and
    Gynecology 118: 1033–1040
Crissman J, Flanagan R 1980 Verrucous carcinoma of the uterine cervix. Journal of
    Reproductive Medicine 25: 139–141
Cruse P J, Foord R 1980 The epidemiology of wound infection. A 10-year prospective
    study of 62 939 wounds. Surgical Clinics of North America 60: 27–47
Delgado G 1978 Stage IB squamous cancer of the cervix: the choice of treatment.
    Obstetrical and Gynecological Survey 33: 174–183
Delgado G, King E M 1982 Radical hysterectomies for IB cervical cancer less than 3
    cm. (In press)
Dodd G D, Rutledge R, Wallace S 1970 Postoperative pelvic lymphocysts. American
    Journal of Roentgenology 108: 312–323
Einhorn N, Bygdeman M, Sjoberg B 1980 Combined radiation and surgical treatment
    for carcinoma of the uterine cervix. Cancer 45: 720–723
Forney J P 1980 The effect of radical hysterectomy on bladder physiology. American
    Journal of Obstetrics and Gynecology 138: 374–382
Fuller A F, Elliott N, Kosloff C, Lewis J L Jr 1982 Lymph node metastases from
    carcinoma of the cervix, stages IB and IIA: implications for prognosis and
    treatment. Gynecologic Oncology 13: 165–174
Genton E, Turpie A G G 1980 Venous thromboembolism associated with gynecologic
    surgery. Clinical Obstetrics and Gynecology 23: 209–241
Green T H Jr 1966 Ureteral suspension for prevention of ureteral complications
    following radical Wertheim hysterectomy. Obstetrics and Gynecology 28: 1–11
Green T H, Morse W J Jr 1969 Management of invasive cervical cancer following
    inadvertent simple hysterectomy. Obstetrics and Gynecology 33: 763–769
Hansen M K 1981 Surgical and combination therapy of cancer of the cervix uteri
    stages Ib and IIa. Gynecologic Oncology 11: 275–287
Heller P B, Lee R B, Lemon M H, Park R C 1981 Lymph node positivity in cervical
    cancer. Gynecologic Oncology 12: 328–335
Herbst A L 1980 Interview with editor: DES update. CA — A Cancer Journal for
    Clinicians 30: 326–332
Hodel K, Rich W M, Austin P, DiSaia P J 1982 The role of ovarian transposition in
    conservation of ovarian function in radical hysterectomy followed by pelvic
    radiation. Gynecologic Oncology 13: 195–202
Hoskins W J, Ford J H Jr, Lutz M H, Averette H E 1976 Radical hysterectomy and
    pelvic lymphadenectomy for the management of early invasive cancer of the cervix.
    Gynecologic Oncology 4: 278–290
Hsu C-T, Cheng Y-S, Su S-C 1972 Prognosis of uterine cervical cancer with extensive
    lymph node metastases. American Journal of Obstetrics and Gynecology 114:
    954–962
Hughes R R, Brewington K C, Hanjani P, Photopulos G, Dick D, Votava C et al
    1980 Extended field irradiation for cervical cancer based on surgical staging.
    Gynecologic Oncology 9: 153–161
Jennings R H, Barclay D L 1972 Verrucous carcinoma of the cervix. Cancer 30:
    430–434
Kaser O, Ikle F A, Hirsch H A 1973 Atlas der gynakologischen operationen unter
    berucksichtigung. Gynakologisch-Urologischer Eingriffe 3. Aufluger Thieme,
    Stuttgart

Kelso J W, Funnell J D 1973 Combined surgical and radiation treatment of invasive carcinoma of the cervix. American Journal of Obstetrics and Gynecology 116: 205–213

Kelso J W, Funnell J D, Puckett T G, Strebel G F 1979 Combined surgical and radiation therapy for invasive carcinoma of the cervix. Southern Medical Journal 72: 648–651

Kolbenstvedt A, Kolstad P 1976 The difficulties of complete pelvic lymph node dissection in radical hysterectomy for carcinoma of the cervix. Gynecologic Oncology 4: 244–254

Koller O 1964 A comparison between the results of irradiation therapy alone and individualized radiological and surgical treatment of cervical carcinoma stage I. Acta obstetrica et gynecologica scandinavica 43: 68–74

Kotz H L, Geelhoed G W 1981 Lethal thromboembolism and its prevention in pelvic surgery: a review. Gynecologic Oncology 12: 271–280

Kurrle G R 1970 The role of irradiation in the treatment of carcinoma cervix uteri — a review of 997 cases. Australian and New Zealand Journal of Obstetrics and Gynaecology 10: 230–237

Lagasse L D, Smith M L, Moore J G, Morton D G, Jacobs M, Johnson G H et al 1974 The effect of radiation therapy on pelvic lymph node involvement in stage I carcinoma of the cervix. American Journal of Obstetrics and Gynecology 119: 328–334

Langley I I, Moore D W, Tarnasky J W, Roberts P H R 1980 Radical hysterectomy and pelvic lymph node dissection. Gynecologic Oncology 9: 37–42

Lee M S, Kim J C, Saxena V S, Kartha P, Zusag T, Hendrickson F R 1980 Late effects of para-aortic irradiation in carcinoma of the uterine cervix and endometrium. Radiology 135: 771–773

Lerner H M, Jones H W III, Hill E C 1980 Radical surgery for the treatment of early invasive cervical carcinoma (stage IB): review of 15 years' experience. Obstetrics and Gynecology 56: 413–418

Liu W, Meigs J V 1955 Radical hysterectomy and pelvic lymphadenectomy. American Journal of Obstetrics and Gynecology 69: 1–32

Low J A, Mauger G M, Carmichael J A 1981 The effect of Wertheim hysterectomy upon bladder and urethral function. American Journal of Obstetrics and Gynecology 139: 826–834

Lu T, Macasaet M A, Nelson J H Jr 1976 The barrel-shaped cervical carcinoma. American Journal of Obstetrics and Gynecology 124: 596–600

Mann W J, Orr J W Jr, Shingleton H M, Austin J M Jr, Hatch K D, Taylor P T 1981 Perioperative influences on infectious morbidity in radical hysterectomy. Gynecologic Oncology 11: 207–212

Martimbeau P W, Kjorstad K E, Kolstad P 1978 Stage IB carcinoma of the cervix, the Norwegian Radium Hospital, 1968–1970: results of treatment and major complications. I. Lymphedema. American Journal of Obstetrics and Gynecology 131: 389–394

Martimbeau P W, Kjorstad K E, Iversen T 1982 Stage IB carcinoma of the cervix, the Norwegian Radium Hospital: results of treatment and major complications. II. Results when pelvic nodes are involved. Obstetrics and Gynecology, in press

Meigs J V 1951 Radical hysterectomy with bilateral pelvic lymph node dissections. A report of 100 patients operated on five or more years ago. American Journal of Obstetrics and Gynecology 63: 854–866

Million R R 1979 Radiotherapeutic approaches. International Journal of Radiation Oncology, Biology and Physics 5: 1027–1028

Morley G W, Seski J C 1976 Radical pelvic surgery versus radiation therapy for stage I carcinoma of the cervix (exclusive of microinvasion). American Journal of Obstetrics and Gynecology 126: 785–798

Morrow C P 1980 Is pelvic radiation beneficial in the postoperative management of stage IB squamous cell carcinoma of the cervix with pelvic node metastasis treated by radical hysterectomy and pelvic lymphadenectomy? Gynecologic Oncology 10: 105–110 van Nagell J R Jr, Schiwietz D P 1976 Surgical adjuncts in radical hysterectomy and pelvic lymphadenectomy. Surgery, Gynecology and Obstetrics 143: 735–737

van Nagell J R, Donaldson E S, Parker J C, van Dyke A H, Wood E G 1977 The prognostic significance of cell type and lesion size in patients with cervical cancer treated by radical surgery. (abstract) Gynecologic Oncology 5: 142–151

Nelson A J, Fletcher G H, Wharton J T 1975 Indications for adjunctive conservative extrafascial hysterectomy in selected cases of carcinoma of the uterine cervix. American Journal of Radiology 123: 91–99

Nelson J H Jr, Boyce J, Macasaet M, Lu T, Bohorquez J F, Nicastri A D et al 1977 Incidence, significance and follow-up of para-aortic lymph node metastases in late invasive carcinoma of the cervix. American Journal of Obstetrics and Gynecology 128: 336–340

Nieminen U, Mattsson T, Widholm O 1974 Radical surgery combined with radiotherapy in the treatment of cervical carcinoma. Annales Chirurgiae et Gynaecologiae Fenniae 63: 134–140

Nieminen U, Pollanen L, Saarikoski S 1970 Radical surgery and radiotherapy in the management of 173 cases of carcinoma of cervix uteri. Acta obstetrica et gynecologica scandinavica 49: 347–349

Nordqvist S R B, Jaramillo B, Sudarsanam A, Charyulu K, Averette H E 1979 Selective therapy for early cancer of the cervix. II. Surgically nonexplored cases. Gynecologic Oncology 7: 257–263

O'Leary J A, Symmonds R E 1966 Radical pelvic operations in the geriatric patient; a 15-year review of 133 cases. Obstetrics and Gynecology 28: 745–753

O'Quinn A G, Fletcher G H, Wharton J T 1980 Guidelines for conservative hysterectomy after irradiation. Gynecologic Oncology 9: 68–79

Orr J W Jr, Shingleton H M, Hatch K D, Mann W J, Austin J M Jr, Soong S-J 1982 Correlation of perioperative morbidity and conization-radical hysterectomy interval. (In press)

Park R C, Patow W E, Rogers R E, Zimmerman E A 1973 Treatment of stage I carcinoma of the cervix. Obstetrics and Gynecology 41: 117–122

Parker R T, Wilbanks G D, Yowell R K, Carter F B 1967 Radical hysterectomy and pelvic lymphadenectomy with and without preoperative radiotherapy for cervical cancer. American Journal of Obstetrics and Gynecology 99: 933–943

Partridge E E, Murad T, Shingleton H M, Austin J M, Hatch K D 1980 Verrucous lesions of the female genitalia. II. Verrucous carcinoma. American Journal of Obstetrics and Gynecology 137: 412–424

Perez C A, Camel H M, Kao M S, Askin F 1980 Randomized study of preoperative radiation and surgery or irradiation alone in the treatment of stage IB and IIA carcinoma of the uterine cervix: preliminary analysis of failures and complications. Cancer 45: 2759–2768

Pilleron J P, Durand J C, Hamelin J P 1974 Prognostic value of node metastasis in cancer of the uterine cervix. American Journal of Obstetrics and Gynecology 119: 458–462

Piver M S 1977 The value of pretherapy para-aortic lymphadenectomy for carcinoma of the cervix uteri. Surgery, Gynecology and Obstetrics 145: 17–18

Piver M S, Chung W S 1975 Prognostic significance of cervical lesion size and pelvic node metastases in cervical carcinoma. Obstetrics and Gynecology 46: 507–510

Piver M S, Barlow J J, Krishnamsetty R 1981 Five-year survival (with no evidence of disease) in patients with biopsy-confirmed aortic node metastasis from cervical carcinoma. American Journal of Obstetrics and Gynecology 139: 575–578

Piver M S, Rutledge F, Smith J P 1974 Five classes of extended hysterectomy for women with cervical cancer. Obstetrics and Gynecology 44: 265–272

Powell J L, Burrell M O, Franklin E W III 1981 Radical hysterectomy and pelvic lymphadenectomy. Gynecologic Oncology 12: 23–32

Rampone J F, Klem V, Kolstad P 1973 Combined treatment of stage IB carcinoma of the cervix. Obstetrics and Gynecology 41: 163–167

Rotman M, John M J, Moon S H, Choi K N, Stowe S M, Abitbol A et al 1979
Limitations of adjunctive surgery in carcinoma of the cervix. International Journal
of Radiation Oncology, Biology, Physics 5: 327–332

Rutledge F N, Seski J 1979 More or less radical surgery. International Journal of
Radiation Oncology, Biology, Physics 5: 1881–1884

Rutledge F N, Fletcher G H, MacDonald E J 1965 Pelvic lymphadenectomy as an
adjunct to radiation therapy in treatment for cancer of the cervix. American
Journal of Roentgenology 93: 607–614

Rutledge F N, Wharton J T, Fletcher G H 1976 Clinical studies with adjunctive
surgery and irradiation therapy in the treatment of carcinoma of the cervix. Cancer
38: 596–602

Rutledge F N, Galakatos A E, Wharton J T, Smith J P 1975 Adenocarcinoma of the
uterine cervix. American Journal of Obstetrics and Gynecology 122: 236–235

Sall S, Pineda A A, Calanog A, Heller P, Greenberg H 1979 Surgical treatment of
stages IB and IIA invasive carcinoma of the cervix by radical abdominal
hysterectomy. American Journal of Obstetrics and Gynecology 135: 442–446

Selim M A, Kurohara S S 1970 Significance of gravidity in cancer of the cervix uteri.
American Journal of Obstetrics and Gynecology 106: 731–735

Seski J C, Diokno A C 1977 Bladder dysfunction after radical abdominal
hysterectomy. American Journal of Obstetrics and Gynecology 128: 643–651

Seydel H G 1975 The risk of tumor induction in man following medical irradiation
for malignant neoplasm. Cancer 35: 1641–1645

Shingleton H M, Palumbo L Jr 1968 Ureteral complications of radical hysterectomy:
effects of preoperative radium and ureteral catheters. Surgery Forum 19: 410–412

Sinclair R H, Pratt J H 1972 Femoral neuropathy after pelvic operation. American
Journal of Obstetrics and Gynecology 112: 404–407

Spanos W J, Greer B E, Hamberger A D, Rutledge F N 1981 Prognosis of squamous
cell carcinoma of the cervix with endometrial involvement. Gynecologic Oncology
11: 230–234

Stage A H, Crawford E J, Robinson L S, Brooks G G 1974 Combined
radiologic/operative therapy in the treatment of cervical malignancy. American
Journal of Obstetrics and Gynecology 120: 960–968

Surwit E, Fowler W C Jr, Palumbo P, Koch G, Gjertsen W 1976 Radical
hysterectomy with or without preoperative radium for stage IB squamous cell
carcinoma of the cervix. Obstetrics and Gynecology 48: 130–133

Talbert L M, Palumbo L, Shingleton H M, Bream C A, McGee J 1965 Urologic
complications of radical hysterectomy for carcinoma of the cervix. Southern
Medical Journal 58: 11–17

Underwood P B Jr, Wilson W C, Kreutner A, Miller M C III, Murphy E 1979
Radical hysterectomy: a critical review of 22 years' experience. American Journal
of Obstetrics and Gynecology 134: 889–898

Webb G A 1975 The role of ovarian conservation in the treatment of carcinoma of the
cervix with radical surgery. American Journal of Obstetrics and Gynecology 122:
476–484

Webb M J, Symmonds R E 1979a Wertheim hysterectomy: a reappraisal. Obstetrics
and Gynecology 54: 140–145

Webb M J, Symmonds R E 1979b Radical hysterectomy: influence of recent
conization on morbidity and complications. Obstetrics and Gynecology 53:
290–292

Weed J C 1967 Treatment of stage I and stage II carcinoma of the cervix. Pacific
Medicine and Surgery 75: 319–325

Weed J C, Holland J B 1977 Combined irradiation and extensive operations in the
treatment of stages I and II carcinoma of the cervix uteri. Surgery, Gynecology
and Obstetrics 144: 869–872

Welander C E, Pierce V K, Nori D, Hilaris B S, Kosloff C, Clark D G C et al 1981
Pretreatment laparotomy in carcinoma of the cervix. Gynecologic Oncology 12:
336–347

Wharton J T, Rutledge F N 1980 Adjunctive surgical procedures with irradiation therapy for carcinoma of the cervix. In: Fletcher G H (ed) Textbook of radiotherapy. Lea & Febiger, Philadelphia, p 773–789

Yajima A, Noda K 1979 The results of treatment of microinvasive carcinoma (stage IA) of the uterine cervix by means of simple and extended hysterectomy. American Journal of Obstetrics and Gynecology 135: 685–6898

Zander J, Baltzer J, Lohe K J, Ober K G, Kaufmann C 1981 Carcinoma of the cervix: an attempt to individualize treatment; results of a 20-year cooperative study. American Journal of Obstetrics and Gynecology 139: 752–759

5

Radiation therapy

Radiotherapy is an important method of primary treatment of patients with cervical cancer. While opinions differ as to its place in the treatment of young patients with early stage cervical cancer, virtually all oncologists consider it to be the treatment of choice in patients with large volume or advanced stage disease.

Although gynaecologists or other primary care physicians refer patients for treatment and may render follow-up care, their ability to communicate with the radiotherapist is restricted since few doctors receive enough instruction in radiation physics or biology to understand the effects of radiotherapy on malignant and normal tissues.

FUNDAMENTALS OF RADIATION PHYSICS

Ionising radiation is radiation which during tissue absorption has sufficient energy to eject one or more orbital electrons from an atom or molecule, resulting in the production of abnormal atomic and molecular species. There are basically two types of ionising radiation: electromagnetic and particulate. X-rays and gamma rays are forms of electromagnetic radiation and differ only in the manner in which they are produced. X-rays are produced extranuclearly by an electrical device that accelerates a beam of electrons to a high energy and directs this beam to strike a target, usually tungsten or gold, whereby the electron kinetic energy is converted to X-rays. Gamma rays are produced intranuclearly and represent excess energy emitted from the unstable nuclei of radioactive isotopes (i.e. cobalt–60). These electromagnetic radiations possess the characteristics of both an energy wave and a packet of energy called a 'photon'. Photons of low energy are those with a long wavelength and a low oscillatory frequency. Conversely, electromagnetic radiations with short wavelengths and high frequencies possess high photon energies. Photons of higher energy are capable of penetrating tissue to a greater depth before they interact with tissue to cause ionisations (Fig. 5.1). When X-rays or gamma rays are absorbed by tissue, their energy is unevenly deposited in discrete packets some

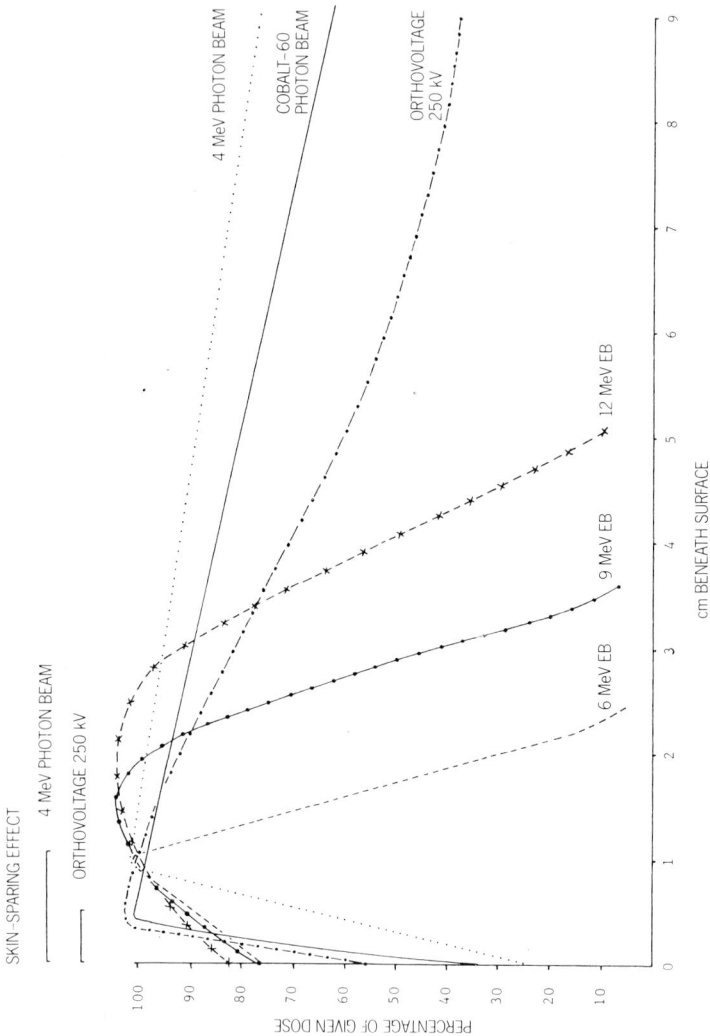

Fig. 5.1 The depth at which the maximum dose of ionising radiation occurs is related to the photon. While 100% of the given dose of superficial radiation (not pictured) is at the skin-air interface, less of the given dose occurs with higher energy sources such as orthovoltage (approximately 50%), cobalt (30%) or 4 MeV photons (20%) and accounts for the skin-sparing effect. A greater percentage of a given dose is realised at greater depths of tissue penetration i.e. at 9 cm only 40% of the given dose of orthovoltage is available to cause ionising events. This percentage is increased substantially with cobalt-60 photons (60%), 4 MeV photons (75%) and higher with 18 MeV or 22 MeV photons. This combination of events (skin-sparing effect of higher energy and increased depth of penetration) allows the radiotherapist to treat tumour-bearing tissues with higher doses. EB = electron beam. (Modified from Hellman, 1982)

distance apart in the absorber. Each absorptive event is capable of breaking chemical bonds and initiating actions at the molecular level which culminate in a biological event. In regard to biological effects, electromagnetic radiation produces ionisation in tissue if the corresponding wavelength is less than 10^{-6}cm.

There are three ways that electromagnetic radiations interact with absorbing tissues. The first is via a process called *photoelectric absorption* wherein all of the photon's energy is expended when it intereacts with an inner shell orbital electron, thereby ejecting that electron from its parent nucleus. The second process is referred to as the *Compton effect*. In this case the incident photon interacts with an orbital electron, resulting in the ejection of that electron (as in the case of photoelectric effect) but with incomplete energy transfer. This results in a scatter photon whose kinetic energy has been reduced by the ejection of the electron. The scatter photon may then go on to interact again. The ejected electron may also proceed to further interact within the absorber to alter other atoms or vital chemical bonds. The third possible process is *pair production*. In this case a high-energy photon (in excess of 1.02 MeV) may undergo a reaction in the vicinity of the nucleus in which a portion of the photon energy is used to create an electron (e−) positron (e+) pair. The remaining energy is provided as kinetic energy to the two newly-created particles. These energetic particles may ultimately annihilate each other and in the process create two 0.51 MeV photons emitted in opposite directions, or may travel in opposite directions, causing ionisation along their paths of travel.

As stated earlier, electromagnetic radiations interact with the absorbing medium (i.e. tissue) in a random fashion causing ionisations which may be near or far apart. Thus, ionisation of critical molecules in living cells is a random event and the probability of such a critical event is proportional to photon number.

Particulate radiations used for radiation therapy are subatomic particles (electrons, protons, alpha particles, neutrons, negative pi–mesons, and atomic nuclei) which have been accelerated to high energy for tissue penetration. All of these particles, with the exception of neutrons, possess two characteristics uniquely different from electromagnetic radiations, namely mass and charge. Because of these characteristics, particulate radiations have greater potential to cause ionisations along their path of travel through the absorber, and this potential is directly related to particle mass size and charge value. The depth of tissue penetration by particulate radiations is not only dependent upon the particle's mass and charge, but also upon the initial energy of the particle. For example, an alpha particle with its large mass (2 protons and 2 neutrons) and strong (2+) positive charge must be accelerated to very high energy in order to penetrate significant tissue depth. The most commonly used particulate radiation in clinical practice is the electron. Linear accelerators are used to produce electron beams of variable energy. The electron's ionisation potential is somewhat greater than that of an equivalent energy photon and can be easily regulated with regard to depth of tissue penetration (Fig. 5.1). Thus, electron beam radiation is used advantageously for the treatment of tumours located near or within superficial areas of the body.

Quantities of radiation are commonly expressed in units defined as Roentgen, rad, or Grey. A Roentgen, defined as a unit of radiation exposure, is not used in therapeutic radiology. Its primary use is in the field of radiation health safety where radiation sources are monitored for their radiation output level. One Roentgen is that amount of X- or gamma radiation which produces one electrostatic unit of charge in one cubic centimetre of dry air. The rad is a unit of absorbed dose commonly used in therapeutic radiology and represents the energy absorbed per gram of absorber material due to ionising radiation of either electromagnetic or particulate type. By definition, one rad represents 100 ergs of energy absorbed per gram of absorber substance or 0.01 Joule per kilogram. The currently recommended nomenclature for measurement of absorbed radiation dose, however, is the Grey. One Grey is equal to one Joule of energy absorbed per kilogram of substance (1 Grey = 100 rad).

FUNDAMENTALS OF RADIATION BIOLOGY

Mammalian cells may be injured by ionising radiation in one of two ways: (1) by the direct interaction of photons or particles with essential molecules causing their ionisation or, (2) by the ionisation of non-essential cellular components which in turn transfer and dissipate their radical electrical energies to vital molecular species. It is commonly accepted that nuclear DNA is the critical target for both of these processes of radiation injury.

Since water comprises approximately 80% of most mammalian cells, it is a more likely candidate for photon or particle radiation interaction. When water is ionised, a number of free radicals are produced which may combine with oxygen to give rise to molecular species which have life-spans and chemical characteristics capable of injury to critical target molecules within the cell. It is commonly accepted that most of the cell injury caused by electromagnetic radiation is due to indirect actions mediated by ionised water in the presence of oxygen and that without the presence of molecular oxygen, this effect is markedly diminished. This has been the basis for radiation treatment of human tumours under hyperbaric oxygen conditions. Particle radiations produce a more dense area of ionisations along their path of travel in tissue, and thus have a higher probability of interacting with critical target molecules. Because of their high ionisation potential, particulate radiations such as neutrons, protons, alpha particles, pi–mesons, and atomic nuclei cause cell injury primarily through direct interaction with critical target molecules.

All proliferating human cells traverse the mitotic cell cycle (Fig. 5.2) whose components include the mitotis or cell division phase (M), the synthesis phase (G_1), the DNA synthesis phase (S), and preparation for cell division phase (G_2). Cells are most sensitive to the effects of ionising radiation during mitosis and least sensitive during the latter portion of the DNA synthesis phase. Non-cycling cells (G_0), usually present in tumours, are in a non-metabolising state and are resistant to radiation. Cells undergoing rapid division, or those with long mitotic futures (stem cells) are the most radiosensitive. The radiation enhancement effect of oxygen, which occurs only if oxygen is present concurrently with the radiation, is constant across all phases of the cell cycle.

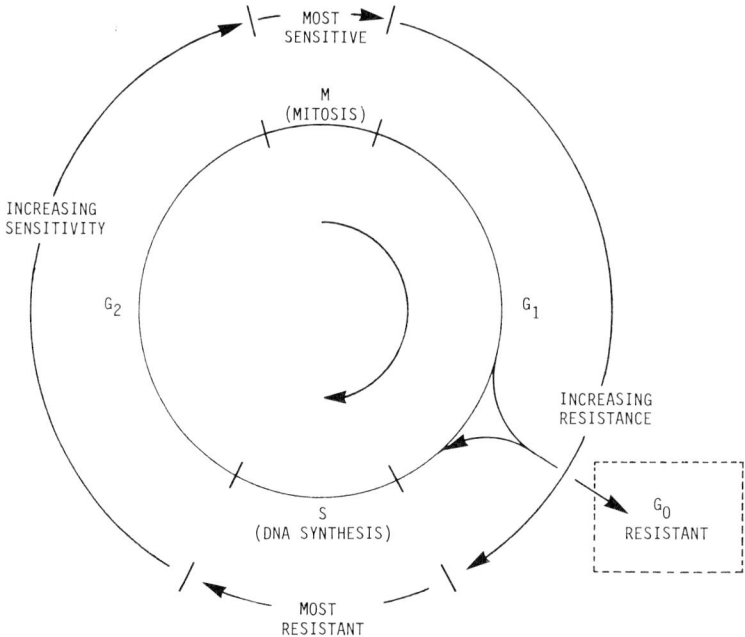

Fig. 5.2   The radiosensitivity of cells differs during the cell cycle. Increasing radioresistance is present during the G_1 and S phase, however, cells proceeding through G_2 have an increased sensitivity to ionising radiation and those in mitosis are the most sensitive. Most tumours have a large number of cells in G_0 (non-dividing), however, these cells may be recalled into the cycle following cell kill during fractional radiotherapy.

For a given dose increment of radiation, a constant proportion rather than an absolute number of cells are killed (Fig. 5.3). D_0 is that dose of radiation required to reduce the surviving fraction of treated cells to 37% of their original number on the exponential curve. The smaller the D_0, the more sensitive the cells are to radiation injury. The D_0 for most mammalian cells falls between 100 and 200 rad. In vitro and in vivo experimental studies suggest little difference in radiosensitivity between normal and tumour cells of the same tissue origin. Additionally, the survival curves of most mammalian cells have a shoulder (D_q) in the low radiation dose region which allows for repair of sublethal damage and results in reduced efficiency of cell killing.

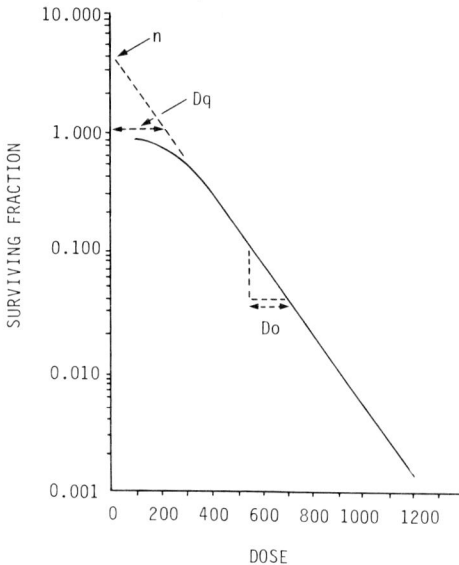

Fig. 5.3 The effective cell kill following is a constant proportion and not an absolute number. The D_0 dose is that which reduces the surviving fraction to 37% on the exponential curve. The fall-off of the curve at lower doses (Dq) is related to the repair of sublethal damage.

It is clinically apparent that radiation fractionation (dose delivered over multiple exposures) is more effective than a single dose in eradicating tumours and minimising normal tissue damage. The advantage of fractionation in tumour regression can be explained by reoxygenation. The apparent critical diffusion distance of oxygen is 100 μm to 150μm from the vascular surface. Hypoxic tumour cells are radioresistant (Fig. 5.4) and all tumours larger than 200 μm have associated zones of hypoxia and necrosis. However, between the proliferating cells (those 100 μm away) and the hypoxic cells (those 200 μm away) there exists a region of tumour cells in an oxygen tension that allows them to be clonogenic, yet renders relative protection from the effects of ionising radiation. This relatively hypoxic region of cells would not be killed by radiation in a single dose; however, fractionated doses kill sensitive cells (those 100 μm away from oxygen supply) and the interval of fractionation allows those relatively resistant cells (between 100 and 200 μm) to re-oxygenate and thereby become sensitive to the radiation delivered in succeeding fractions. Clinically this corresponds to the tumour regression apparent during teletherapy. A clinical radiobiological research model to explain time-dose radiation effects in solid tumours has been developed by Whitmore (1969). In this model, four fundamental processes are described as influencing factors that take place during fractionated radiation treatment of solid tumours:

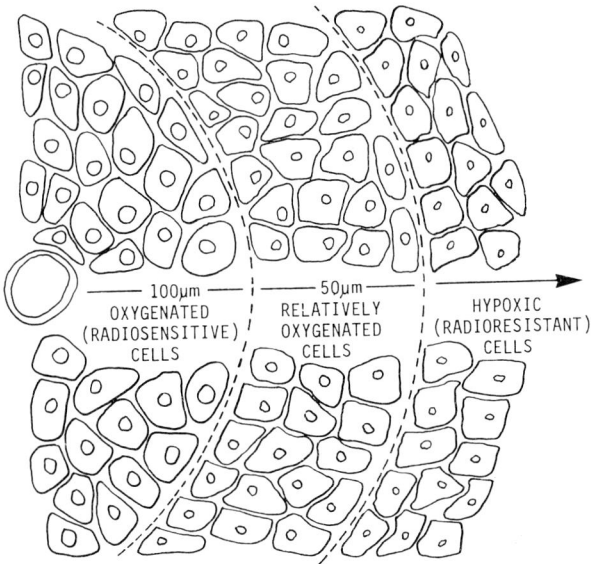

Fig. 5.4 Well-oxygenated cells (those less than 100 μm from a vessel) are more radiosensitive than hypoxic cells. During radiation fractionation, the sensitive cells die, allowing re-oxygenation of both the relative hypoxic cells and hypoxic cells. Repeated fractional doses will thereby be able to affect more cells that are oxygenated than a single dose.

tumour cell repair, reoxygenation, repopulation, and resortment. The fundamental thesis of this model is that properly selected radiation time-dose fractionation schemes can take advantage of the physical and physiological changes that occur within the tumour volume during treatment to provide greater tumour cell kill.

In normal tissues, small fractionated doses of radiation are better tolerated than a large single dose because it allows repair of sublethal damage. Sublethal damage results when a cell has received ionising events to some but not all of the critical target sites. Many of these sites are not irreparably damaged and the cell may survive if given time for repair. In addition, normal cells are more capable of dividing and of regrowth, a process termed repopulation.

CLINICAL APPLICATION OF RADIATION THERAPY

The therapeutic index for radiation therapy (i.e. dose to kill tumour versus the dose to kill normal cells) in patients with cervical carcinoma is narrow. Fletcher (1973) indicated that the curative dose of radiation increases directly as the size of the tumour increases (Table 5.1). This becomes important when one considers the tolerance of the surrounding pelvic structures (Table 5.2). While the vagina, cervix, uterus and ureters (with intact blood supply) are relatively radioresistant, the dose

Table 5.1 Squamous cell carcinoma of the cervix dose-tumour-volume relationship: average dose radiation required to obtain 90% control in area treated (from Fletcher 1973)

Tumour volume	Dose (rad)
< 2 cm	5000
2 cm	6000
2-4 cm	7000
4-6 cm	7500–8000
6 cm	8000–10 000

Table 5.2 Radiation tolerance levels of abdomino-pelvic organs

Organ	Risk TD 5/5* (rad)	TD 50/5** (rad)	Type of injury
Bladder	6000	8000	Ulcer, contracture
Bone	6000	15 000	Necrosis, fracture
Intestine	4500	6000	Ulcer, stricture, fistula
Muscle	6000	8000	Fibrosis
Ovary	300	1250	Sterilization
Rectum	5500	8000	Ulcer, stricture, fistula
Skin	5500	7000	Atrophy, ulcer, fibrosis
Spinal cord	5000	6000	Necrosis, transection
Ureters	7500	10 000	Stricture
Uterus	10 000	20 000	Necrosis, perforation
Vagina	9000	10 000	Ulcer, fistula

*Total radiation dose (rad) which results in a 5% complication rate in patients followed for 5 years
**Total radiation dose (rad) which results in a 50% complication rate in patients followed for 5 years

that predicts a 50% risk of bladder or rectal injury is not greatly different from that necessary to cure large cervical squamous cell carcinomas. While tolerance doses allow cure, they initiate progressive arteritis and fibrosis in the normal tissue which may predispose to complications and interfere with healing if surgery is later required. Renal and hepatic tissues are non-proliferating and tolerate radiation poorly. While bone has a relatively high tolerance, prior radiation hinders repair if fractures occur.

Radiosensitivity should not be equated to radiocurability. The former relates to the innate sensitivity of the particular tumour cell, while the latter implies a favourable tumour-normal tissue relationship such that curative doses of radiation therapy can be administered without creating excessive damage to the surrounding normal tissue. Cervical carcinomas are radiocurable because therapeutic schemas have been developed to protect the normal tissues.

RADIOTHERAPY SCHEME — TECHNICAL CONSIDERATIONS

The radiation therapist must consider many factors to enhance the chance for cure and to minimise the risk of complications (Table 5.3).

Table 5.3 Factors to be considered in treatment planning

Technical	Clinical
Total radiation dose	Tumour volume
Daily dose	Cell type and grade
Time of delivery	Anatomical factors
Total number of fractions	Age
Field size	Nutritional status
Sequence of therapy	Systemic disease
Energy source	Previous surgery

The total dose necessary to cure a patient with a 2 cm tumour differs from that which would sterilise a 6 cm tumour. Additionally, the total dose usually represents a combination of teletherapy and brachytherapy. To aid in the measurement of pelvic dose certain reference points have been introduced so as to optimise tumour dosage while minimising radiation dose to normal pelvic structures (Fig. 5.5).

The development of higher energy radiation equipment (cobalt–60, linear accelerators) has allowed for the delivery of greater depth doses. Durrance (1969) indicated that the risk of central pelvic recurrence in patients with stage I or II carcinoma of the cervix was decreased by 50% after the introduction of supervoltage units. Recently Kurohara (1979) compared a series of patients treated by orthovoltage and supervoltage. The use of the latter was associated with increased patient survival in all stages. Most authors indicate that this increased control of pelvic tumour is associated with a relative increased risk of distal metastases. This work has been confirmed by Katz (1980), who in an autopsy series of cervical cancer deaths indicated less ureteral involvement in those patients who were treated more recently.

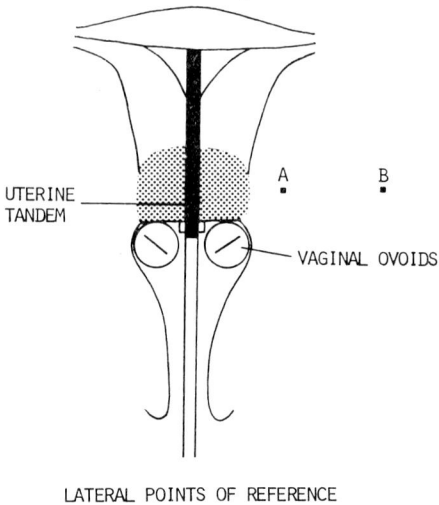

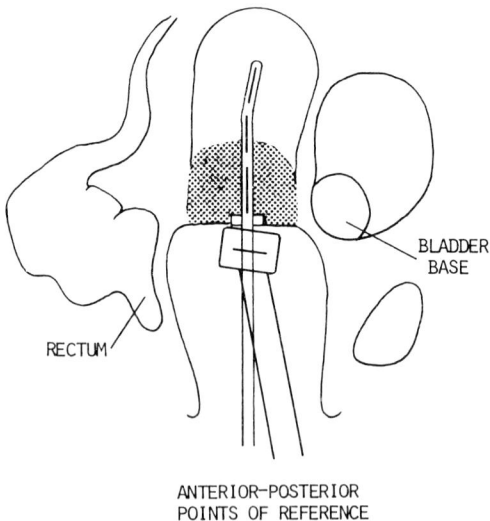

LATERAL POINTS OF REFERENCE

ANTERIOR-POSTERIOR
POINTS OF REFERENCE

Fig. 5.5 Reference points used during pelvic radiotherapy include point A (2 cm lateral from the midline and 2 cm above the lateral vaginal fornix) which corresponds to the paracervical tissues near the ureter and point B (3 cm lateral to point A) which represents the pelvic sidewall. The doses to the base of the bladder and rectum are important reference points in the anterior-posterior plane. These reference points may be distorted in women with large cervical tumours.

The incorporation of larger treatment volume increases complications. Although individualised therapy is important, the usual pelvic field consists of anterior and posterior opposing ports (15 cm × 15 cm or 16 cm × 16 cm) treated daily with a total of 180 to 200 rad. The usual upper border of this field is L_5 and would incorporate the common iliac nodes (Fig. 5.6). Incorporating larger treatment volumes

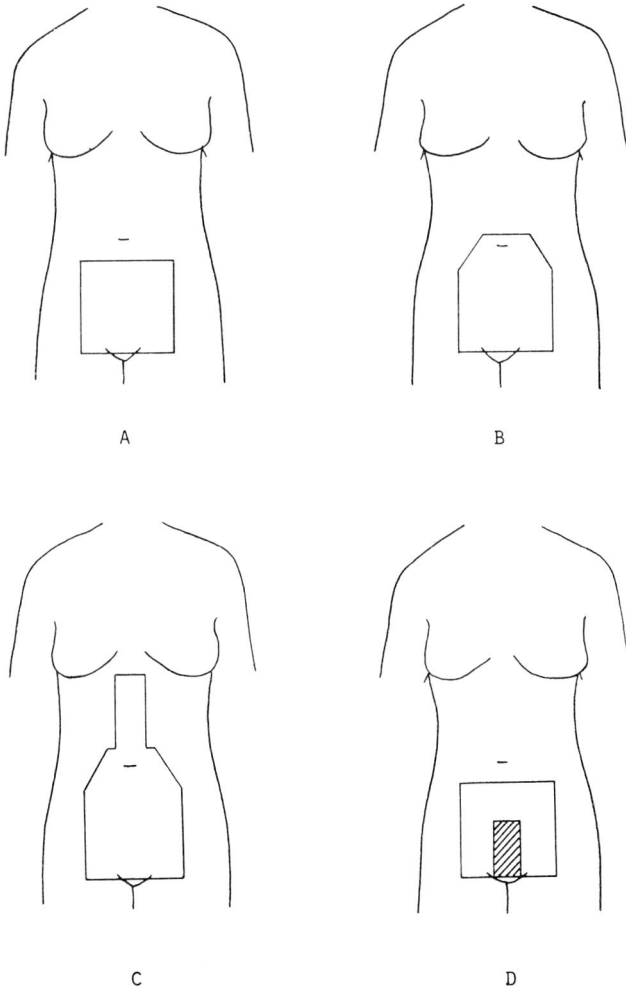

A

B

C

D

Fig. 5.6   The usual pelvic point (A) would include all pelvic tissue to the mid-common iliac vessels. B represents an extension of this field to L_{4-5} to include the entire common iliac nodal group, as well as the nodal areas at the bifurcation of the aorta. The treatment of metastases in the para-aortic nodes necessitates extending the radiation field to T_{12} (C). Most treatment schemes necessitate a midline shield (D) in order to decrease the total dose to the rectum and bladder.

such as the periaortic nodes requires a decrease in total dose in order to avoid serious complications. The utilisation of lateral pelvic ports in larger patients (those with an anterior-posterior diameter greater than 20–22 cm) may improve dosimetry.

The treatment sequence depends on the tumour volume. Patients with early invasive cervical disease (focal micro-invasion, micro-invasion, microcarcinoma) have a low risk of lymphatic involvement and the therapist may elect to treat them with intracavitary sources alone (Fig. 5.7). Hamberger (1978) reported a 100% cure in 41 patients with stage IA (less than 3 mm invasion) cervical cancer treated with this scheme. In the 93 patients with stage IB (less than 1 cm in size) disease, none had central recurrence. The survival rate was 96% and was associated with a low incidence (1%) of serious complications. Patients with larger tumours usually begin treatment with the delivery of 2000–5000 rad by teletherapy. The homogeneous characteristics of teletherapy cause tumour regression and reduce the anatomical distortion that is often associated with advanced tumours. An intracavitary radium or caesium source is then placed and loaded. Following the intracavitary treatment, midline shields are placed to protect the central pelvic structures and a parametrial boost of teletherapy is delivered. While combinations vary, most centres attempt to deliver 7000 to 8000 rad to point A and 6000 rad to point B (Fig. 5.8) while maintaining the bladder and rectal dose at 6000 rad.

Many schemes of intracavitary radiation have been proposed. It is understood that the simple addition of rad from brachytherapy and teletherapy is not correct; however, attempts to standardise the biological equivalence of intracavitary and external therapy have not been successful and the optimal method of conversion remains unknown. Thus many schemes currently utilised are based on clinical experience in which the dosage to specified pelvic reference points is kept within a narrow range which allows for cure and minimal complications. The dosimetry calculations after placement of the intracavitary device are usually determined after obtaining anterior-posterior and lateral pelvic films that relate spatial relationships between the tumour, bladder and rectum. More recent reports indicate that computerised tomography may more accurately determine appropriate three-dimensional dosimetry, however, more thorough investigation is necessary before this relatively expensive process can be advocated.

Regardless of the method of localisation, the appropriate application and packing of the intracavitary device is important. Slight displacement or malposition can result in a marked alteration of tumour dose (Fig. 5.9). In fact, central pelvic failure in patients with stage I–II

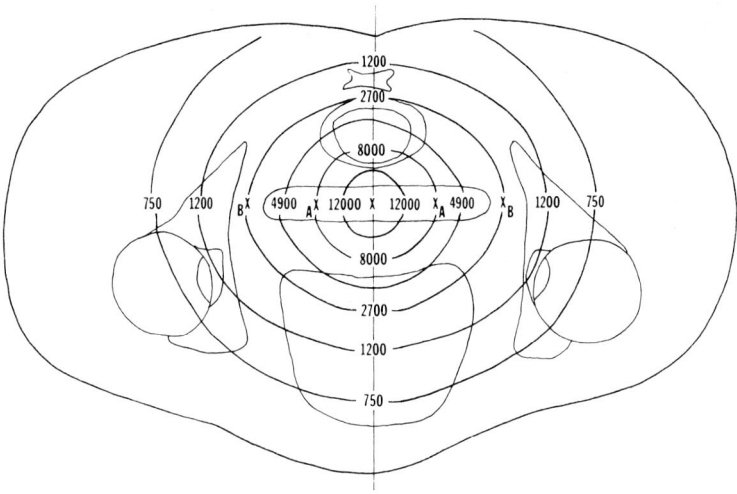

Fig. 5.7 Typical dosimetry of patients treated with intracavitary therapy alone. This scheme allows for high local dose to the cervix and paracervical area (point A), however, the pelvic sidewall dose (point B) is small. This form of therapy is not to be used in patients with a high risk of nodal metastases. (Modified from Cooper and Barish, 1981)

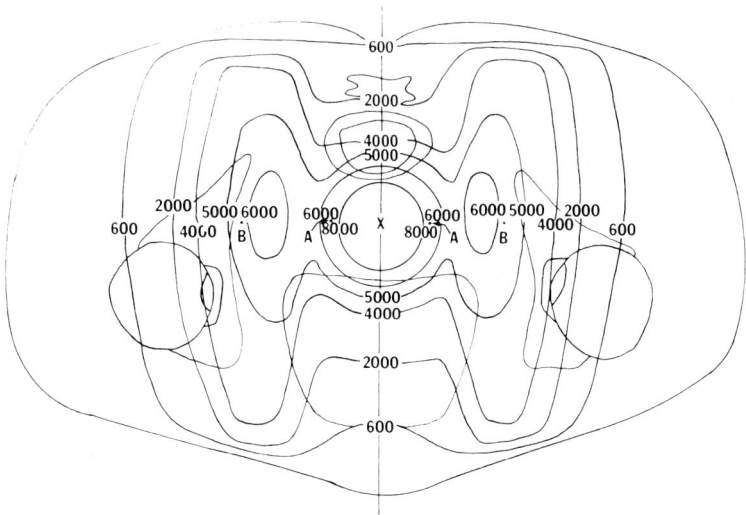

Fig. 5.8 Dosimetry with combined teletherapy and brachytherapy. Dose to the paracervical tissues (point A) is usually kept at 6000–7000 rad and the dose to the pelvic sidewall (point B) is usually 5000 to 6000 rad. Bladder and rectal dose are maintained at levels to minimise the risk of complications. (Modified from Cooper and Barish, 1981)

tumours can often be found retrospectively to be related to malplacement of the applicator.

It is important to minimise the delay in intracavitary therapy as prolonged delays (more than 14 days) may allow tumour regrowth and may be associated with failure.

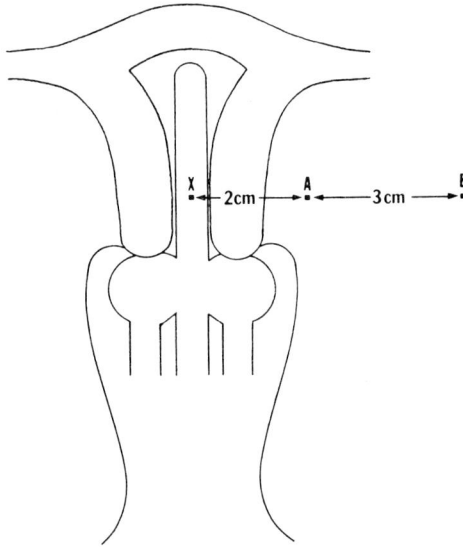

Fig. 5.9 The dose at a particular point from the radiation source varies with the inverse of the distance squared. For example, the dose above is 15 000 rad at point X, the dose at point A (1/4 of X) would be 3750 rad and the dose at point B (1/25 of X) would be 600 rad. With a 1 cm displacement to the left, the dose at point A (1/9 of X) would fall to 1666 rad. Because the intracavitary sources include the tandem and the vaginal ovoids, malposition or slippage would result in marked alteration of dosimetry.

Clinical considerations

Anatomical variations must be taken into consideration. Narrow vaginal vaults or asymmetrical scarred vaginal fornices of some women may not permit use of an intracavitary device. However, emphasis on the teletherapy component may result in further vaginal stricturing. Tumour involving the lower vagina (stage IIIA) may require a perineal port. The inferior portion of the usual pelvic port is at the level of the obturator foramen and lowering this port to include the lower vagina may result in acute vulvitis. However, a perineal port allows for adequate therapy while minimising complications.

Patients with stage IV disease are treatment problems. Many have extrapelvic disease or large volume disease, precluding cure with radiation alone. A special group, those with stage IVA disease, are occasionally treated by primary pelvic exenteration. However Million's

(1972) report of a 30% survival in selected patients with histological evidence of bladder invasion with only a 4% vesicovaginal fistula rate would encourage us to use radiotherapy as the initial treatment.

The prognostic importance of cell type is not established (Table 2.7, Ch. 2). Conflicting reports concerning the prognostic significance of cell type may be partially explained by the fact that the diagnosis of most patients treated with radiation is made with a small biopsy, which may not represent the major cell type of the tumour.

Adenocarcinoma, and particularly mixed adenosquamous carcinoma, has been said to be radioresistant and to have a worse prognosis stage by stage than does squamous cell carcinoma (Wheeless 1970, Julian 1977). In a controlled study (1981), we were unable to show any difference in curability of both of these tumour types if a correction was made for size (volume) of tumour. The excellent cure rates reported by Rutledge (1975) using radiation therapy alone or in combination with conservative hysterectomy for adenocarcinomas suggests that the cell type or histology is relatively unimportant, and that tumour volume is more important in predicting cure.

The effect of age on survival and complications has been the subject of numerous publications and is controversial. Many authors suggest a decreased normal tissue tolerance in older patients, particularly those with vascular disease, and some have advocated a decreased fraction dose (less than 160 rad) in order to decrease the risks of serious complications. Mann's (1980) report on stage I patients at this institution indicated that survival was not different in patients under or over 40 years treated with radiation or radical surgery. Kjorstad (1977) reported better survival in younger patients. However, Stanhope (1980) indicated that survival was decreased in patients less than 35 years old in all stages except IA and IV. He suggested that this might be due to altered immunological defences or increased tumour virulence in young women with cervical cancer.

Since much of the small bowel lies in the pelvic teletherapy field, one would expect some degree of radiation enteritis to occur in most patients. The acute radiation ileitis that occurs with pelvic radiotherapy may cause a patient to digest less food and be unable to store nutrients that reach the small intestine. Some degree of malnutrition during therapy may be expected and can become disabling, although the acute radiation reaction subsides following therapy. Donaldson (1981) compared two groups of patients receiving abdominal radiotherapy. The first group received total parenteral nutrition (TPN); the second group received it only if they had lost 10% of their body weight. He found no difference in toleration of radiation therapy or in long-term results between the two groups. Valerio (1978) was unable to demonstrate improved tolerance to radiation therapy using TPN. Copeland (1978), however, treated 39 seriously malnourished patients with TPN during radiation therapy and reported that 95% of the patients were able to complete the planned course of therapy; this was higher than he would have predicted without TPN. It remains to be shown whether aggressive nutritional support as an adjunct to aggressive cancer therapy can enhance tumour response and patient survival. Certainly, cachexia is no longer a contra-indication to radiation therapy, since it can be corrected by TPN.

Treatment evaluation of associated medical problems is essential. It has been observed that anaemia contributes to increased hypoxia, and in fact, patients with uncorrected anaemia have an increased risk of failing treatment (Table 5.4). For this reason, we suggest pretreatment transfusion.

Table 5.4 Pelvic recurrence related to anaemia (stage IIB–III) (after Bush 1978)

	Control		Transfused
Haemoglobin (g/100ml)	< 12	> 12	> 12
No. of patients	20	48	67
% recurrence	50	23	16

Medical problems such as diabetes or hypertension are often associated with significant vascular disease and may contribute to tumour hypoxia as well as decreasing blood supply to normal pelvic tissues. Rogers (1960) indicated a poor survival in patients with significant arteriosclerosis and Nordqvist (1979) found a decreased rate of survival in patients with stage IB or IIA who had diabetes or other cardiovascular diseases. Pre-treatment evaluation should include a search for objective evidence regarding the degree of vascular disease, by general physical examination and especially by fundoscopic examination. Although complication rates may be increased in these women, the goal of radiation therapy should remain curative.

Pelvic inflammatory disease (PID) produces reactive vasculitis which, when combined with radiation, has been reported to be associated with an increased rate of bowel complications. However, this information on PID is often obtained by history, making it difficult to determine the exact role of infection in predisposing to bowel complications. While active tubal infection may require pre-treatment laparotomy and bilateral salpingo-oöphorectomy, the surgical procedure itself carries added risk. In fact, Piver (1976) indicated that salpingo-oöphorectomy might be contra-indicated during surgical staging procedures because it increased the risk of serious small bowel complications. If a pelvic operative procedure is performed prior to radiation, it would seem prudent to interpose the sigmoid colon or omentum between the small bowel and the raw operative surfaces in order to minimise the risk of small bowel adhesions.

Untreated patients with bilateral ureteral obstruction and uraemia need special attention. Taylor (1981) reported that aggressive medical or surgical management, prior to or during radiotherapy, is beneficial. The mean survival (17 months) of patients with such management was greatly increased over those without it (25 days). It has been our practice to relieve ureteral obstruction with transvesical or percutaneous stents in attempts to avoid the possible necessity of dialysis for vascular volume overload or hyperkalaemia.

A modern radiotherapy programme incorporating appropriate megavoltage and intracavitary therapy and attention to these specific problem areas can attain cure in 85% to 90% of patients with stage I disease, in 65% to 70% of patients with stage II disease and 40% to 50% in patients with stage III disease. Ten to 30% of patients with stage IV disease may be cured. Overall serious complications are present in less than 10% of patients.

SPECIAL CIRCUMSTANCES

Large volume, late stage disease is associated with poor survival. However, a significant number of these patients will have tumour confined to the pelvis and these patients, with a large hypoxic tumour component, may benefit from the use of radiosensitising drugs. Piver (1977) and Hreschchyshyn (1979) have reported an increased response rate and survival in patients receiving adjunctive hydroxyurea. This drug kills cells during the S phase, a time of relative radioresistance, and blocks G_1 cells at the S phase interface when they are relatively radiosensitive, thereby increasing the number of cells vulnerable during radiotherapy. Other radiosensitisers such as misonidazole are currently under investigation. The role of hyperthermia, which kills cells during the S phase, is undetermined in the treatment of cervical cancer. Watson's (1978) report on the use of hyperbaric oxygen concluded that it resulted in fewer pelvic recurrences; however, radiation tolerance in normal tissues was apparently decreased and the rate of complication was high.

Carcinoma of the cervical stump is less commonly encountered than in the earliest years of this century, when supracervical hysterectomy was an acceptable operation. While the treatment scheme may be altered, an intracavitary tandem can be used if the endocervical canal is at least 2 cm in length and in any event vaginal ovoids can be used. Rousseau (1972) reported equal survival, stage for stage, in patients with cervical stump cancers. While the possibility of high radiation dose to the small bowel exists because of expected adhesions, the possibility of an increase in serious complications may be more theoretical than real.

The finding of invasive cervical cancer in a total hysterectomy surgical specimen should prompt immediate consultation and referral, as these patients can be successfully treated with radiation therapy (Table 5.5). Reports from Andras (1973) and Davy (1977) indicate an excellent survival in patients with clear surgical margins who were treated promptly with radiation. Survival is decreased if the surgical margins are involved, i.e. apparent stage II disease or greater and if there was a prolonged delay between hysterectomy and radiotherapy.

Table 5.5 Survival of patients treated with radiation following an inadequate surgical procedure (Combined figures from Andras 1973 and Davey 1977)

Specimen	No. of patients	Survival (%)
Surgical margins free	113	85
Surgical margins involved		
treated within 6 months	54	44
treated after 6 months	50	33

The discovery of a coexisting second malignancy may require treatment modification. In many cases it is justified to treat the cervical cancer aggressively, except in those cases where the second malignancy has an extremely poor prognosis, in which case therapy for the cervical cancer should be directed towards palliation of symptoms. Vaginal bleeding, the most common symptom, may be effectively palliated by intracavitary radiation. An alternate treatment programme might include a reduced teletherapy field, high dose fractions, short duration teletherapy or transvaginal radiation.

The discovery of a high incidence of para-aortic nodal spread (Table 3.11, Ch. 3) in patients with cervical cancer has created a new problem for the radiotherapist, i.e., how to treat patients with this finding (Fig. 5.6). The treatment of extended fields has resulted in high complication rates (Table 5.6). While the long-term benefit in terms of survival has not yet been determined, most reports indicate some increase in survival with treatment. Before a patient is selected for extended radiotherapy one should consider supraclavicular (scalene) node biopsies, as the finding of metastases in supraclavicular nodes precludes radiotherapeutic cure and these patients become candidates for chemotherapy. Additionally, the larger treatment fields necessary to encompass larger volume tumour may require a reduction in total dose, adding to the risk of pelvic failure. Prior to initiating extended field

Table 5.6 Extended field radiation for para-aortic node metastases

Author	Year	No. of patients	RT dose (rad)	Complications (%)	Survival (%)	Type of exploration
Guthrie	1974	10	5400	–	44[a]	Transperitoneal
Schellhas	1975	9	6000	0	–	Extraperitoneal
Berman	1977	4	4000–5200	25	–	Transperitoneal
		7	4000–5200	0	–	Extraperitoneal
Nelson	1977	48	6000	48	45[a]	Transperitoneal
Wharton	1977	24	5500	42	13	Transperitoneal
Sudarsanam	1978	21	4000–4320	–	20	Transperitoneal
Averette	1979	29	4400–5000	14	–	Transperitoneal
Bonanno	1980	18	6000	26	21	Transperitoneal
Hughes	1980	22	4500–5100	9	29	Transperitoneal
Ballon	1981	19	4320–5120	0	23[b]	Extraperitoneal
Buchsbaum	1981	23	4750–5540	–	22	Transperitoneal
Piver	1981	21	6000	62	10	Transperitoneal
		10	4400–5000	10		
Welander	1981	31	4400	20	26	Transperitoneal
Tewfik	1982	23	5000–5500	28[c]	33	Transperitoneal

[a]2-year survival, [b]projected 5-year survival, [c]intestinal complication

radiotherapy, investigation of the upper gastro-intestinal tract should be performed to detect active gastric or duodenal ulcers, which may be adversely affected by radiation dosages of 4500 rad or higher.

The information obtained from these investigations is difficult to compare but it indicates that few patients with macroscopic disease in aortic nodes survive, that a total dose exceeding 4500 rad to the para-aortic nodal area is associated with serious gastro-intestinal complications and para-aortic nodal biopsy by a retroperitoneal approach reduces the risk of small bowel adhesions and is associated with fewer complications. The place for adjunctive radiosensitisers or intraoperative electron beam therapy to aortic node metastases requires further investigation.

Patients found to have metastases in pelvic lymph nodes at radical hysterectomy present a unique problem. While the use of postoperative radiotherapy has been advocated and widely used, its benefit (Table 5.7) has not been adequately demonstrated and requires further prospective investigation. Because of the increased rate of complications associated with pelvic radiation following radical hysterectomy, we advocate its use only in patients with three or more involved nodes or those with bilaterally positive nodes, since these patients are clearly at high risk for recurrence. Post-surgical radiation therapy might also be used in other patients who are at risk for failure; Abdulhayoglu (1980) advocated whole-pelvis radiation therapy in patients without nodal involvement but with other high-risk factors such as tumour involvement of the outer third of the cervical stroma, undifferentiated tumours and tumours with definite lymph-vascular space (LVS) involvement. We have used it for LVS involvement, and also for patients with close (less than 1 cm) margins of resection, however we cannot make a statement regarding the benefits of adjunctive radiation for these purposes.

Table 5.7 Radical abdominal hysterectomy. Survival with positive pelvic nodes with or without post-operative radiotherapy

Author	Year	Operation only		Post-operative rt.	
		Pts	Surv. %	Pts	Surv. %
Guttmann	1970	–	–	50	76
Rampone	1973	–	–	81	63
Piver	1975	39	56	–	–
Keys	1976	–	–	39	69
Morrow*	1980	144	59	30	60
Martimbeau	1982	–	–	120	53
Fuller	1982	39	56	32	47
Totals		222	58.1	352	60.5

*Collected series: Alabama (Birmingham), Mayo, Miami, Chicago, Michigan

Patients with pelvic recurrence following radical hysterectomy may benefit from radiation therapy. Our material indicates that 27% of patients who have recurrence after initial surgical treatment will survive if appropriate radiation therapy is utilised. This cure rate is almost identical to that of Krebs (1982) who reported a 25% survival in patients treated with radiation for a post-surgical recurrence.

COMPLICATIONS

The complications of radiation therapy are logically divided into those occurring acutely during therapy related to radiation reaction and those occurring later related to the continued effects of arteritis and fibrosis. While the acute complications are usually managed by medications or short interruption of the radiation therapy, the long-term complications are usually more serious.

The introduction of megavoltage teletherapy has made serious skin problems less frequent. However if these are present, particularly in the intertriginous areas, drying agents such as cornstarch may be helpful. Acute paniculitis or subcutaneous fibrosis is rare if the skin dose is 5000 rad or less.

Gastro-intestinal complaints are common during therapy. Nausea and vomiting may be relieved by using a low gluten, low protein, low lactose diet. Phenothiazines or other anti-emetics should be utilised as necessary. Diarrhoea secondary to acute ileitis can be treated symptomatically with such medications as diphenoxylate hydrochloride with atropine (Lomotil® or Imodium®); however, if the diarrhoea is severe and unresponsive to medical therapy, radiation should be temporarily interrupted. Some authors have advocated salicylates to treat the diarrhoea, since these drugs decrease local prostaglandin synthesis and thereby alleviate the symptoms.

Acute haemorrhagic cystitis is rare (less than 3%) and usually self-limiting. However, symptoms of urgency or frequency require investigation. Bladder fistulae and hydronephrosis are said to be more common in women who have cystitis during therapy. Clinical infection and bacteriuria should be treated with antibiotics.

Acute complications of patients undergoing intracavitary therapy are rare. Psychologically, patients appear to tolerate immobilisation better when placed on scheduled doses of a tranquilliser such as diazepam. Subcutaneous low-dose heparin reduces the risk of occult deep vein thrombosis and should be started prior to intracavitary placement.

The development of fever during treatment is a serious problem. Van Herek (1965) reported 260 patients with fever, usually associated with intracavitary therapy. The survival in patients with fever was lessened, stage for stage, when compared to those without. Survival of those patients with fevers of long duration was less than that of those with fevers of short duration. Davy (1974) confirmed the bad prognostic significance of fever and reported a 14% survival of patients with stage I and II cervical cancer if the fever had a genital origin. These treatment failures may be related to hypoxia in a necrotic tumour, uterine perforation and tumour dissemination during intracavitary placement, therapy delay or alteration of the treatment scheme if the intracavitary source is removed, or to altered host-resistance.

We would hesitate to use an intracavitary source in the presence of pyometra but would effect uterine drainage and proceed with external teletherapy. If fever develops during the intracavitary brachytherapy treatment phase, the patient is evaluated for extrapelvic causes. If none are found, antibiotic coverage for Gram-negative and anaerobic bacteria is begun. It is rarely necessary to remove the intracavitary system.

The loss of ovarian function and distortion of the vagina are a concern, especially in young patients with early stage disease. Abitbol & Davenport (1974) indicated that the triad of significant vaginal narrowing, marked pelvic fibrosis and pelvic pain were present in the majority of patients following radiation for cervical cancer. While the efficacy of oestrogen therapy and vaginal dilatation is unproved, we have advocated the two modalities in an effort to decrease these problems. It must be remembered, however, that oestrogen is freely absorbed from the irradiated vagina, and should not be administered to women with an absolute contra-indication for the drug, i.e. those with history of a deep venous thrombosis or with breast cancer.

Gastro-intestinal complications

Serious late gastro-intestinal complications are seen in as many as 8% of patients following radiation therapy. Proctosigmoiditis often associated with persistent rectal bleeding may respond to a low-residue diet and steroid enemas. If refractory to conservative measures, a diverting colostomy may be beneficial; however, after diversion, as many as 50% of patients will continue to bleed and may require bowel resection. Fortunately, rectovaginal fistulae or rectal strictures are infrequent (about 2% or less). If a fistula occurs, biopsies should be performed at the fistulous site to determine the presence or absence of cancer. Primary surgical repair of rectovaginal fistulae is quite difficult to achieve and is successful only if new blood supply (such as with use of a bulbocavernosus flap) is transposed into the area of injury. Bricker (1979) has recently reported successful closure of such fistulae by sigmoid colon transposition. In spite of these operative possibilities, many of these patients will require a permanent diverting colostomy, however.

The terminal ileum, with its relatively fixed position and tenuous blood supply, is the segment of small bowel most commonly involved in late complications. The risk of injury is increased in patients who have bowel adhesions following a previous abdominal surgical procedure or in those with significant vascular disease. Van Nagell (1974) reported individuals with a small body habitus to be particularly prone to small bowel complications. Small bowel obstruction occurs in 1% to 4% of patients following radiotherapy. These patients usually have a long history of symptoms suggestive of partial small bowel obstruction. Before surgical intervention, which should be performed prior to a catastrophic event such as perforation, the surgeon must aggressively treat vascular volume deficits and metabolic abnormalities. The proper surgical procedure to prevent small bowel perforation is controversial. Wheeless (1973) and Smith (1966) recommend simple bypass procedures such as an ileo-ascending colostomy. More recently, Schmitt (1981) indicated that intestinal resection may be the procedure of choice as fewer patients would require further surgical procedure to treat complications of the bypassed segment. We have tended to perform the simplest procedure, i.e. a bypass, unless bowel necrosis was evident.

The development of a small bowel fistula is more serious and requires immediate medical therapy directed at volume replacement, caloric replacement and correction of sepsis. Despite the use of parenteral hyperalimentation, few small bowel radiation fistulae will close spontaneously. Prior to surgical intervention, a fistulogram and small bowel series should be performed to determine the presence or absence of complex, i.e. large and small bowel, fistulae or distal small bowel obstruction. A simple bypass procedure is not recommended since it predisposes the patient to a second operation, often made necessary by an incompetent ileocaecal valve and continued fistulous drainage. We prefer to resect the involved segment, and to avoid a primary anastomosis in radiated bowel.

The seriousness of an operation for gastro-intestinal complications following radiation is evident in Smith's (1966) report, in which postoperative deaths occurred in 11% of patients following the first operation, 27% of patients following a second operation and 43% following a third operative procedure. Evidence of recurrent or persistent cancer should be actively sought since it may alter the treatment plan.

Urinary complications

The incidence of serious urinary complications ranges from 1% to 5% and increases markedly in patients receiving more than 8000 rad to the base of the bladder. The presence of hydronephrosis or ureteral stricture should prompt investigation for recurrent cancer. If cancer is present and the patient is not a candidate for exenteration, no surgical therapy is indicated. If no cancer is present, therapeutic alternatives include no therapy, transvesical or percutaneous ureteral stents, ureterolysis, transuretero-ureterotomy, ureteral reimplantation or conduit diversion. In these instances, we determine kidney function with an isotope scan. Patients with poor unilateral renal perfusion may be observed without treatment if the remaining kidney has adequate function; however, if the obstructed kidney has good perfusion, a transuretero-ureterotomy, performed outside of the radiation field, may be beneficial. In patients with bilateral obstruction due to radiation, we would recommend a transverse colon conduit since attempts to reimplant the ureters into the radiated bladder is fraught with high complication rates.

Some patients with radiation-induced vesico-vaginal fistulae have had primary repair using a vulvar pedicle graft or interposed omentum to provide new blood supply to the area. While some fistulae can be successfully managed in this way, more patients require permanent urinary diversion.

Bone injury

With low-energy teletherapy, radionecrosis of the femoral head was a potential complication. The introduction of supervoltage equipment has reduced the incidence of radionecrosis of bone to a negligible level. However, if fractured, previously irradiated bones heal poorly.

Carcinogenesis

The possible increased risk of inducing tumours in patients receiving pelvic radiotherapy has created some debate. Fehr (1973) indicated that the risk for the later development of sarcoma of the bony pelvis was very low and with megavoltage therapy should be rarely encountered. The risk of leukaemia following radiation is slightly increased but not dramatically so. Other forms of tumours such as uterine sarcomas, or carcinomas, occur in radiated fields. We have observed several such uterine fundal tumours, and at least one soft part sarcoma in a pelvic (posterior) radiation field. One might speculate that even the squamous carcinomas occurring in the pelvis many years following radiation for cancer of the cervix are radiation-induced second primaries and not recurrences.

BIBLIOGRAPHY

Abdulhayoglu G, Rich W M, Reynolds J, DiSaia P J 1980 Selective radiation therapy in stage IB uterine cervical carcinoma following radical pelvic surgery. Gynecologic Oncology 10: 84–92

Abitbol M M, Davenport J H 1974a Sexual dysfunction after therapy for cervical carcinoma. American Journal of Obstetrics and Gynecology 119: 181–189

Abitbol M M, Davenport J H 1974b The irradiated vagina. Obstetrics and Gynecology 44: 249–256

Alert J, Jimenez J, Beldarrain L, Montalvo J, Roca C 1980 Complications from irradiation of carcinoma of the uterine cervix. Acta radiologica et oncologica 19: 13–15

Alfert H J, Gillenwater J Y 1972 The consequences of ureteral irradiation with special reference to subsequent ureteral injury. Journal of Urology 107: 369–371

Allen W E Jr, Reddi R P 1980 Simplified irradiation dosimetry in carcinoma of the cervix (external irradiation and one radium insertion). Journal of the National Medical Association 72: 361–370

Andras E J, Fletcher G H, Rutledge F 1973 Radiotherapy of carcinoma of the cervix following simple hysterectomy. American Journal of Obstetrics and Gynecology 115: 647–655

Aron B S, Schlesinger A 1974 Complications of radiation therapy: the genitourinary tract. Seminars in Roentgenology 9: 65–74

Averette H E, Jobson V W 1979 The role of exploratory laparotomy in the staging and treatment of invasive cervical carcinoma. International Journal of Radiation Oncology, Biology and Physics 5: 2137–2138

Ballon S C, Berman M L, Lagasse L D, Petrilli E S, Castaldo T W 1981 Survival after extraperitoneal pelvic and paraaortic lymphadenectomy and radiation therapy in cervical carcinoma. Obstetrics and Gynecology 57: 90–95

Beecham C T, Beiler D D 1976 Treatment of cervical carcinoma. American Journal of Obstetrics and Gynecology 124: 281–284

Beecham J B, Halvorsen T, Kolbenstvedt A 1978 Histologic classification, lymph node metastases and patient survival in stage IB cervical carcinoma. Gynecologic Oncology 6: 95–105

Berman M L, Lagasse L D, Watring W G, Ballon S C, Schlesinger R E, Moore J G et al 1977 The operative evaluation of patients with cervical carcinoma by an extraperitoneal approach. Obstetrics and Gynecology 50: 658–664

Bloomer W D, Hellman S 1975 Normal tissue responses to radiation therapy. New England Journal of Medicine 293: 80–83

Boice J D, Hutchison G B 1980 Leukemia in women following radiotherapy for cervical cancer, ten-year follow-up of an international study. Journal of National Cancer Institute 65: 115–129

Bonanno J P, Boyce J, Fruchter R, Khulpateea N, Macasaet M, Remy J C 1980 Involvement of para-aortic lymph nodes in carcinoma of the cervix. Journal of American Osteopathic Association 79: 567–571

Boronow R C 1971 Management of radiation-induced vaginal fistulas. American Journal of Obstetrics and Gynecology 110: 1–8

Boronow R C, Hickman B T 1977 A comparison of two radiation therapy-treatment plans for carcinoma of the cervix. II. Complications and survival rates. American Journal of Obstetrics and Gynecology 128: 99–105

Boronow R C, Rutledge F 1971 Vesicovaginal fistula, radiation and gynecologic cancer. American Journal of Obstetrics and Gynecology 111: 85–90

Bosch A, Frias Z 1977 Complications after radiation therapy for cervical carcinoma. Acta Radiologica (Ther.) 16: 53–61

Bosch A, Marcial V A 1967 Evaluation of the time interval between external irradiation and intracavitary curietherapy in carcinoma of the uterine cervix: influence on curability. Radiology 88: 563–567

Brady L W 1979 Surgery or radiation therapy for stage I and IIA carcinoma of the cervix. International Journal of Radiation Oncology. Biology and Physics 5: 1877–1879

Bricker E M, Johnston W D 1979 Repair of postirradiation rectovaginal fistula and stricture. Surgery, Gynecology and Obstetrics 148: 499–506

Buchsbaum H J 1979 Extrapelvic lymph node metastases in cervical carcinoma. American Journal of Obstetrics and Gynecology 133: 814–824

Buchsbaum H J, Tewfik A, Lifshitz S, Latourette H B 1981 Radiation therapy of para-aortic lymph nodes in cervical carcinoma. In press

Burns B C, Upton R T 1969 Management of urinary tract complications of treatment for carcinoma of the uterine cervix. In: Cancer of the uterus and ovary. Year Book Medical Publishers, Chicago, p 257–268

Bush R S, Jenkin R P, Allt W E et al 1978 Definitive evidence for hypoxic cells influencing cure in cancer therapy. British Journal of Cancer 37: 302–306

Calame R J 1969 Recurrent carcinoma of the cervix. American Journal of Obstetrics and Gynecology 105: 380–385

Cheung A Y C 1980 Extended field irradiation for invasive carcinoma of the cervix. Gynecologic Oncology 9: 280–291

Chism S E, Park R C, Keys H M 1975 Prospects for para-aortic irradiation in treatment of cancer of the cervix. Cancer 35: 1505–1509

Ciatto S, Pirtoli L, Cionini L 1980 Radiotherapy for postoperative failures of carcinoma of the cervix uteri. Surgery, Gynecology and Obstetrics 151: 621–624

Cochrane J P, Yarnold J R, Slack W W 1981 The surgical treatment of radiation injuries after radiotherapy for uterine carcinoma. British Journal of Surgery 68: 25–28

Cooper G Jr, Williams D H 1962 Epidermoid carcinoma of the cervix: orthovoltage and supervoltage irradiation. American Journal of Roentgenology, Radium Therapy and Nuclear Medicine 88: 971–975

Cooper J S, Barish R J 1981 Individualized radiotherapy for cervical cancer. Contemporary Obstetrics and Gynecology 18: 139–147

Copeland E M 1978 Intravenous hyperalimentation as an adjunct to cancer patient management. CA — A Cancer Journal for Clinicians 28: 322–330

Copeland E M, Daly J M, Dudrick S J 1977 Nutrition as an adjunct to cancer treatment in the adult. Cancer Research 37: 2451–2456

Coutsoftides T, Fazio V W 1979 Small intestine cutaneous fistulas. Surgery, Gynecology and Obstetrics 149: 333–336

Daly J M, Dudrick S J, Copeland E M 1980 Intravenous hyperalimentation: effect on delayed cutaneous hypersensitivity in cancer patients. Annals of Surgery 192: 587–592

Davy M 1974 The prognosis of carcinoma of the cervix with particular reference to infection. Australian and New Zealand Journal of Obstetrics and Gynaecology 14: 1–5

Davy M, Bentzen H, Jahren R 1977 Simple hysterectomy in the presence of invasive cervical cancer. Acta obstetrica et gynecologica scandinavica 56: 105–108

Delgado G 1978 Stage IB squamous cancer of the cervix: the choice of treatment. Obstetrical and Gynecological Survey 33: 174–183

DeWys W D, Kubota T T 1981 Enteral and parenteral nutrition in the care of the cancer patient. Journal of the American Medical Association 246: 1725–1727

Dische S, Saunders M I 1980 Tumour regression and prognosis: a clinical study. British Journal of Cancer 41: 11–13

Dische S, Bennett M H, Saunders M I, Anderson P 1980 Tumour regression as a guide to prognosis: a clinical study. British Journal of Radiology 53: 454–461

Donaldson S S, Wesley M N, DeWys W D et al 1981 A prospective randomized clinical trial of the value of total parenteral nutrition in children with cancer. American Journal of Diseases of Children, in press

Durrance F Y 1969 Treatment for carcinoma of the cervix following inadequate surgical therapy. In: Cancer of the uterus and ovary. Year Book Medical Publishers, Chicago, p 229–240

Durrance F Y, Fletcher G H, Rutledge F 1969 Analysis of central recurrent disease in stages I and II squamous cell carcinomas of the cervix on intact uterus. American Journal of Roentgenology, Radium Therapy and Nuclear Medicine 106: 831–838

Easley J D, Fletcher G H 1971 Analysis of the treatment of stage I and stage II carcinomas of the uterine cervix. American Journal of Roentgenology, Radium Therapy and Nuclear Medicine 111: 243–248

Editorial 1961 Dosage limitation in the combined treatment by irradiation and surgery of carcinoma of the uterine cervix. American Journal of Roentgenology, Radium Therapy and Nucelar Medicine 86: 775–776

Emami B, Watring W G, Won T, Anderson B, Piro A J 1980 Para-aortic lymph node radiation in advanced cervical cancer. International Journal of Radiation Oncology, Biology and Physics 6: 1237–1241

Evans J C, Bergsjo P 1965 The influence of anemia on the results of radiotherapy in carcinoma of the cervix. American Journal of Roentgenology, Radium Therapy and Nuclear Medicine 84: 709–716

Fehr P E, Prem K A 1974 Postirradiation sarcoma of the pelvic girdle following therapy for squamous cell carcinoma of the cervix. American Journal of Obstetrics and Gynecology 116: 192–200

Finck F M, Denk M 1970 Cervical carcinoma: relationship between histology and survival following radiation therapy. Obstetrics and Gynecology 35: 339–343

Fletcher G H 1973 Clinical dose-response curves of human malignant epithelial tumours. British Journal of Radiology 46: 1–12

Fletcher G H 1979 Predominant parameters in the planning of radiation therapy of carcinoma of the cervix. Bulletin of Cancer: 561–572

Fletcher G H 1980 Female pelvis: squamous cell carcinoma of the uterine cervix. In: Textbook of radiotherapy. Lea and Febiger, Philadelphia, p 720–788

Fletcher G H, Rutledge F N 1972 Extended field technique in the management of the cancers of the uterine cervix. American Journal of Roentgenology, Radium Therapy and Nuclear Medicine 114: 116–122

Fuller A F, Elliott N, Kosloff C, Lewis J L Jr 1982 Lymph node metastases from carcinoma of the cervix, stages IB and IIA: implications for prognosis and treatment. Gynecologic Oncology 13: 165–174

Futoran R J, Nolan J F 1976 Stage I carcinoma of the uterine cervix in patients under 40 years of age. American Journal of Obstetrics and Gynecology 125: 790–797

Goellner J R 1976 Carcinoma of the cervix: clinico-pathologic correlation of 196 cases. American Journal of Clinical Pathology 66: 775–785

Goldson A L, Delgado G, Hill L T 1978 Intraoperative radiation of the para-aortic nodes in cancer of the uterine cervix. Obstetrics and Gynecology 52: 713–717

Goodgame J T Jr 1980 A critical assessment of the indications for total parenteral nutrition. Surgery, Gynecology and Obstetrics 151: 433–441

Graham J B, Villalba R J 1963 Damage to the small intestine by radiotherapy. Surgery, Gynecology and Obstetrics 116: 665–668

Gray M J, Kottmeier H L 1957 Rectal and bladder injuries following radium therapy for carcinoma of the cervix at the Radiumhemmet. American Journal of Obstetrics and Gynecology 74: 1294–1303

Green T H, Morse W J 1969 Management of invasive cervical cancer following inadvertent simple hysterectomy. Obstetrics and Gynecology 33: 763–769

Gunn W G 1980 Radiation therapy for the aging patient. CA — A Cancer Journal for Clinicians 30: 337–347

Guthrie R T, Buchsbaum H J, White A J, Latourette H B 1974 Para-aortic lymph node irradiation in carcinoma of the uterine cervix. Cancer 34: 166–168

Guttmann R 1970 Significance of postoperative irradiation in carcinoma of the cervix: a ten-year survey. American Journal of Roentgenology 108: 102–108

Hall E J 1978 Radiobiology for the radiologist. Harper and Row, Hagerstown, Maryland

Halpin T F, Frick H C, Munnell E W 1972 Critical points of failure in the therapy of cancer of the cervix: a reappraisal. American Journal of Obstetrics and Gynecology 114: 755–764

128   CANCER OF THE CERVIX

Hamberger A D 1980 Long term results of radium therapy in cervical cancer. International Journal of Radiation Oncology, Biology and Physics 6: 647–648

Hamberger A D, Fletcher G H, Wharton J T 1978 Results of treatment of early stage I carcinoma of the uterine cervix with intracavitary radium alone. Cancer 41: 980–985

Hancock B W, Bruce L, Heath J, Sugden P, Ward A M 1979 The effects of radiotherapy on immunity in patients with localized carcinoma of the cervix uteri. Cancer 43: 118–123

Harris J R, Hellman S 1981 (authors' reply to G. Kleinfeld) CA — A Cancer Journal for Clinicians 31: 185–187

Heller P B, Lee R B, Leman M H, Park R C 1981 Lymph node positivity in cervical cancer. Gynecologic Oncology 12: 328–335

Hellman S 1982 Principles of radiation therapy. In: DeVita E T (ed) Cancer principles and practice of oncology. J.B. Lippincott Company, Philadelphia, Ch 7, p 104

Hibbitts K R, Raeside D E, Adams G D, Bogardus C R Jr, Darrow B A 1981 Optimal radiotherapy treatment planning for carcinoma of the cervix uteri. Radiology 138: 215–217

Hiilesmaa V K, Vesterinen E, Nieminen U, Grohn P 1981 Carcinoma of the uterine cervix stage III: a report of 311 cases. Gynecologic Oncology 12: 99–106

Hintz B L, Kagan A R, Chan P, Gilbert H A, Nussbaum H, Rao A R et al 1980 Radiation tolerance of the vaginal mucosa. International Journal of Radiation Oncology, Biology and Physics 6: 711–716

Hintz B L, Kagan A R, Gilbert H A, Rao A R, Chan P, Nussbaum H 1981 Systemic absorption of conjugated estrogenic cream by the irradiated vagina. Gynecologic Oncology 12: 75–82

Hreschchyshyn M M, Aron B S, Boronow R C, Franklin E W III, Shingleton H M, Blessing J A 1979 Hydroxyurea or placebo combined with radiation to treat stages IIIB and IV cervical cancer confined to the pelvis. International Journal of Radiation Oncology, Biology and Physics 5: 317–322

Hsu C-T, Cheng Y-S, Su S-C 1972 Prognosis of uterine cervical cancer with extensive lymph node metastases. American Journal of Obstetrics and Gynecology 114: 954–962

Huddleston A L, Taylor P T, Elkon D, Normansell M L, Constable W C 1980 Dose variations in pelvic radiotherapy. British Journal of Radiology 53: 734–735

Hughes R R, Brewington K C, Hanjani P, Photopulos G, Dick D, Votava C et al 1980 Extended field irradiation for cervical cancer based on surgical staging. Gynecologic Oncology 9: 153–161

von Hugo R, Hafter R, Hiller K F, Lochmuller H, Selbmann H K, Graeff H 1981 Prevention of deep-vein thrombosis in patients with gynecological cancer undergoing radiotherapy. A comparison of calcium heparin and a semisynthetic heparin analogue. Geburtshilfe und Frauenheilkunde 41: 179–183

Hutchison G B 1968 Leukemia in patients with cancer of the cervix uteri treated with radiation. A report covering the first 5 years of an international study. Journal of the National Cancer Institute 40: 951–982

Jackson B T 1976 Bowel damage from radiation. Proceedings of the Royal Society of Medicine 69: 683–686

Jampolis S, Andras E J, Fletcher G H 1975 Analysis of sites and causes of failures of irradiation in invasive squamous cell carcinoma of the intact uterine cervix. Radiology 115: 681–685

Janson P O, Jansson I, Skryten A, Damber J E, Lindstedt G 1981 Ovarian endocrine function in young women undergoing radiotherapy for carcinoma of the cervix. Gynecologic Oncology 11: 218–223

Jenkins V K, Dillard E A Jr, Olson M H, Perry R R 1980 Lymphocyte response and radiation therapy for patients with gynecologic cancer. Gynecologic Oncology 9: 209–219

Jiminez J, Alert J, Beldarrain L, Montalvo J, Roca C 1979 Carcinoma of the uterine cervix. Acta radiologica et oncologica 18: 465–469

Jobson V W, Girtanner R E, Averette H E 1980 Therapy and survival of early invasive carcinoma of the cervix uteri with metastases to the pelvic nodes. Surgery, Gynecology and Obstetrics 151: 27–29

Joelsson I, Raf L, Soderberg G 1971 Stenosis of the small bowel as a complication in radiation therapy of carcinoma of the uterine cervix. Acta radiologica 10: 593–604

Johnsson J E 1977 Squamous cell carcinoma of the uterine cervix. Acta radiologica (Ther.) 16: 33–52

Julian C G, Daikoku N H, Gillespie A 1977 Adenoepidermoid and adenosquamous carcinoma of the uterus. American Journal of Obstetrics and Gynecology 128: 106–116

Kagan A R, Nussbaum H, Gilbert H, Chan P Y M, Rao A, Saltz A et al 1979 A new staging system for irradiation injuries following treatment for cancer of the cervix uteri. Gynecologic Oncology 7: 166–175

Kao M-S, Srisuro C, Camel H M 1977 Complications following parametrial radiogold treatment for cervical carcinoma. Obstetrics and Gynecology 50: 665–669

Katz H J, Davies J N P 1980 Death from cervic uteri carcinoma: the changing pattern. Gynecologic Oncology 9: 86–89

Keys H, Park R C 1976 Treatment and survival of patients with cancer of the cervix and nodal metastases. International Journal of Radiation Oncology, Biology and Physics 1: 1091–1097

Kinsella T J, Bloomer W D 1980 Tolerance of the intestine to radiation therapy. Surgery, Gynecology and Obstetrics 151: 273–284

Kinsella T J, Bloomer W D 1981 New therapeutic strategies in radiation therapy. Journal of the American Medical Association 245: 1669–1674

Kiricuta I, Goldstein A M B 1972 The repair of extensive vesicovaginal fistulas with pedicled omentum: a review of 27 cases. Journal of Urology 108: 724–727

Kirkinen P, Kauppila A, Kontturi M 1980 Treatment of ureteral strictures after therapy for carcinoma of the uterus. Obstetrical and Gynecological Survey 151: 487–490

Kjorstad J E 1977 Carcinoma of the cervix in the young patient. Obstetrics and Gynecology 50: 28–30

Kottmeier H L 1964 Complications following radiation therapy in carcinoma of the cervix and their treatment. American Journal of Obstetrics and Gynecology 88: 854–866

Kottmeier H L, Gray M J 1961 Rectal and bladder injuries in relation to radiation dosage in carcinoma of the cervix. American Journal of Obstetrics and Gynecology (July): 74–82

Krebs H B, Helmkamp B F, Sevin B-U, Nadji M, Averette H E 1982 Recurrent cancer of the cervix following radical hysterectomy and pelvic node dissection. Obstetrics and Gynecology 59: 422–427

Kurohara S S, DiSaia P, Kurohara J, Grossman I, George F W III, Morrow C P 1979 Uterine cervical cancer: treatment with megavoltage radiation results and afterloading intracavitary techniques. American Journal of Roentgenology 133: 293–297

Lagasse L D, Creasman W T, Shingleton H M, Ford J H, Blessing J A 1980 Results and complications of operative staging in cervical cancer: experience of the gynecologic oncology group. Gynecologic Oncology 9: 90–98

Lagasse L D, Smith M L, Moore J G, Morton D G, Jacobs M, Johnson G H et al 1974 The effect of radiation therapy on pelvic lymph node involvement in stage I carcinoma of the cervix. American Journal of Obstetrics and Gynecology 119: 328–334

Lang E K, Wood M, Brown R, Pirkle T N, Johnson B, Enright J R et al 1973 Complications in the urinary tract related to treatment of carcinoma of the cervix. Southern Medical Journal 66: 228–236

Lee K R, Mansfield C M, Dwyer S J III, Cox H L, Levine E, Templeton A W 1980 CT for intracavitary radiotherapy planning. American Journal of Roentgenology 135: 809–813

Lee M S, Kim J D, Saxena V S, Kartha P, Zusag T, Hendrickson F R 1980 Late effects of para-aortic irradiation in carcinoma of the uterine cervix and endometrium. Radiology 135: 771–773

Lepanto P, Littman P, Mikuta J, Davis L, Celebre J 1975 Treatment of para-aortic nodes in carcinoma of the cervix. Cancer 35: 1510–1513

Mann J W Jr, Levy D, Hatch K D, Shingleton H M, Soong S-J 1980 Prognostic significance of age in stage I carcinoma of the cervix. Southern Medical Journal 73: 1186–1188

Martimbeau P W, Kjorstad K E, Kolstad P 1978 Stage IB carcinoma of the cervix, the Norwegian Radium Hospital, 1968–1970: results of treatment and major complications. I. Lymphedema. American Journal of Obstetrics and Gynecology 131: 389–394

Martimbeau P W, Kjorstad K E, Iversen T 1982 Stage IB carcinoma of the cervix, The Norwegian Radium Hospital. Results of treatment and major complications. II. Results when pelvic nodes are involved. Obstetrics and Gynecology, in press

Martins A, Sternberg S S, Attiyeh F F 1980 Radiation-induced carcinoma of the rectum. Diseases of the Colon and Rectum 23: 572–575

Maruyama Y, van Nagell J R Jr, Utley J, Vider M L, Parker J C 1974 Radiation and small bowel complications in cervical carcinoma therapy. Radiology 112: 699–703

Meleka F M, Calame R J 1980 Cancer of uterine cervix: parameters related to failure in radiation treatment. New York State Journal of Medicine (April): 734–738

Mercado R, Sala J M 1968 Comparison of conventional and supervoltage radiation in the management of cancer of the cervix. Radiology 90: 967–970

Meyer J E 1981 Radiography of the distal colon and rectum after irradiation of carcinoma of the cervix. American Journal of Roentgenology 136: 691–699

Million R R 1979 Radiotherapeutic approaches. International Journal of Radiation Oncology, Biology and Physics 5: 1027–1028

Million R R, Rutledge F, Fletcher G H 1972 Stage IV carcinoma of the cervix with bladder invasion. American Journal of Obstetrics and Gynecology 113: 239–246

Morley G W, Seski J C 1976 Radical pelvic surgery versus radiation therapy for stage I carcinoma of the cervix (exclusive of microinvasion). American Journal of Obstetrics and Gynecology 126: 785–798

Morrow C P (Moderator, panel report) 1980 Is pelvic radiation beneficial in the postoperative management of stage IB squamous cell carcinoma of the cervix with pelvic node metastasis treated by radical hysterectomy and pelvic lymphadenectomy? Gynecologic Oncology 10: 105–110

Muram D, Curry R H, Drouin P 1982 Cytologic follow-up of patients with invasive cervical carcinoma treated by radiotherapy. American Journal of Obstetrics and Gynecology 142: 350–354

van Nagell J R Jr, Barber H R K (eds) 1982 Modern concepts of gynecologic oncology. John Wright-PSG, Boston

van Nagell J R, Kielar R, Donaldson E S et al 1979 Correlation between retinal and pelvic vascular status: a determinant factor in patients undergoing pelvic irradiation for gynecologic malignancy. American Journal of Obstetrics and Gynecology 134: 551–555

van Nagell J R, Parker J C, Maruyama Y et al 1977 The effect of pelvic inflammatory disease on enteric complications following radiation therapy for cervical cancer. American Journal of Obstetrics and Gynecology 128: 767–771

van Nagell J R Jr, Maruyama Y, Parker J C Jr, Dalton W L 1974 Small bowel injury following radiation therapy for cervical cancer. American Journal of Obstetrics and Gynecology 118: 163–167

van Nagell J R Jr, Parker J C Jr, Maruyama Y, Utley J, Luckett P 1974 Bladder or rectal injury following radiation therapy for cervical cancer. American Journal of Obstetrics and Gynecology 119: 727–732

Nahhas W A, Nisce L Z, D'Angio G J, Lewis J L Jr 1971 Lateral ovarian transposition. Obstetrics and Gynecology 38: 785–788

Nelson J H Jr, Boyce J, Macasaet M, Lu T, Bohorquez J F, Nicastri A D et al 1977 Incidence, significance and follow-up of para-aortic lymph node metastases in late invasive carcinoma of the cervix. American Journal of Obstetrics and Gynecology 128: 336–340

Nieminen U, Pollanen L, Saarikoski S 1970 Radical surgery and radiotherapy in the management of 173 eases of carcinoma of cervix uteri. Acta obstetrica et gynecologica scandinavica 49: 347–349

Nordqvist S R B, Jaramillo B, Sudarsanam A, Charyulu K, Averette H E 1979 Selective therapy for early cancer of the cervix. II. Surgically nonexplored cases. Gynecologic Oncology 7: 257–263

Pagnini C A, Palma P D, DeLaurentiis G 1980 Malignancy grading in squamous carcinoma of uterine cervix treated by surgery. British Journal of Cancer 41: 415–421

Palmer J P, Spratt D W 1956 Pelvic carcinoma following irradiation for benign gynecological diseases. American Journal of Obstetrics and Gynecology 72: 497–505

Parsons J T, Thar T L, Bova F J, Million R R 1980 An evaluation of split-course irradiation for pelvic malignancies. International Journal of Radiation Oncology, Biology and Physics 6: 175–181

Paunier J-P, Delclos L, Fletcher G H 1967 Causes, time of death and sites of failure in squamous-cell carcinoma of the uterine cervix on intact uterus. Radiology 88: 555–562

Peckham B M, Kline J C, Schultz A E, Cameron J R, Vermund H 1969 Radiation dosage and complications in cervical cancer therapy. American Journal of Obstetrics and Gynecology 104: 485–494

Perez C A, Breaux S, Madoc-Jones H, Camel H M, Purdy J, Sharma S et al 1979 Correlation between radiation dose and tumor recurrence and complications in carcinoma of the uterine cervix: stages I and IIA. International Journal of Radiation Oncology, Biology and Physics 5: 373–382

Pilleron J P, Durand J C, Hamelin J P 1974 Prognostic value of node metastasis in cancer of the uterine cervix. American Journal of Obstetrics and Gynecology 119: 458–462

Pitkin R M, Van Voorhis L W 1971 Postirradiation vaginitis: an evaluation of prophylaxis with topical estrogen. Radiology 99: 417–421

Piver M S, Chung W S 1975 Prognostic significance of cervical lesion size and pelvic node metastases in cervical carcinoma. Obstetrics and Gynecology 46: 507–510

Piver M S, Lele S 1976 Enterovaginal and enterocutaneous fistulae in women with gynecologic malignancies. Obstetrics and Gynecology 48: 560–563

Piver M S, Barlow J J, Krishnamsetty R 1981 Five-year survival (with no evidence of disease) in patients with biopsy-confirmed aortic node metastasis from cervical carcinoma. American Journal of Obstetrics and Gynecology 139: 575–578

Piver M S, Barlow J J, Vongtama V, Blumenson L 1977 Hydroxyurea as a radiation sensitizer in women with carcinoma of the uterine cervix. American Journal of Obstetrics and Gynecology 129: 379–383

Piver M S, Barlow J J, Vongtama V, Webster J 1974 Hydroxyurea and radiation therapy in advanced cervical cancer. American Journal of Obstetrics and Gynecology 120: 969–972

Polish R A 1980 Prediction of radiation-related small-bowel damage. Radiology 135: 219–221

Prempree T, Patanaphan V, Sewchand W, Scott R M 1980 Parametrial implants in the treatment of stage IIIB carcinoma of the cervix. II. Analysis of success and failure. Cancer 46: 1485–1491

Punnonen R, Gronroos M, Rauramo L, Voutilainen A, Aho A J, Hartikainen P 1976 Complications following radiotherapy in gynaecological carcinoma: comparison between X-ray and megavoltage therapy. Annales chirurgiae et gynaecologiae 65: 62–67

Rafla S 1971 Major surgery after radical radiotherapy. Cancer 27: 314–322

Rampone J F, Klem V, Kolstad P 1973 Combined treatment of stage IB carcinoma of the cervix. Obstetrics and Gynecology 41: 163–167

Reber H A, Roberts C, Way L W, Dunphy J E 1978 Management of external gastrointestinal fistulas. Annals of Surgery 188: 460–467

Rogers C C, Levitt S Y, Crosby W C, Brandt E N Jr 1967 Effect of hypertension and arteriosclerosis on response to radiation therapy of carcinoma of the cervix: a retrospective clinical study. Radiology 89: 733–736

Roswit B, Malsky S T, Reid C B 1972 Severe radiation injuries of the stomach, small intestine, colon and rectum. American Journal of Roentgenology 114: 460–475

Rotman M, John M 1979 Para-aortic irradiation in cervical carcinoma. International Journal of Radiation Oncology, Biology and Physics 5: 2139–2141

Rotman M, Rogow L, DeLeon G, Heskel N 1977 Supportive therapy in radiation oncology. Cancer 39: 744–750

Rousseau J, Fenton J, Debertrand P, Mathieu G 1972 Carcinoma of the cervix. Radiology 103: 413–418

Rousseau J, Fenton J, Mathieu G, Dulac G, Picco C 1976 Late sequelae and complications in exclusive high voltage radiotherapy for carcinoma of the cervix uteri. J Radiol Electrol 57: 409–419

Rubin P 1979 Current concepts in cancer — updated cervix cancer — introduction. International Journal of Radiation Oncology, Biology and Physics 5: 1009–1011

Rubin P, Casarett G W 1968 Clinical radiation pathology. W. B. Saunders, Philadelphia, vol II, p 919–933

Rubin P, Prabhasawat D 1961 Characteristic bone lesions in post-irradiated carcinoma of the cervix: metastases versus osteonecrosis. Radiology 76: 703–717

Rutledge F N, Galakatos A E, Wharton J T, Smith J P 1975 Adenocarcinoma of the uterine cervix. American Journal of Obstetrics and Gynecology 122: 236–245

Sala J M, deLeon A D 1963 Treatment of carcinoma of the cervical stump. Radiology 81: 300–306

Schellhas H F 1975 Extraperitoneal para-aortic node dissection through an upper abdominal incision. Obstetrics and Gynecology 46: 444–447

Schmitt E H III, Symmonds R E 1981 Surgical treatment of radiation induced injuries of the intestine. Surgery, Gynecology and Obstetrics 153: 896–900

Scott R M, Brizel H E, Wetzelberger C 1966 The etiology of treatment failures in early stage carcinoma of the cervix. American Journal of Roentgenology 96: 565–568

Seydel H G 1975 The risk of tumor induction in man following medical irradiation for malignant neoplasm. Cancer 35: 1641–1645

Shierholz J D, Buchsbaum H J, Lifshitz S, Latourette H B 1977 Pyometra complicating radiation therapy of uterine malignancy. Journal of Reproductive Medicine 19: 100–102

Shingleton H M, Gore H, Bradley D H, Soong S-J 1981 Adenocarcinoma of the cervix. I. Clinical evaluation and pathologic features. American Journal of Obstetrics and Gynecology 139: 799–814

Slater J M, Fletcher G H 1971 Ureteral strictures after radiation therapy for carcinoma of the uterine cervix. American Journal of Roentgenology 111: 269–272

Smith J P, Golden P E, Rutledge F 1966 Surgical management of intestinal injuries following irradiation for carcinoma of the cervix. In: Cancer of the uterus and ovary. Year Book Medical Publishers, Chicago, p 241–256

Smith P G 1977 Leukemia and other cancers following radiation treatment of pelvic disease. Cancer 39: 1901–1905

Soeters P B, Ebeid A M, Fischer J E 1979 Review of 404 patients with gastrointestinal fistulas; impact of parenteral nutrition. Annals of Surgery 190: 189–202

Stanhope C R, Smith J P, Wharton J T, Rutledge F N, Fletcher G H, Gallager H S 1980 Carcinoma of the cervix: the effect of age on survival. Gynecologic Oncology 10: 188–193

Strockbine M F, Hancock J E, Fletcher G H 1970 Complications in 831 patients with squamous cell carcinoma of the intact uterine cervix treated with 3000 rad or more whole pelvis irradiation. American Journal of Roentgenology 108: 293–304

Sudarsanam A, Charyulu K, Belinson J, Averette H, Goldberg M, Hintz B et al 1978 Influence of exploratory celiotomy on the management of carcinoma of the cervix. Cancer 41: 1049–1053

Swan D S, Roddick J W 1973 A clinical-pathological correlation of cell type classification for cervical cancer. American Journal of Obstetrics and Gynecology 116: 666–670

Swan R W 1974 Stagnant loop syndrome resulting from small-bowel irradiation injury and intestinal by-pass. Gynecologic Oncology 2: 441–445

Swan R W, Fowler W C Jr, Boronow R C 1976 Surgical management of radiation injury to the small intestine. Surgery, Gynecology and Obstetrics 142: 325–327

Tak W K, Munzenrider J E, Mitchell G W Jr 1979 External irradiation and one radium application for carcinoma of the cervix. International Journal of Radiation Oncology, Biology and Physics 5: 29–36

Taylor P T, Andersen W A 1981 Untreated cervical cancer complicated by obstructive uropathy and oliguric renal failure. Gynecologic Oncology 11: 162–174

Tepmongkol P, Skulchan V 1980 Complications after radiation for carcinoma of cervix. Journal of the Medical Association of Thailand 63: 238–244

Tewfik H, Buchsbaum H J, Lifshitz S, Latourette H B 1982 Para-aortic lymph node irradiation in carcinoma of the cervix after exploratory laparotomy and biopsy-proven positive aortic nodes. International Journal of Radiation Oncology, Biology and Physics 8: 13–18

Thomas W O Jr, Harris H H, Enden J A 1969 Postirradiation malignant neoplasms of the uterine fundus. American Journal of Obstetrics and Gynecology 104: 209–219

Underwood P B Jr, Lutz M H, Smoak D L 1977 Ureteral injury following irradiation therapy for carcinoma of the cervix. Obstetrics and Gynecology 49: 663–669

Valerio D, Overett L, Malcolm A et al 1978 Nutritional support for cancer patients receiving abdominal and pelvic radiotherapy: a randomized preoperative clinical experiment of intravenous versus oral feeding. Surgery Forum 29: 145–147

Van Herik M 1965 Fever as a complication of radiation therapy for carcinoma of the cervix. American Journal of Roentgenology 93: 104–109

Villasanta U 1972 Complications of radiotherapy for carcinoma of the uterine cervix. American Journal of Obstetrics and Gynecology 114: 717–726

Volterrani F, Prosperini G, Sigurta D, Vona S, Musumeci R, Milani A et al 1979 Present status of treatment for invasive cervical carcinoma. Tumori 65: 611–624

Watson E R, Halnow K E, Kische S et al 1978 Hyperbaric oxygen and radiotherapy: a medical research council trial in carcimoma of the cervix. British Journal of Radiology 51: 879–887

Weed J C, Holland J B 1977 Combined irradiation and extensive operations in the treatment of stages I and II carcinoma of the cervix uteri. Surgery, Gynecology and Obstetrics 144: 869–872

Welander C E, Pierce V K, Nori D, Hilaris B S, Kosloff C, Clark D G C et al 1981 Pretreatment laparotomy in carcinoma of the cervix. Gynecologic Oncology 12: 336–347

Wentz W B, Reagen J W 1959 Survival in cervical cancer with respect to cell type. Cancer 12: 384–388

Wentz W B, Reagen J W 1970 Clinical significance of postirradiation dysplasia of the uterine cervix. American Journal of Obstetrics and Gynecology 106: 812–817

Wharton J T, Jones H W III, Day T G Jr, Rutledge F N, Fletcher G H 1977 Preirradiation celiotomy and extended field irradiation for invasive carcinoma of the cervix. Obstetrics and Gynecology 49: 333–338

Wheeless C R Jr 1973 Small bowel bypass for complications related to pelvic malignancy. Obstetrics and Gynecology 42: 661–666

Wheeless C R Jr, Graham R, Graham J B 1970 Prognosis and treatment of adenoepidermoid carcinoma of the cervix. Obstetrics and Gynecology 35: 928–932

Whitmore G F 1969 Summary of conference in time and dose relationships in radiation biology as applied to radiotherapy. BLN Report 50203 (C–57): 353–358

Widholm O, Mattsson T 1972 Urinary tract infections in association with radium therapy for gynecological cancer. Acta obstetrica et gynecologica scandinavica 51: 247–250

Xynos F P, Benjamin I, Sapiente R, Waheed R, Nalesnik W J 1980 Adriamycin and hydroxyurea as radiopotentiators in the treatment of squamous cell carcinoma of the cervix implanted in nude mice: a preliminary report. Gynecologic Oncology 9: 170–176

Yamagata S, Green G H 1976 Radiation-induced immune changes in patients with cancer of the cervix. British Journal of Obstetrics and Gynaecology 83: 400–408

Zander J, Baltzer J, Lohe K J, Ober K G, Kaufmann C 1981 Carcinoma of the cervix: an attempt to individualize treatment; results of a 20-year cooperative study. American Journal of Obstetrics and Gynecology 139: 752–759

6

Post-treatment surveillance

Post-treatment surveillance is designed to detect recurrent or persistent disease. Although carried out universally, the timing of visits and duration of follow-up is based on tradition rather than fact. Although it is arguable that surveillance has little value, as most patients with recurrence will not survive, close surveillance may be beneficial in other ways (Table 6.1). Clinical examination and careful questioning may allow early detection of therapy complications, other medical problems or other primary malignancies. Intermittent reassurance by the physician allows the patient to live a more normal life if the visits reduce her anxiety concerning possible recurrence.

Table 6.1 Justifications for post-treatment surveillance

1. To detect recurrence
2. To detect and manage complications of therapy
3. To detect other medical problems
4. To detect other primary cancers
5. To reassure the patient

FREQUENCY OF VISITS

The majority of recurrences are apparent soon after treatment. Munnell (1960) reported that 82% of cervical cancer recurrences were evident within 2 years of therapy. Halpin (1972) reported that 60% recurred within 2 years and 82% recurred within 4 years. Kurohara (1971) stated that more than 70% of patients have recurrence within 2 years and 85% of recurrences were discovered prior to 5 years. Van Nagell (1979) indicated that 76% of post-therapy recurrences were detected within 2 years. Muram (1982) detected 51% of recurrences in the first year and 78% of recurrences within 2 years. Krebs (1982) reported that 83% of recurrences following radical hysterectomy were detected within 2 years. Our information confirms these findings and indicates that the time elapsing before recurrence relates to the size of the original lesion, i.e. large tumours tend to recur earlier than small tumours. Tumours 2 cm or less in size recurred at a median time of 1.6 years. Three-centimetre tumours recurred at a median time of 1 year; tumours larger than 3 cm recurred at a median time of 0.4 years. The median time to recurrence for surgical patients was 1 year; for radiation patients, it was 1.3 years. The latter comparison, however, is not corrected for size of lesion and the patients treated by radiation probably had larger tumours.

Examinations within the first 6 months following radiation therapy are important not only to detect recurrence but also for prognosis. Hardt (1982) reported a 5% recurrence rate in patients whose tumour had completely regressed within 1 month of therapy. Those with an intermediate response had a recurrence/persistence rate of 27% while those with an incomplete response had an 85% recurrence/persistence rate. Seventy-five per cent of the incomplete responders had central pelvic recurrence. Dische (1980) indicated that the degree of tumour regression in patients examined at the end of radiotherapy correlated with survival. Those patients with a 75–100% regression had a median survival of 77 months while those with less than a 25% regression had a median survival of 17 months. Marcial (1970) indicated excellent survival in patients who had complete tumour regression within 3 months following therapy.

We currently advocate an examination at the completion of therapy and at least every 3 months during the first 2 years following treatment. We urge patients to return for examination at least every 6 months during the next 3 years and yearly thereafter. Patients with unusual symptoms or signs are advised to attend sooner and not wait for their next appointment.

At each visit the physician should ask appropriate questions and examine the patient (Table 6.2). Although 10% to 40% of patients with recurrent cervical cancer are asymptomatic, recurrence is preceded by vaginal bleeding in 6–15% of patients, by pain (back, sciatic, pelvic) in 20–50% of patients, by weight loss, anorexia or malaise in 1–25% of

Table 6.2 Recommended surveillance after treatment

Question patient related to symptoms:
Vaginal bleeding or discharge
Back, sciatic or pelvic pain
Weight loss, anorexia
Cough, dyspnoea, haemoptysis
Lower extremity swelling

Examination:
Nodal (supraclavicular and inguinal) palpation
Abdominal palpation
Vaginal speculum examination
Cervicovaginal cytology
Bimanual rectovaginal examination

patients, by leg oedema in 5–12% of patients and by cough, dyspnoea or haemoptysis in 1–5% of patients.

Physical examination should include supraclavicular and inguinal node palpation as this may be the initial abnormal finding in 1–4% of patients with recurrence. Abdominal palpation may detect masses or hepatic enlargement. An abnormal bimanual examination is the initial evidence of recurrence in 20–25% of patients. Any visible vaginal lesion should be biopsied. However, the physician must be careful if vaginal vault necrosis is present; Burns (1966) indicated that necrosis may precede a vesicovaginal fistula in over 79% of patients developing this urinary complication and careless random biopsies may further predispose to this problem. If an abnormal bimanual examination is present without a mucosal lesion, fine-needle aspiration or transvaginal biopsies are indicated. Fine-needle aspiration can be performed on an outpatient basis. Shepherd (1981) used this technique in 50 patients with cervical cancer. The aspirate indicated the presence of tumour in 96% of patients and was more accurate than cervical cytology or punch biopsy. The procedure can be performed with little risk in patients with central or parametrial lesions; however, due to the proximity to major blood vessels, pelvic sidewall lesions should be sampled with caution. Proper interpretation of the aspirate requires an experienced cytopathologist (see Table 3.5, Ch. 3.)

CYTOLOGY

Abnormal cervical smears as a predictor of recurrence are assigned varying degrees of importance by different investigators. For instance, positive smears are said to be the first sign of recurrence in 3% to 50% of patients and may precede clinical evidence of recurrence by 3 to 24 months. Their value in the early detection is in patients with central pelvic recurrence, which may be present in 13% to 28% of those patients having recurrence after radical hysterectomy (Table 6.3).

Table 6.3 Stage IB, IIA site of recurrence in patients treated by radical hysterectomy

Author	Year	No. of pts	No. of rec.	% rec.	Site of recurrence C.P. %	L.P. %	E.P. %
Webb	1980	564	68	18.4	13.2	42.6	44.1
Krebs	1982	312	40	12.8	27.5	37.5	35.0
Authors	1982	200	30	15.0	20.0	23.3	56.7
Totals		1076	138	12.8	18.8	37.0	44.2

C.P. = Central pelvic, L.P. = Lateral pelvic, E.P. = Extrapelvic

However, Jampolis (1975) reported that the incidence of central pelvic recurrence following radiation varies according to initial stage (Table 6.4). The failure rate in the central pelvis varies between 3% and 8% in his series, although the recurrence rates are higher when the patient has received radiation in suboptimal dosages due to poor dosimetry or obsolete equipment. Because these patients are potentially curable with additional therapy, we feel that such a simple. inexpensive diagnostic test as cervical cytology should be used routinely to increase the opportunity for early detection of recurrence.

Table 6.4 Site of recurrence in patients treated by radiation (modified from Jamopolis 1975)

Stage	No. of pts	No. of rec.	% rec.	C.P. %	C.P. +R %	R%	R + D %	D%
IB	316	31	10	0	23	0	29	48
IIA	178	34	19	3	9	6	15	66
IIB	204	69	34	0	14	6	19	61
IIIA	160	63	39	8	22	11	11	48
IIIB	58	24	41	0	50	8	4	38
Totals	916	221	24	2.7	20.8	6.8	15.8	53.9

C.P. = Central pelvic, C.P. + R = Central + regional, R = Regional, R + D = Regional + distal, D = Distal

The differentiation between dysplastic cells, invasive cancer and repair cells is extremely difficult in the vaginal cytological preparation taken after radiotherapy. However, the finding of dysplastic cells in the smear of a previously irradiated patient should alert the physician to the possibility of recurrence. Wentz (1970) reported a 56% chance of recurrence in patients who had such atypical cytology; if the dysplastic cells were formed within 3 years of treatment, 71% developed recurrence. McLennan (1975) noted radiation dysplasia in 21% of his patients and reported that its incidence was higher in patients with persistent or recurrent disease, i.e. it often coexisted with invasive cancer. Colposcopy may be of limited use following radiation, and if non-diagnostic, examination under anaesthesia with Lugol's staining and multiple biopsies of non-staining or palpably abnormal areas is required to determine if the invasive cancer persists or has recurred. The excision of the involved mucosa may be all the treatment required if the final diagnosis is radiation dysplasia.

Although these examinations are primarily intended to detect recurrent or persistent cervical cancer, it should be remembered that these patients may develop a second primary cancer. In fact, 1% to 8% of cervical cancer patients later succumb as a result of another tumour. The possible increased risk of leukaemia enhanced by radiation or chemotherapy, as well as the usual ongoing risk of breast and gastro-intestinal cancer, should prompt examination of the breast, instructions to the patient in breast self-examination, appropriate haematological studies and a stool specimen for occult blood at yearly intervals. Although rectal bleeding is most commonly due to radiation proctitis, it should nevertheless be investigated by proctosigmoidoscopy and barium enema studies.

DIAGNOSTIC TESTS

Little information exists concerning the benefits to the patient of radiological and other detection procedures in the post-treatment surveillance period. Photopulos (1977) evaluated 73 treated patients with a group of diagnostic tests consisting of intravenous pyelography (IVP), chest X-rays, barium enema, cystoscopy, proctoscopy and bone scan. Nine patients (12%) had abnormal surveys and eight of these women died of recurrent cancer. The survey was abnormal in three of 63 patients not suspected of having recurrence and in six patients of 10 with suspected recurrence. While the false-negative rate was only 7%, he concluded that with the exception of the IVP and chest X-rays, the tests should not be routinely used in patients without clinical evidence of recurrence, since most recurrences were diagnosed by physical examination.

Although others have advocated yearly chest X-rays as part of routine surveillance of treated cervical cancer patients, we have not obtained them regularly, and reserve their use for patients with pulmonary symptoms or signs of pelvic recurrence. This is based on the fact that an isolated chest recurrence is unusual in cancer of the cervix. Very rarely, one may encounter an isolated solitary chest lesion (Fig. 6.1) which can be excised with control of the disease; however, chest metastases usually portend a poor prognosis.

Unilateral obstruction on IVP may be indicative of a pelvic sidewall recurrence following radical hysterectomy, but in our experience is rarely encountered in patients with a normal bimanual pelvic examination. Ureteral obstruction following radiation therapy is associated with recurrence in over 90% of cases. While recommendations vary, some have suggested obtaining routine follow-up IVPs as frequently as every 6 months. Because central or lateral pelvic recurrence following primary surgical treatment may be cured with radiation, we are inclined to recommend an IVP at 6 months and at 1 year in those patients considered to be at high risk for failure. However, following radiation therapy, we would not recommend any routine schedule for IVPs but obtain them if there are symptoms

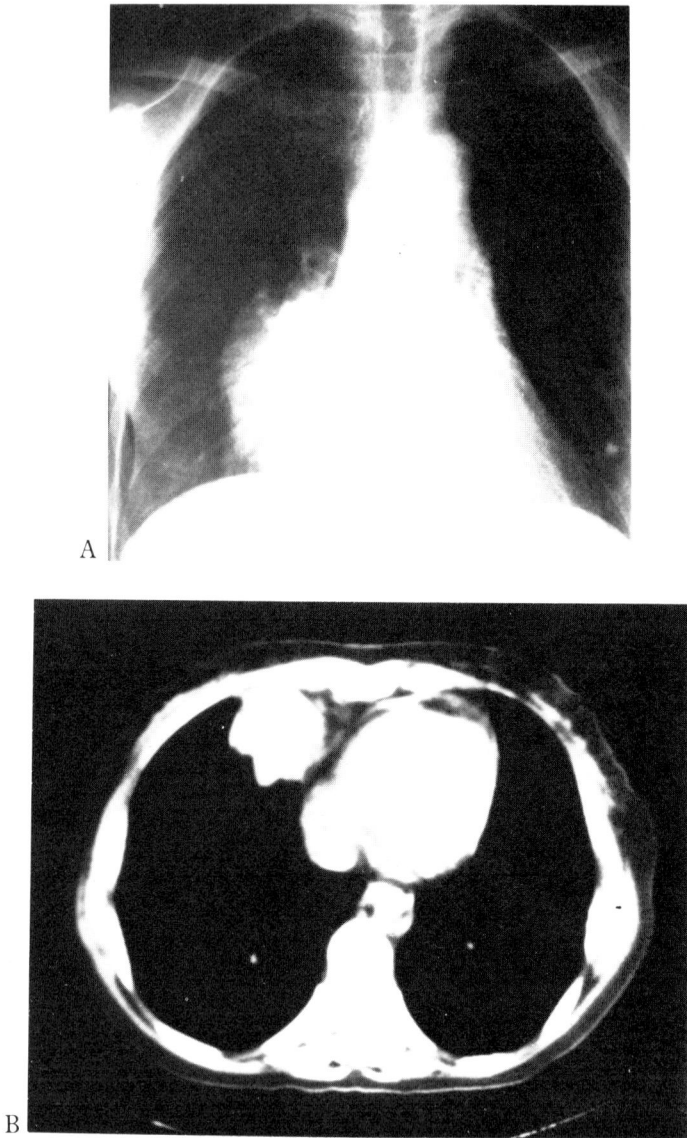

Fig. 6.1 Recurrent carcinoma in the thorax of a 55-year-old woman with cervical squamous carcinoma
A. A large mass is present at the right cardiophrenic angle
B. A computerised axial tomogram reveals the mass to be in the anterior portion of the right lobe, away from the pericardium and mediastinum

suggesting ureteral obstruction or pelvic findings suggesting recurrence. Since some patients have radiation-induced ureteral strictures in the absence of recurrent cancer, one should always confirm the nature of the obstruction by fine-needle aspiration or, if necessary, by laparotomy, as intervention may preserve existing renal function.

While Walsh (1981) reported computed tomography to be a sensitive test to aid in the diagnosis of recurrence, further prospective evaluation is necessary before its use can be advocated on a routine basis, if for no other reason than because of its expense. Lacking a curative chemotherapeutic agent for cervical cancer, it benefits the patient little to detect retroperitoneal tumour or liver metastases. If effective agents are identified in the future, one should also be more aggressive in preventing death from renal obstruction, in order to allow administration of drug therapy.

Other diagnostic studies such as cystocopy, proctoscopy, barium enema and lymphangiography should only be utilised in symptomatic patients, as part of the evaluation for suspected recurrence.

BIBLIOGRAPHY

Adcock L L 1979 Radical hysterectomy preceded by pelvic irradiation. Gynecologic Oncology 8: 152–163
Badib A O, Kurohara S S, Webster J H, Pickren J W 1968 Metastasis to organs in carcinoma of the uterine cervix. Cancer 21: 434–439
Bramm H G, Griffith R P, Griffith T H, Shasteen W J 1979 Retroperitoneal fibrosis simulating carcinoma of the cervix. Obstetrics and Gynecology 53: 77S-78S
Burns B C, Upton R T 1969 Management of urinary tract complications of treatment for carcinoma of the uterine cervix. In: Cancer of the uterus and ovary. Year Book Medical Publishers, Chicago, p 257–268
Calame R J 1969 Recurrent carcinoma of the cervix. American Journal of Obstetrics and Gynecology 105: 380–385
Campos J 1970 Persistent tumor cells in the vaginal smears and prognosis of cancer of the radiated cervix. Acta cytologica 14: 519–522
Dische S, Bennett M H, Saunders M I, Anderson P 1980 Tumour regression as a guide to prognosis: a clinical study. British Journal of Radiology 53: 454–461
Durrance F Y, Fletcher G H, Rutledge F N 1969 Analysis of central recurrent disease in stages I and II squamous cell carcinomas of the cervix on intact uterus. American Journal of Roentgenology 106: 831–838
Fehr P E, Prem K A 1974 Malignancy of the uterine corpus following irradiation therapy for squamous cell carcinoma of the cervix. American Journal of Obstetrics and Gynecology 119: 685–692
Freiman D B, Ring E J, Oleaga J A, Carpiniello V C, Wein A J 1978 Thin needle biopsy in the diagnosis of ureteral obstruction with malignancy. Cancer 42: 714–716
Futoran R J, Nolan J F 1976 Stage I carcinoma of the uterine cervix in patients under 40 years of age. American Journal of Obstetrics and Gynecology 125: 790–797
Gary R K, Sala J M, Spratt J S Jr 1964 The detection and treatment of postirradiationally recidivated cancers of the cervix uteri. Radiology 83: 208–218
Ginaldi S, Wallace S, Jing B-S, Bernardino M E 1981 Carcinoma of the cervix: lymphangiography and computed tomography. American Journal of Roentgenology 136: 1087–1091

Greenwald E F, Breen J L, Gregori C A 1980 Cardiac metastases associated with gynecologic malignancies. Gynecologic Oncology 10: 75–83

Grumbine F C, Rosenshein N B, Zerhouni E A, Siegelman S S 1981 Abdominopelvic computed tomography in the preoperative evaluation of early cervical cancer. Gynecologic Oncology 12: 286–290

Halpin T F, Frick H C, Munnell E W 1972 Critical points of failure in the therapy of cancer of the cervix: a reappraisal. American Journal of Obstetrics and Gynecology 114: 755–764

Hardt N, van Nagell J R, Hanson M, Donaldson E, Yoneda J, Maruyama Y 1982 Radiation-induced tumor regression as a prognostic factor in patients with invasive cervical cancer. Cancer 49: 35–39

Holm H H, Pedersen J F, Kristensen J K, Rasmussen S N, Hancke S, Jensen F 1975 Ultrasonically guided percutaneous puncture. Radiologic Clinics of North America 13: 493–503

Jampolis S, Andras E J, Fletcher G H 1975 Analysis of sites and causes of failures of irradiation in invasive squamous cell carcinoma of the intact uterine cervix. Radiology 115: 681–685

Katz H J, Davies J N P 1980 Death from cervic uteri carcinoma: the changing pattern. Gynecologic Oncology 9: 86–89

Kraus H, Schumann R 1979 Cytologic presentation of recurrent carcinoma of the uterine cervix and corpus after radiotherapy. Acta cytologica 23: 114–118

Krebs H B, Helmkamp B F, Sevin B–U, Nadji M, Averette H E 1982 Recurrent cancer of the cervix following radical hysterectomy and pelvic node dissection. Obstetrics and Gynecology 59: 422–427

Kurohara S S, Vongtama V Y, Webster J H, George F W 1971 Post-irradiational recurrent epidermoid carcinoma of the uterine cervix. American Journal of Roentgenology 111: 249–259

Kwon T H, Prempree T, Tang C–K, Villasanta U, Scott R M 1981 Adenocarcinoma of the uterine corpus following irradiation for cervical cancer. Gynecologic Oncology 11: 102–113

Lojeck M A, Fer M F, Kasselberg A G, Glick A D, Burnett L S, Julian C G et al 1980 Cushing's syndrome with small cell carcinoma of the uterine cervix. American Journal of Medicine 69: 140–144

Marcial V A, Bosch A 1970 Radiation-induced tumor regression in carcinoma of the uterine cervix: prognostic significance. American Journal of Roentgenology 108: 113–123

McIlhaney J S Jr, Kaplan A L 1969 Recurrences of carcinoma of the cervix after ten years. Southern Medical Journal (September): 1119–1122

McLennan M T, McLennan C E 1975 Significance of cervicovaginal cytology after radiation therapy for cervical carcinoma. American Journal of Obstetrics and Gynecology 121: 96–100

Martins A, Sternberg S S, Attiyeh F F 1980 Radiation-induced carcinoma of the rectum. Diseases of the Colon and Rectum 23: 572–575

Meyer J E 1981 Radiography of the distal colon and rectum after irradiation of carcinoma of the cervix. American Journal of Roentgenology 136: 691–699

Montanari G D, Marconato A, Montanari G R, Grismondi G L 1968 Granulation tissue on the vault of the vagina after hysterectomy for cancer: diagnostic problems. Acta cytologica 12: 25–29

Munnell E W, Bonney W A Jr 1960 Critical points of failure in the therapy of cancer of the cervix. American Journal of Obstetrics and Gynecology 81: 521–534

Muram D, Curry R H, Drouin P 1982 Cytologic follow-up of patients with invasive cervical carcinoma treated by radiotherapy. American Journal of Obstetrics and Gynecology 142: 350–354

Muram D, Oxorn H, Curry D H, Drouin P, Walters J H 1981 Postradiation ureteral obstruction: a reappraisal. American Journal of Obstetrics and Gynecology 139: 289–293 van Nagell J R Jr, Rayburn W, Donaldson E S, Hanson M, Gay E C, Yoneda J et al 1979 Therapeutic implications of patterns of recurrence in cancer of the uterine cervix. Cancer 44: 2354–2361

Nordqvist S R B, Sevin B–U, Nadji M, Greening S E, Ng A B P 1979 Fine-needle aspiration cytology in gynecologic oncology. I. Diagnostic accuracy. Obstetrics and Gynecology 54: 719–724

Palmer J P, Spratt D W 1956 Pelvic carcinoma following irradiation for benign gynecological diseases. American Journal of Obstetrics and Gynecology 72: 497–505

Photopulos G J, Shirley R E L Jr, Ansbacher R 1977 Evaluation of conventional diagnostic tests for detection of recurrent carcinoma of the cervix. American Journal of Obstetrics and Gynecology 129: 533–535

Photopulos G J, McCartney W H, Walton L A, Staab E V 1979 Computerized tomography applied to gynecologic oncology. American Journal of Obstetrics and Gynecology 135: 381–383

Rampone J F, Klem V, Kolstad P 1973 Combined treatment of stage IB carcinoma of the cervix. Obstetrics and Gynecology 41: 163–167

Rayburn W F, van Nagell J R Jr 1980 Cervicovaginal cytology in the diagnosis of recurrent carcinoma of the cervix uteri. Surgery, Gynecology and Obstetrics 151: 15–16

Rhamy R K, Stander R W 1962 Pyelographic analysis of radiation therapy in carcinoma of the cervix. American Journal of Roentgenology 87: 41–43

Rubin P, Prabhasawat D 1961 Characteristic bone lesions in postirradiated carcinoma of the cervix: metastases versus osteonecrosis. Radiology 76: 703–717

Ruponen S, Gronroos M, Makinen E, Rauramo L 1974 Prognostic value of urography in irradiated cervical carcinoma. Annales chirurgiae et gynaecologiae fenniae 63: 127–129

Sheldon R S, Decker D G, Lee R A 1971 Recurrence of carcinoma of the cervix 25 years after primary surgical treatment: report of a case. American Journal of Obstetrics and Gynecology 110: 1140–1141

Shepherd J H, Cavanagh D, Ruffolo E, Praphat H 1981 The value of needle biopsy in the diagnosis of gynecologic cancer. Gynecologic Oncology 11: 309–320

Shingleton H M, Fowler W C Jr, Pepper F D Jr, Palumbo L 1969 Ureteral strictures following therapy for carcinoma of the cervix. Cancer 24: 77–83

Slater J M, Fletcher G H 1971 Ureteral strictures after radiation therapy for carcinoma of the uterine cervix. American Journal of Roentgenology 111: 269–272

Suit H D, Gallager H S 1964 Intact tumor cells in irradiated tissue. Archives of Pathology 78: 648–651

Tao L C, Pearson F G, Delarue N C, Langer B, Sanders D E 1980 Percutaneous fine-needle aspiration biopsy. I. Its value to clinical practice. Cancer 45: 1480–1485

Thomas W O Jr, Harris H H, Enden J A 1969 Postirradiation malignant neoplasms of the uterine fundus. American Journal of Obstetrics and Gynecology 104: 209–219

Ulmsten U 1975 Obstruction of the upper urinary tract after treatment of carcinoma of the uterine cervix. Acta obstetrica et gynecologica scandinavica 54: 297–301

Underwood P B Jr, Lutz M H, Smoak D L 1977 Ureteral injury following irradiation therapy for carcinoma of the cervix. Obstetrics and Gynecology 49: 663–669

Van Voorhis L W 1970 Carcinoma of the cervix. II. A critical evaluation of patient follow-up. American Journal of Obstetrics and Gynecology 108: 115–121

Wahlstrom T, Lindgren J, Korhonen M, Seppala M 1979 Distinction between endocervical and endometrial adenocarcinoma with immunoperoxidase staining of carcinoembryonic antigen in routine histological tissue specimens. Lancet 2: 1159–1160

Walsh J W, Amendola M A, Hall D J, Tisnado J, Goplerud D R 1981 Recurrent carcinoma of the cervix: CT diagnosis. American Journal of Roentgenology 136: 117–122

Webb M J, Symmonds R E 1980 Site of recurrence of cervical cancer after radical hysterectomy. American Journal of Obstetrics and Gynecology 138: 813–817
Wentz W B, Reagan J W 1970 Clinical significance of postirradiation dysplasia of the uterine cervix. American Journal of Obstetrics and Gynecology 106: 812–817
Zornoza J, Lukeman J M, Jing B S, Wharton J T, Wallace S 1977 Percutaneous retroperitoneal lymph node biopsy in carcinoma of the cervix. Gynecologic Oncology 5: 43–51

7

Recurrent cervical cancer

Earlier detection of cervical cancer by routine cytological screening, improved equipment and technique for radiation therapy and better selection of candidates for primary surgical treatment have resulted in a higher cure rate of patients with cervical cancer. Although this success is gratifying, the physician who treats these patients will be faced with persistence or recurrence in almost half of all patients treated for cervical cancer.

Disease discovered within the first 3 to 6 months following therapy is often termed persistent cancer, while tumours found after that time are referred to as recurrent. The tumouricidal effects of radiation therapy continue after the completion of therapy, therefore most oncologists hesitate to diagnose persistent cervical cancer during the first 3 months after therapy. However, if examination during or immediately after therapy indicates no response or tumour growth, the diagnosis of persistent cervical cancer may be established earlier. The terms are sometimes confusing and might be clarified by calling a tumour persistent when there is not a complete clinical remission or when progressive disease is documented during or immediately after therapy. Recurrent tumours would include those that later become evident after a period of complete clinical remission. Disease discovered after a primary surgical approach should be termed persistent if margins or nodes were involved and recurrent if the above is not true.

The disease-free interval depends on multiple factors including the adequacy of initial treatment, tumour susceptibility, host resistance, the original stage and volume of tumour and the adequacy of follow-up. The majority (more than 80%) of recurrences will be discovered within 3 years of initial therapy. Early-stage or low-volume tumours tend to recur later than those tumours which were initially of advanced stage or high volume.

Although one might postulate that an earlier diagnosis of recurrence would increase the rate of curability, this has not been substantiated. Although Roddick (1968) reported early diagnosis leading to an increased rate of resectability, he failed to note an increased rate of cure.

Brunschwig (1967) reported an increased survival in patients treated with exenterative surgery among those patients with a late recurrence (more than 6 months). Creasman (1972) reported increased resectability and increased 2-year survival rates in patients who suffered recurrence 2 years or more following first treatment, presumably on the basis of the biological activity of the tumour. However, Deckers (1972) reported no significant difference in survival for patients undergoing exenterative surgery for late (more than 5 years after treatment) recurrent cervical cancer.

The extent of recurrent or persistent disease dictates the form of therapy that may be offered. Patients initially treated with a surgical procedure, especially if inadequate (total hysterectomy), may be at increased risk for central pelvic recurrence. Initial treatment with radiation therapy results in excellent central pelvic control; however the incidence of distal metastases may be increased when compared to those patients initially treated surgically.

The pelvic fibrosis following radiation therapy makes the pelvic examination for detection of recurrence difficult, even for the most experienced examiner. The problem was demonstrated by Kottmeier (1954) who reported 80 patients without a histological diagnosis of recurrent tumour but 'obvious recurrent tumor on bimanual examination'. Many of these patients survived 15 years without progression. Although a laparotomy may be required to confirm the diagnosis of recurrence, treatment without a tissue diagnosis of recurrent cancer is unacceptable.

CHOICE OF TREATMENT

Therapy for patients with recurrent cervical cancer is dictated by the mode of initial treatment. Most patients with advanced disease and some with stage I disease have received radiotherapy as primary treatment while others have received radiation for treatment of a surgical recurrence. To date, there exists no effective chemotherapeutic agent or regimen for the treatment of cervical cancer, therefore a post-radiation recurrence mandates a radical or ultraradical surgical approach if cure is the goal. The majority of reports concerning exenterative surgery are from the United States; when compared to salvage operations in patients with other types of cancer, pelvic exenteration ranks favourably in allowing for survival with high expectations for rehabilitation. If the lesion is not amenable to surgery, the ultimate prognosis is poor as few patients with recurrent cervical cancer will survive 5 years.

Most authors consider total hysterectomy inadequate therapy for patients with recurrent cervical cancer. Following tolerance doses of megavoltage radiotherapy this procedure carries a high risk of urinary complications while rarely offering a chance for cure.

A select group of patients with small-volume central pelvic recurrence may be successfully treated with radical hysterectomy. In selected patients, the 5-year survival approaches 30% to 50%; however, because of the difficulty of assessing volume of tumour, the procedure may fail, whereas a more radical procedure might have resulted in cure. Additionally, radical hysterectomy following tolerance doses of megavoltage radiotherapy is associated with a high rate (20–50%) of serious urinary complications. Successful surgical techniques designed to diminish these complications such as less ureteral dissection can result in less than optimal surgical margins. Since this may be the last chance for cure, gynaecologic oncologists at this institution feel that pelvic exenteration should be the surgical treatment of choice in patients with centrally recurrent cervical cancer following primary radiation therapy.

Exenterative procedures may be partial (conservation of the bladder or rectum) or total (Fig. 7.1–7.3). Controversy exists as to the

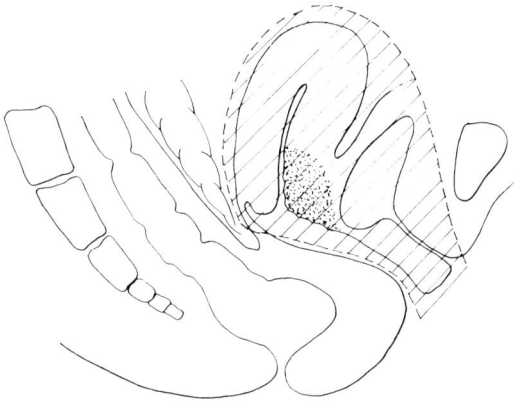

Fig. 7.1 Anterior exenteration involves the surgical removal of the bladder, uterus and cervix and is considered in patients with a deep cul-de-sac. It is imperative that frozen sections be obtained at the time of exploration. If tumour is present in the posterior vagina margin, total exenteration is the preferred operation.

advisability of partial exenterative procedures, and early reports indicating poor survival with partial exenteration continue to be quoted. More recently, however, the available literature would indicate that the procedure can be performed successfully (Table 7.1). As with radical hysterectomy, the problem of adequacy of the surgical margins with partial exenterations is the key issue. The surgeon should remember that despite normal appearing bladder or rectal mucosa,

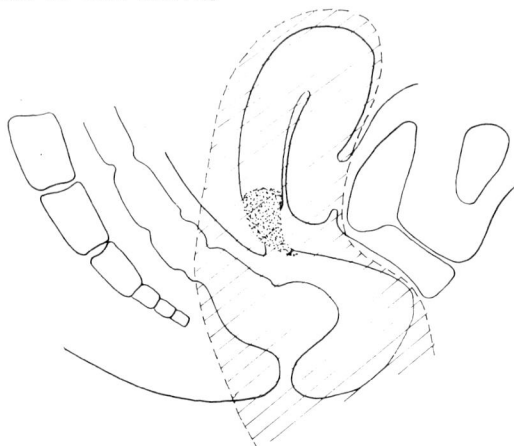

Fig. 7.2 Posterior exenteration involves the surgical removal of the rectum, uterus and cervix. Following radiation therapy, urinary complications are high.

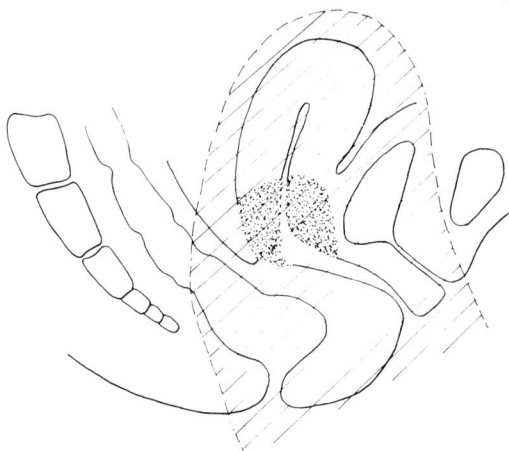

Fig. 7.3 Total exenteration involves the removal of bladder, urethra, cervix, uterus, vagina and rectum. The anal canal may be preserved in some women, allowing re-anastomosis of the sigmoid colon.

Table 7.1 Survival related to the type of exenteration in patients with recurrent cervical cancer

Author	Year	Anterior exenteration			Total exenteration		
		No. of patients	Surgical mortality (%)	5-year survival (%)	No. of patients	Surgical mortality (%)	5-year survival (%)
Ingersoll	1966	18	–	11.1	53	–	26.4
Brunschwig	1967	95	10.5	18.9	217	20.3	17.1
Inguilla	1967	32	25.0	21.9	51	49.0	5.9
Ketchum	1970	9	–	44.0	81	–	25.0
Creasman	1974	27*	–	33.3	59	–	20.3
Symmonds**	1975	59	–	42.0	36	–	41.0
Authors	1982	48	5.3	60.0	53	12.7	29.0

*Partial exenteration, **SCC only

occult invasion of the submucosa of these organs may be found in some patients undergoing exenteration. Since no patient with a positive surgical margin survives, it is not justifiable to do a partial exenteration unless adequate margins can be obtained.

We currently feel an anterior exenterative procedure may benefit those patients with central pelvic recurrence, minimal vaginal extension anteriorly and a deep cul-de-sac (Fig. 7.1). Significant vaginal extension (beyond the upper third) and posterior vaginal extension increases the likelihood of involvement of the rectovaginal septum margin, either by direct extension or by paravaginal lymphatic extension.

The proximity of the irradiated uterine cervix and the lower urinary tract increases the risk of bladder and ureteral fistulae following posterior exenteration. This fact, coupled with the inability to obtain a wide surgical margin between the cervix and the bladder, makes this procedure quite limited in usefulness for cancer of the cervix.

Total exenteration is the most commonly used surgical procedure for patients with central recurrence. Some patients with tumour involving the lower third of the vagina require an additional perineal resection including a radical vulvectomy and groin dissection. Although this latter procedure leads to an occasional cure, it is associated with increased postoperative morbidity.

PREOPERATIVE CONSIDERATIONS

Because of the extent of exenterative surgery, numerous psychological and physiological considerations must be undertaken prior to operation.

Surgical mortality increases with age (Table 7.2). Older patients are

Table 7.2 Pelvic exenteration age-related operative mortality (Authors 1982)

Age group	No. of patients	% of age group	Cumulative percentage
≤ 40 years	24	0	0
41–50 years	36	5.6	3.3
51–60 years	38	13.2	7.1
> 61 years	27	18.5	9.6

prone to have other medical conditions predisposing them to serious complications. In our opinion, this procedure should rarely be considered in those patients who are over 70 years of age.

A history of recent weight loss should prompt careful evaluation for metastatic disease. Weight loss, in the absence of metastatic disease, is not considered a contra-indication, but malnourished patients are subject to increased operative complications and may benefit from preoperative hyperalimentation.

While obesity may render the procedure technically more difficult, in itself it is not an absolute contra-indication to a surgical approach. The surgeon must be aware of and able to manage the particular intraoperative and postoperative complications associated with obesity.

Medical illness such as diabetes, hypertension, vascular disease or pulmonary disease, should be carefully considered in the patient's initial evaluation; however, only in the extreme situation where it appears that the medical disease will limit the patient's survival should the patient not be considered a candidate for surgery.

The presence of sciatic pain and leg oedema usually contra-indicate a surgical approach as few of these patients have a resectable tumour and resection yields few 5-year survivors.

An important aspect of preoperative assessment is the ability of the patient and her family to withstand the psychological stress of the operative procedure and the 3- to 4-month recovery period. The importance of extensive preoperative counselling of both the patient and her family cannot be overemphasised. An emotional or psychiatric disorder which interferes significantly with the patient's ability to care for herself is a relative contra-indication to exenterative surgery.

Because of the impact of extrapelvic disease on prognosis, each candidate should undergo extensive preoperative evaluation prior to exploration (Table 7.3). A chest X-ray not only helps to establish the

Table 7.3 Preoperative evaluation prior to exenteration

Chest X-ray
Intravenous pyelogram*
Barium enema
Cystoscopy
Proctoscopy
Liver enzymes
Renal function studies
Lymphangiogram, abdominal pelvic ultrasound scan or computed tomography
Scalene node biopsy

*May be deleted if computed tomography is obtained

presence or absence of pulmonary metastasis but is helpful in the preoperative diagnosis of coexisting pulmonary disease and serves as a baseline for postoperative surveillance.

Evaluation of the urinary tract is important because of the proximity of the bladder and ureters to the cervix. The probability of resecting the tumour is directly related to the degree of abnormality on the intravenous pyelogram (IVP). As many as 60% of patients with unilateral obstruction have an unresectable tumour. This figure approaches 90% with bilateral ureteral obstruction. Additionally, patients with resectable tumours and abnormal pyelograms apparently have a poorer long-term prognosis when compared to patients undergoing exenteration with normal intravenous pyelography. Although each patient must be considered individually, obstructive uropathy is a relative contra-indication to exenterative surgery. The usual cause of obstructive uropathy following treatment is recurrent cancer, however the burden is on the physician to prove the obstruction is secondary to tumour and not to radiation fibrosis. If an exenterative procedure is considered in a patient with high-grade unilateral ureteral obstruction, a preoperative renal scan to determine the residual function of the obstructed kidney becomes essential. Incorporating a non-functioning kidney into a urinary conduit predisposes the patient to serious infectious complications. In this situation, consideration should be given to alternatives such as nephrectomy or permanent ureteral ligation.

Tumour extension to the bladder does not contra-indicate a surgical approach, however the report from Kiselow (1967) relates its prognostic significance. His finding of a statistically significant decrease in survival in patients with (32.2%) when compared to those without (54.5%) bladder involvement would suggest that cystoscopic examination of the lower urinary tract is an essential part of the preoperative evaluation, despite the fact that few exenterative procedures include bladder conservation.

According to Kiselow, tumour invading the rectum or colon also has an unfavourable effect on prognosis. Its presence was associated with a decrease in survival from 50.6% to 25.7%. Radiation changes may make a proctoscopic examination difficult. The finding of intact rectal mucosa does not necessarily allow the surgeon to plan rectal conservation, because as many as 61% of patients may have occult tumour involvement of the muscularis of the rectum. Theoretically, patients with tumour involvement of the posterior or anterior vagina may be at risk for submucosal involvement of the rectum or rectovaginal septum either by direct extension or through paravaginal lymphatic metastases.

Barium studies of the colon are essential to establish the presence of coexisting disease, benign or malignant. While the incidence of coexistent malignancy is small (Mortel 1972), a procedure of this magnitude is not likely to be considered in the presence of another primary malignancy.

While liver metastases in patients with recurrent cancer of the uterine cervix are unusual, their presence indicates disseminated disease and contra-indicates a surgical approach. Serum liver function studies serve as a screen for hepatic metastases, however computed tomography may also be beneficial. Any abnormalities require investigation via percutaneous aspiration or intraoperatively prior to exenteration.

The spine is the most common site of bone metastases and the previously mentioned radiographic studies are usually adequate to determine the presence or absence of metastases.

Although radiation therapy is capable of sterilising 50% of nodal disease, the possibility of lymphatic involvement either within or outside the original treatment field should be investigated in patients with apparent central pelvic recurrence. The most commonly involved nodes outside the primary treatment field are those in the para-aortic area. Supraclavicular and inguinal nodes may be involved later but are more accessible to examination and biopsy. The latter may represent metastatic lymphatic spread via the vulvar lymphatics from disease in the lower vagina or retrograde metastasis from obstructed pelvic nodes. Current diagnostic methods utilised in screening for nodal metastasis include computerised axial tomography (CAT), ultrasonography and lymphangiography. Because of the detrimental influence of positive nodes on prognosis and the fact that these tests are associated with little morbidity, at least one should be performed prior to laparotomy (Fig. 7.4). The individual test is only reliable when strict criteria are used to determine the positivity or negativity of nodes. Additionally, the variability in the reported false-negative and false-positive rates of these diagnostic tests suggests that the results correlate with the experience of the individual who interprets them. Because the experience may differ

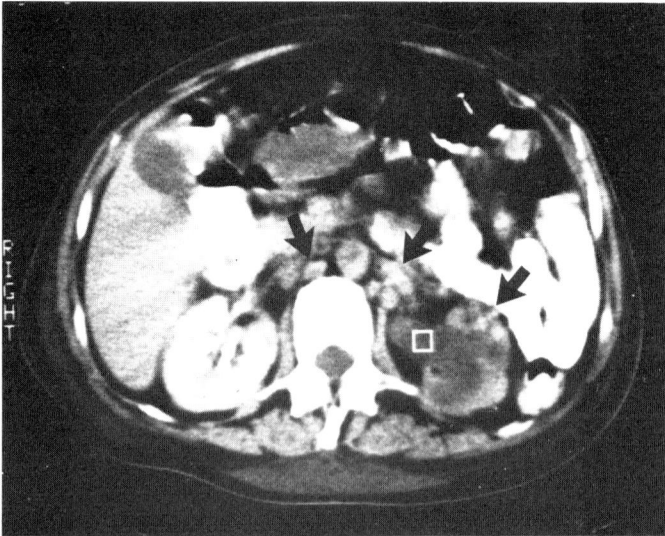

Fig. 7.4 CAT scan of a woman with recurrent squamous cell carcinoma indicating high-grade left ureteral obstruction (arrow) and retroperitoneal lymphadenopathy (arrows).

between institutions, it is important that the physician know which test might be most appropriate at his institution.

Ultrasonography is reputed to detect enlarged 3 cm pelvic nodes and 2 cm periaortic nodes while computerised tomography is said to resolve 1 cm enlarged nodes in both the pelvic and para-aortic space. The resolution of the CAT scan may help quantify lateral tumour extension and aid in determining resectability or the necessity for levator resection (Fig. 7.5); however, one must be careful in interpreting these results so

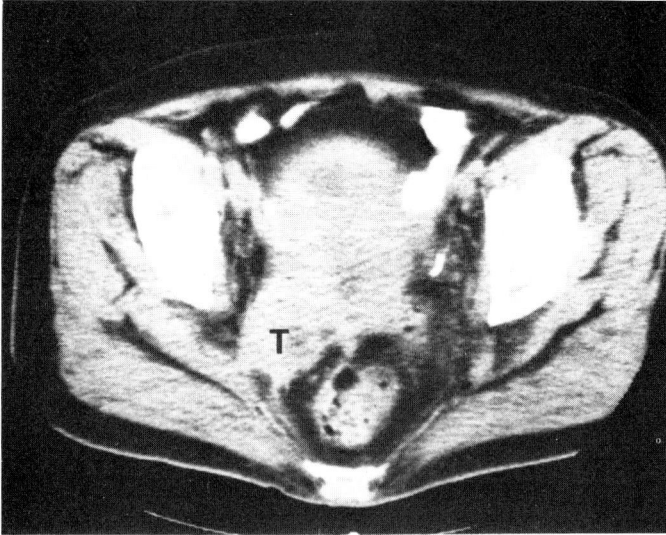

Fig. 7.5   Pelvic CAT scan indicating recurrent tumour (T) extending to the right pelvic sidewall. Following documentation by fine-needle aspiration, she was not considered a candidate for exenteration.

as not to confuse fibrosis and tumour extension. Both ultrasonography and CAT scans are relatively new techniques compared to lymphangiography. While there is a larger reported experience with the latter, it should be noted that lymphangiograms are more invasive, more difficult to perform and subject to complications such as lipid pneumonia. Because of the lack of universal criteria, the incidence of false-positive lymphangiograms is difficult to establish; however, reports adhering to specific criteria, such as nodal filling defects, deviation around a mass or complete lymphatic obstruction, usually result in false-positive rates greater than 15%. Importantly, Piver (1973) has reported that previous radiation therapy apparently has little effect in altering the criteria for or lymphangiographic image of positive or negative nodes.

Regardless of the method used to evaluate the nodal areas, any enlarged or 'positive' node requires histological or cytological confirmation prior to denying a surgical procedure. This may be obtained reliably by fine-needle aspiration. However, if fine-needle aspiration is negative or non-diagnostic, then exploration may still be warranted if no other contra-indications exist.

Many authors perform scalene node biopsies as part of their preoperative evaluation. A survey of the literature indicates that approximately 17% of patients with recurrence and periaortic nodal metastases may have subclinical metastatic disease in the scalene nodes (Table 7.4). While the procedure may be performed under local anaesthesia, it should only be performed by those who are willing to accept the possible complications of pneumothorax, vascular or lymphatic injury in the neck.

Table 7.4 Scalene node metastasis in patients with recurrent cancer

Author	Year	No. of patients with positive para-aortic nodes and clinically negative supraclavicular nodes	% positive supraclavicular nodes
Ketchum	1973	22	18.2
Perez-Mesa	1976	17	5.9
Lee	1981	25	24.0
Totals		64	17.2

Although computerised tomography may help delineate the pelvic boundaries of the tumour, examination under anaesthesia should be performed to confirm tumour size and mobility. If the tumour is fixed to the pelvic side wall, adequate surgical margins are unattainable and an exenterative procedure is contra-indicated.

The literature indicates that 2% to 14% of patients will have recurrent cervical cancer limited to the central pelvis. If no absolute contra-indications (Table 7.5) are present, the patient is a candidate for curative surgery.

Preoperative preparation

An important but difficult aspect of pre-operative preparation (Table 7.6) is related to the patient's mental attitude and expectations. Although it may be impossible to explain the magnitude of the procedure, preoperative discussion with the patient and selected family members is important, and the prolonged rehabilitation period should be stressed.

While current information suggests that as many as 50% of hospitalised patients have clinical or laboratory evidence of malnutrition, the incidence in patients with recurrent cancer may be

Table 7.5 Preoperative contra-indications to exenteration in patients with recurrent cervical cancer

Absolute
1. Extra-pelvic disease
2. Triad of unilateral leg oedema, sciatica and ureteral obstruction
3. Tumour-related pelvic sidewall fixation
4. Bilateral ureteral obstruction (if 2° to recurrence)
5. Severe life-limiting medical illness
6. Psychosis or the inability of the patient to care for herself
7. Religious or other beliefs that prohibit the patient from accepting transfusion
8. Inability of physician or consultants to manage any or all intraoperative and postoperative complications
9. Inadequate hospital facilities

Relative
1. Age over 70 years
2. Large tumour volume
3. Unilateral ureteral obstruction
4. Metastasis to the distal vagina

Table 7.6 Preoperative preparation

1. Intensive psychological counselling
2. Nutritional evaluation
3. Mechanical and antibiotic bowel preparation
4. Pulmonary function tests
5. Stomal placement
6. Perioperative antibiotics

higher. Additionally, malnourished patients are subject to increased postoperative morbidity and mortality. Although the diagnosis of a malnourished state may easily be confirmed in patients with recent weight loss, other nutritional parameters such as a low serum albumin (less than 3.0 g/dl), increased tricep skin-fold thickness, low serum transferrin or altered delayed hypersensitivity as determined by skin testing should be evaluated. Malnourished patients may benefit from aggressive preoperative alimentation.

All exenterative procedures require an interruption of the bowel. Although few specific reports concerning infection after exenteration are available, a mechanical and antibiotic bowel preparation instituted prior to a procedure that requires interruption of the gastro-intestinal tract (Judd 1975, Parker 1978) will decrease the risk of intra-abdominal or wound infections.

Additional important studies include arterial blood gases and pulmonary function tests, to aid in the preoperative diagnosis of subtle pulmonary disease, help predict the postoperative recovery after a long operative procedure and allow appropriate diagnosis and management of the postoperative pulmonary complaints or complications.

Postoperative rehabilitation will be greatly influenced by patient adjustment and management of her urinary and/or faecal stoma. Preoperative discussion with the physician, stomal therapist or another patient who has a stoma will help to allay fear and misconceptions. The optimal areas for stomal placement, situated to avoid the beltline and skin-folds, should be designated preoperatively, both in the sitting and standing position.

The preoperative hospitalisation should be minimised, as evidence from the general surgical literature indicates the rate of wound infections increases in direct proportion to the duration of preoperative hospitalisation (Cruse 1980).

Although commonly administered, the use of perioperative parenteral antibiotics has no documented benefit in exenterative surgery. If one is to use antibiotics, the risk of bacterial resistance, pseudomembranous colitis, anaphylactic reactions and fungal infection should be weighed.

The reported risk of a patient developing pulmonary emboli after exenteration is 1–6%. This relatively high risk is probably related both to the duration of the operative procedure and the trauma to pelvic vessels. There exists little information regarding the risks and benefits of prophylactic heparin or other methods of prophylaxis to decrease deep vein thrombosis.

THE EXENTERATIVE OPERATION

The operative procedure may be logically divided into three categories: (1) determining resectability, (2) resection, and (3) reconstruction including the construction of the urinary conduit and pelvic closure.

Our preferred incision is vertical, extended around the umbilicus as necessary. While some authors advocate a transverse incision designed to optimise lateral pelvic exposure, we currently feel the vertical incision gives adequate exposure with a decreased risk of wound complications. Additionally, the vertical incision allows easy dissection of the omentum used to cover the pelvic basin, as well as allowing the surgeon access to create a transverse colon conduit.

The serosal and peritoneal surfaces are inspected and palpated. If intraperitoneal disease is present the procedure is abandoned, as only an occasional patient will survive. The dissection of the para-aortic nodes with intraoperative histological assessment is considered an important portion of the procedure because of the frequency of involvement of nodes in recurrent disease, and the marked difference in prognosis if metastases are present. Metastases to aortic nodes contra-indicate exenteration.

A pelvic lymphadenectomy following therapeutic pelvic radiotherapy is made difficult by dense adhesions and tissue reaction. The technical difficulty is associated with prolonged operative time, increased blood loss and an increased risk of postoperative lymphocysts, leg oedema and thrombophlebitis. However, the prognostic significance of positive pelvic nodes is well documented. The reported 5-year survival of patients with negative pelvic nodes ranges between 35% and 65% while only 10–15% of patients will survive if the nodes contain metastatic disease (Table 7.7). While the therapeutic effect of lymphadenectomy at exenteration is not known, the 5-year survival of patients with untreated

Table 7.7 Survival of patients with recurrent cervical cancer related to lymph node status at pelvic exenteration

Author	Year	No. of pts	Negative lymph nodes 5-year survival (%)	No. of pts	Positive lymph nodes 5-year survival (%)
Ingersoll	1966	39	38.5	33	6.1
Kiselow	1967	88	50.0	28	21.4
Ketchum	1970	69	33.0	21	11.0
Barber	1971	166	17.4	97	5.1
Creasman	1974	29	27.6	14	14.3
Symmonds	1975	68	42.0	30	15.0
Morley	1976	45	78.0	9	0.0
Rutledge	1977	–	–	30	11.0

recurrence is less than that for patients with pelvic node metastases treated with exenteration and lymphadenectomy. Information concerning single node involvement or subclinical disease is not available. Some authors feel that exenteration is contra-indicated in the presence of pelvic node metastasis; others feel that the decision to continue must be individualised. Creasman's (1974) report indicating no difference in survival in patients with negative nodes and those with unknown nodal status has prompted some surgeons to disfavour lymphadenectomy. However this report fails to mention the possible selection process involved. Lymphadenectomy may have been performed in patients with palpably enlarged nodes and not performed in those patients with non-enlarged nodes. Nodal enlargement may be secondary to the infection frequently present with recurrent cervical cancer and the procedure should not be abandoned without histological evidence of involvement. The clinical situation may be more complicated after lymphangiogram where reaction to dye may cause secondary nodal enlargement. Because of its prognostic value and the possible therapeutic benefit of lymphadenectomy, we advocate extensive intraoperative nodal sampling. The complication rate has been small in those procedures where adequate pelvic drainage has been established. Metastatic disease in multiple or bilateral pelvic nodes or in adherent nodes requiring major vessel excision probably precludes cure.

The avascular paravesical and pararectal spaces are then opened to verify resectability. Assessment of the inferior portion of the operative procedure, removing the tumour and vagina as it traverses the levators, is important as tumour extension or skip metastases that require resection of the levator musculature may be associated with a poor prognosis. If unresectable, the procedure can be stopped without a significant risk of bleeding.

Between 33% and 60% of patients explored will have a negative intraoperative evaluation (Table 7.8) and will undergo exenteration. The usual duration of the operative procedure is between 5 and 6 h,

Table 7.8 Intraoperative contra-indications to exenteration

1. Extrapelvic disease
2. Malignant ascites
3. Multiple positive pelvic nodes
4. Tumour invasion of major vessels
5. Documented bowel serosal involvement

with an anterior exenteration requiring less operative time. Prolonged operative time (greater than 8 h) is associated with decreased survival and while this may be related to increased technical difficulty or different surgical technique, the effect on prognosis makes it important to minimise anaesthesia and operative time. While some authors have advocated a multidisciplinary team approach, others have performed the procedure with a single team approach. Regardless of who performs the surgery, there should be an adequate number of experienced surgeons available during the procedure to avoid fatigue as a cause of errors in surgical judgment.

The usual blood loss for total exenteration varies between 2000 and 4000 ml with less in partial procedures. Ketchum (1970) has reported that mortality is increased if the procedure is associated with an interoperative blood loss of greater than 3800 ml. Since 15% to 42% of blood loss is present on gowns and drapes, intraoperative estimates and replacement may be inadequate, predisposing the patient to hypotension; efforts must be directed to quantitate this loss. Intraoperative use of a pulmonary artery catheter allows for dynamic management and appropriate maintenance of the patient's vascular volume. Replacement consists of packed red blood cells and crystalloid since whole blood offers little benefit over component therapy. Fresh frozen plasma, cryoprecipitate and platelets are used as necessary.

Intestinal staples have been used in many exenterative procedures at this institution, with an associated decrease in operative time of 20% and 28% for total and anterior exenteration respectively (Table 7.9). Additional benefits of surgical staple use include a secure anastomosis using a monofilament non-reactive permanent suture material with less intrasurgeon variation and minimal intra-abdominal contamination.

RECURRENT CERVICAL CANCER 159

Table 7.9 Operative time related to type of exenteration, type of intestinal segment and stapler use (115 patients) (Authors 1982)

Type of exenteration	Intestinal segment	Staples	Mean operative time (h)
Anterior*	Ileal†	+	4.9 ± 0.8
	Ileal†	−	6.8 ± 1.3
	Transverse colon	+	5.2 ± 0.7
Total*	Ileal†	+	5.4 ± 0.9
	Ileal†	−	6.4 ± 1.3
	Transverse colon	+	5.9 ± 1.3

*Anterior exenteration significantly shorter than total exenteration ($P < 0.001$)
† Operative time when staples were used is significantly shorter in anterior ($P = 0.0001$) and total ($P = 0.005$) exenteration

While it has been argued that gastro-intestinal staples in the urinary conduit predispose to the development of calculi, the reported incidence is small (2–4%). These calculi usually pass easily and are rarely responsible for decreased renal function or serious infection.

Early attempts at urinary diversion involved a wet colostomy or a rectal bladder. However, the disastrous effects of faecal contamination of the urinary tract prompted the search for alternative methods. Since the first description of the urinary conduit, most authors have used a segment of distal ileum. Advocates of sigmoid colon conduits point out that this type of diversion avoids a primary bowel anastomosis. However, the previous radiotherapy to these two intrapelvic bowel segments has resulted in high rates of urinary complications. While pale serosa or thickened mesentery may indicate marked radiation effect, such changes are not invariably present. The inability to distinguish the degree of radiation injury to bowel has prompted many surgeons to utilise a segment of unirradiated transverse colon for the urinary conduit (Fig. 7.6). At this institution its use had been associated with a decreased risk of postoperative urinary leaks (Table 7.10) and late urinary infections. Avoiding an anastomosis in the irradiated ileum has also been associated with a decreased risk of small bowel obstruction or fistulae (Table 7.11).

Utilisation of silastic ureteral stents anchored to the intestinal segment or ureter by plain catgut sutures can decrease technical errors during conduit construction while offering protection against acute urinary strictures (Fig. 7.7). Their use does not significantly increase the risk of acute postoperative pyelonephritis. While utilising stents precludes an antireflux anastomosis, we feel that there exists little

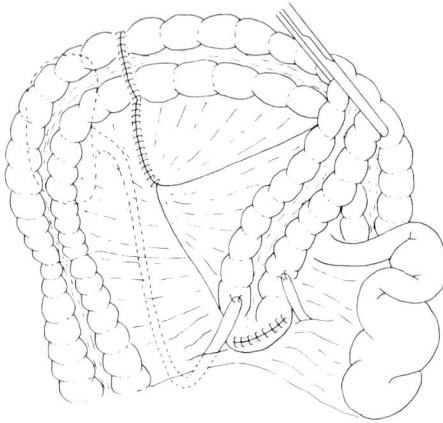

Fig. 7.6 The segment of transverse colon has been isolated and the colon reanastomosed. The ureters enter the peritoneal cavity through the small bowel mesentery. The conduit is then fixed to the posterior peritoneum after the single layer uretero-intestinal anastomosis.

Table 7.10 Urinary leaks following exenteration (Authors 1982)

Type of conduit	No. of pts	% urinary leaks
Ileal	97	10.3
Transverse colon	16	0

Table 7.11 Gastro-intestinal complications related to method of urinary diversion (Authors 1982)

Type of conduit	No. of patients	% small bowel obstruction	% small bowel fistula
Ileal	100	9	10
Transverse colon	17	0	0

documentation that this type of uretero-intestinal anastomosis is superior or worth the extra time in patients who are undergoing exenterative procedures. Appropriate stomal protrusion of 6 to 13 mm above the skin can be accomplished with a rosebud technique that allows for optimal appliance management postoperatively.

Management of the pelvic defect is important. The raw, denuded pelvic cavity with its dense fibrous reaction may predispose to postoperative infections and gastro-intestinal complications. Techniques designed to decrease the contact of small bowel and the pelvic defect consisting of grafts constructed of foreign material such as amnion or marlex have not proved satisfactory. While a pedicle or free peritoneal graft, as described by Morley (1976), provides a suitable alternative to cover the pelvic defect, optimal closure probably involves

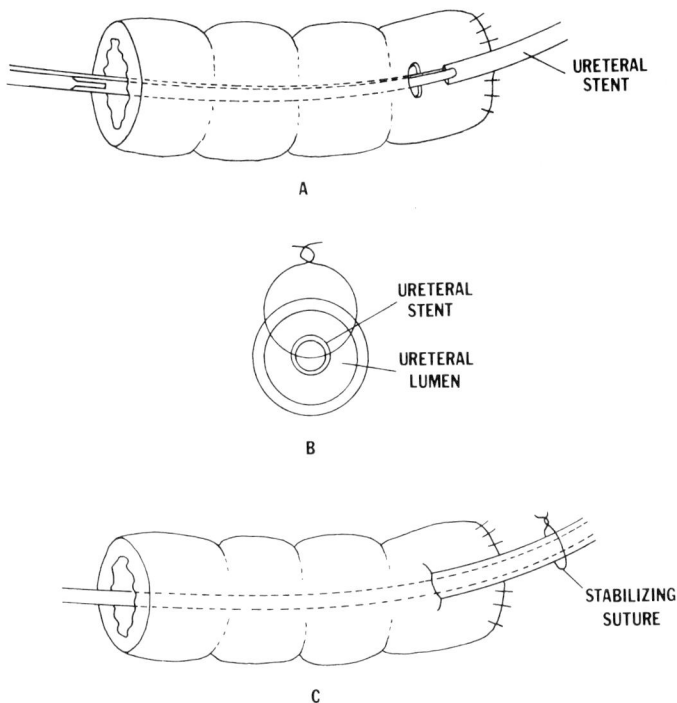

Fig. 7.7 A silastic ureteral stent is pulled through a small incision in the bowel (A) and fixed to the ureter (to avoid expulsion) with a loosely tied 4-0 absorbable suture (B). The ureteral and intestinal mucosal surfaces are sutured. (Drawing modified from Rutledge 1977)

a method that transposes new blood supply into the pelvis. A recently described effective method of pelvic closure involves transposition of an omental pedicle into the pelvis (Fig. 7.8). The use of omental grafts has been associated with a decreased rate of major small bowel complications. If the omentum is inadequate or surgically absent, we would utilise a sigmoid lid or peritoneal graft. Other methods to decrease the size of the pelvic defect and protect the small bowel after total exenteration include that reported by Lagasse (1973). The sigmoid colon is mobilised and anastomosed to a 3 cm rectal stump. Although problems with healing and rectal fistula are evident, the posterior pelvis is protected and 45% of patients heal adequately allowing the diverting colostomy to be temporary.

Vaginal reconstruction with a gracilis or gluteal myocutaneous flap at the time of exenteration offers another theoretical alternative to increase blood supply to the pelvic defect. Objective evidence that this may further decrease postoperative complications is lacking, but it appears to show promise. It does increase operating time and presents certain

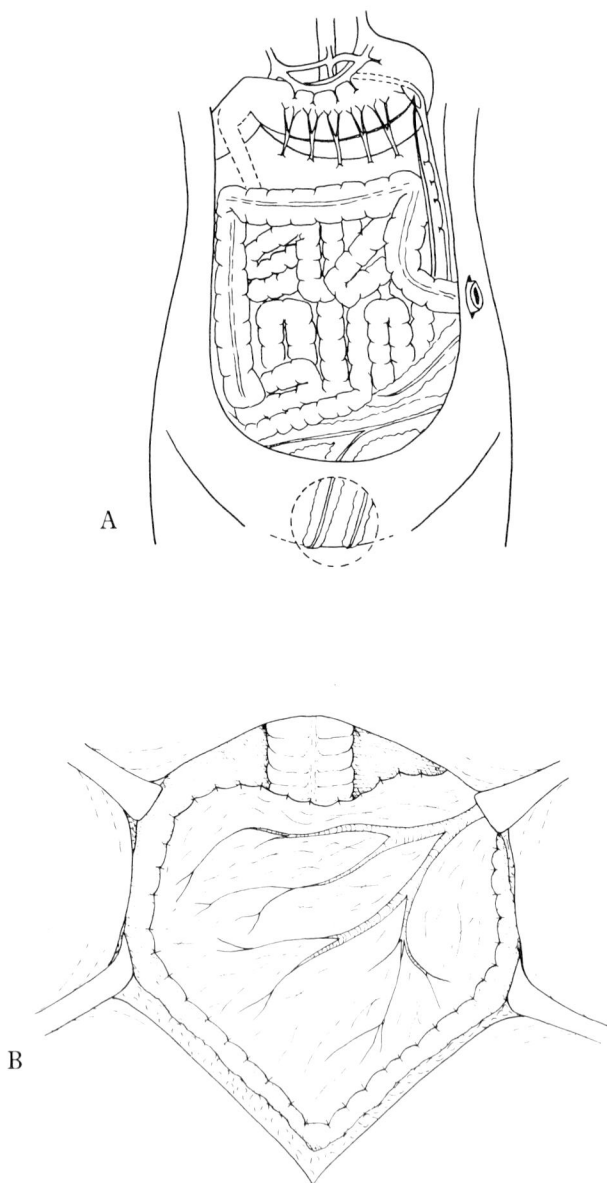

Fig. 7.8 The omental flap has been created (conserving the left gastroepiploic artery) and placed in the gutter (A) to completely cover the denuded pelvis (B). (A modified from Rutledge, 1977; B modified from Wheeless, 1981)

problems and complications, primarily related to blood supply to the flap and wound breakdown of the graft site.

The preferred method of abdominal closure is a Smead-Jones technique utilising a permanent monofilament suture. This type of internal retention suture is reported to offer optimal protection against abdominal dehiscence, a problem that can be expected with increased frequency after pelvic radiotherapy.

The surgical pathologist and the surgeon should review the surgical specimen together prior to fixation as pathological interpretation of the surgical specimen is vital. Important surgical margins should be extensively investigated as tumour-involved margins imply recurrence and death. If an anterior exenteration is undertaken, surgical margins at the cul-de-sac should be obtained intraoperatively. Although there is no evidence that adjuvant chemotherapy will benefit these patients, it might be considered for those with close or involved margins as they are at high risk for recurrence.

Postoperative care

After exenteration, the patient is placed in an intensive care unit for 48 to 72 h as the marked fluid shifts and possibility of occult bleeding require close monitoring of the patient's volume status. Central venous pressure monitoring has been replaced by the pulmonary artery catheter which enables the physician to monitor postoperative cardiac performance as well as volume status. The catheter is more invasive and is subject to more complications than a central venous line, however in over 70 patients at this institution its use has resulted in only one major complication (a haemothorax). The physician should be aware of other potential complications of the pulmonary artery catheter, including pulmonary parenchymal damage, balloon rupture, arrhythmias, infection, thrombophlebitis or inadvertent knotting of the catheter. Other possible complications such as valvular damage or endocardial vegetations have been reported, but only after long-term use.

As many as 38% of patients have significant preoperative blood volume deficits. When combined with extensive intraoperative blood loss, fluid shifts, and the necessity for a prolonged anaesthetic, additional monitoring with an arterial line, we currently feel, is not only beneficial but warranted intraoperatively and during the acute postoperative recovery period.

Large volume blood loss may be associated with a consumptive coagulopathy. In fact, following a one-volume transfusion, clotting elements are reduced by 70% to 75%. Clinical bleeding may not occur until a two-volume transfusion is required where approximately 10% of the original blood clotting elements remain. Since stored blood is essentially devoid of platelets and markedly depleted in factors V and VIII, we prefer to use blood component therapy consisting of packed red blood cells to increase oxygen-carrying capacity and platelets, fresh frozen plasma and cryoprecipitate (containing factors V, VIII, XII and fibrinogen) to correct a coagulopathy. If additional volume restoration is necessary, albumin, with its decreased risk of hepatitis, is preferable to frozen plasma.

The majority of patients are unable to tolerate an adequate oral intake until the 10th to 14th postoperative day. This, coupled with the marked catabolic response to a major surgical procedure, may predispose to the rapid development of malnutrition with its resultant increased risk of poor healing or other major postoperative complications. In an effort to minimise these risks, parenteral hyperalimentation with dextrose and amino acid solutions is begun immediately postoperatively. The use of a jejunostomy feeding tube placed intraoperatively allows for effective long-term hyperalimentation with less expense and risk of complications by utilising an elemental diet. Hypoproteinaemia or extensive retroperitoneal dissection may result in initial intolerance to jejunal feedings, however, parenteral alimentation can usually be discontinued by the fourth postoperative day as most patients are able to receive at least 2500 kcal via the jejunostomy feeding tube. The benefits of hyperalimentation after exenteration are justified by the evidence that it reduces the risk of sepsis and promotes healing in patients who have received preoperative radiation therapy.

Postoperatively, the urinary stents are expelled on the 19th to 21st day coinciding with the resorption of the stabilising suture. No manipulation of these stents should be performed prior to that time.

The pelvis may be examined in the early postoperative period if indicated by sepsis or bleeding. At that time pelvic irrigations with a solution of hydrogen peroxide and saline may begin, and may be utilised on a daily basis as long as they seem beneficial.

Symptomatic pulmonary emboli are reported to occur in 1–5% of patients after exenteration and are not infrequently stated to be the cause of postoperative deaths. Our experience would indicate that thromboemboli are rarely fatal unless accompanied by other major postoperative complications such as gastro-intestinal or urinary fistulae. During and after exenteration the pelvic vessels are traumatised and exposed to local infection, both of which predispose to thrombus formation. To date, little evidence exists that perioperative subcutaneous heparin or other forms of prophylaxis such as pneumatic compression stockings decrease the risk of embolic phenomena. Because of this significant risk and the failure of medical prophylaxis, several authors advocate intraoperative inferior vena caval occlusion.

Perioperative complications

The risk of major complications associated with exenterative surgery has hindered acceptance of this procedure by referring physicians and patients (Table 7.12). The fact that this procedure is only rarely performed in large numbers in individual institutions has not allowed adequate evaluation of technical modifications designed to decrease complications.

Efforts to decrease the incidence of intraoperative hypotension include the isolation and ligation of individual pedicles, especially those small penetrating vessels over the sacrum, at the pelvic sidewall and in the periuretheral area near the pubic symphysis. Additional modifications reported by others include the use of an aortic tourniquet, hypotensive anaesthesia and pelvic packs. Although serious postoperative bleeding may be managed by reoperation, newer radiological techniques utilising arteriographic gelfoam embolisation of bleeding vessels have, in experienced hands, given excellent results and this procedure should be considered since it is likely to be associated with less morbidity than re-exploration.

Most series would suggest that febrile morbidity is present in 75% to 85% of patients after exenteration. A non-infectious aetiology, such as pulmonary atelectasis, is present in 40% to 70% of patients. While some authors maintain patients on a ventilator for 48 to 72 h postoperatively, it has been our decision to proceed with extubation earlier if the patients can maintain adequate arterial oxygenation, are able to generate an acceptable negative inspiratory force (greater than 30 cm of H_2O) and have an acceptable tidal volume (greater than 700 ml). Only on rare occasions has a patient required over 6 h of postoperative ventilation. No patient has required re-intubation in the immediate postoperative period unless she required reoperation.

Pelvic cellulitis is the most common cause of infectious morbidity after pelvic exenteration. Regardless of technique, the vulnerable, denuded and irradiated pelvic defect is routinely contaminated during the operative procedure. Clinically, cellulitis usually presents as a low-grade fever and slowly responds to antibiotics and irrigation of the pelvic defect. Utilisation of the omental carpet and/or myocutaneous grafts has resulted in a clinical reduction in the amount of postoperative pelvic cellulitis. Theoretically, the new blood supply and reduction in size of the pelvic defect will increase local defence mechanisms and improve healing.

Although much less frequent, the development of a pelvic abscess after exenteration is associated with major morbidity. In our experience the overall incidence of pelvic abscess was less than 3%, however all three patients developed major urinary or intestinal complications.

Table 7.12 Complications after pelvic exenteration

	Kiselow 1967 207 pts %	Ketchum 1970 94 pts %	Symmonds 1975 198 pts %	Karlen 1975 87 pts %	Rutledge 1977 296 pts %	Morgan 1980 56 pts %	Authors 137 pts %
ACUTE & INTERMEDIATE							
Cardiovascular							
Cerebrovascular accident	0.5	1.1		1.1			0.1
Coagulopathy					11.1[a]		
Haemorrhage	3.9	20.2	1.5	10.3			
Myocardial infarction		3.2					0.1
Thromboembolism		6.4	2.0				3.6
Thrombophlebitis	4.3	15.6	4.5	4.6			3.6
Infections							
Pelvic cellulitis	18.8[b]	9.6	4.0	9.2		70.0[g]	36.5
Pelvic abscess	[b]	17.0	3.0	2.2			2.2
Pneumonia		10.6				5.4	2.9
Pyelonephritis	3.9	21.3	7.1	16.1		12.5	17.5
Wound infection		29.8	14.6	20.7[c]		23.2	13.9
Sepsis (not defined)	[b]			4.6	20.9[d]	12.5	
Intestinal							
Evisceration	2.9[e]		1.0				0
Fistula/leak	11.6	8.5	5.1	[c]	13.9f		6.6[h]
Obstruction		18.1	6.6	26.4	[f]		3.6
Bleeding				13.8			
Stomal necrosis		2.1					
Psychosis	1.9				1.0		4.4
Pulmonary							
Oedema/failure	1.0	5.3		2.3			

Table 7.12 (*cont.*)

	Kiselow 1967 207 pts %	Ketchum 1970 94 pts %	Symmonds 1975 198 pts %	Karlen 1975 87 pts %	Rutledge 1977 296 pts %	Morgan 1980 56 pts %	Authors 137 pts %
ACUTE & INTERMEDIATE							
Urinary							
Fistula/leak	e	13.8	1.0	10.3			7.3
Obstruction			1.0				
Uraemia (without obstruction)	1.4				5.7		
LATE	191 Pts %	73 Pts %	182 Pts %	65 Pts %	256 Pts %		125 Pts %
Intestinal							
Fistula	5.8	8.2	8.2				1.6
Hernia	2.6			c			
Stoma revision	8.4	8.2		4.6	4.6*		2.4
Obstruction	6.3	21.9	5.5			5.1	5.6
Urinary							
Calculi	1.0	5.5					2.4
Infection	6.3	24.7	3.8	21.5	12.1		14.4
Loss of renal unit or procedure to prevent same	1.6	13.7	1.6				3.2
Stomal revision	7.3			7.7			2.4
Fistula			3.2				0.8
Pelvic abscess or sinus	3.7						

a includes cerebrovascular accidents, coagulopathy, myocardial infarction, thrombophlebitis, haemorrhage, b includes wound infection, pelvic abscess, cellulitis, c includes wound infection, dehiscence and hernia, d all sources, e urinary and gastro-intestinal fistulae, f includes obstruction and fistulae, g cellulitis and abscess, h small bowel, * faecal or urinary stoma

Infectious pulmonary complications are reported in less than 10% of exenterative patients. However, if pneumonia develops, unusual or opportunistic organisms may be the aetiology, as the patient's normal defence mechanisms are likely to be suppressed.

The reported incidence of pyelonephritis following exenteration ranges between 5% and 20%. After one postoperative week almost all urinary conduits are colonised with bacteria, which makes the diagnosis of pyelonephritis difficult. The type of urinary conduit or the introduction of a ureteral stent does not appear to alter the risk of pyelonephritis. The use of perioperative antibiotics has little effect on the development of pyelonephritis; it appears urinary prophylaxis may prevent infection if administered around the time of stent removal.

Previous radiotherapy, with its detrimental effects on healing and contamination from interruption of the gastro-intestinal tract, makes wound infections and dehiscence common. The overall risk of abdominal wound infection varies between 5% and 30%. In our experience, the use of a gastro-intestinal stapler and a preoperative mechanical and antibiotic bowel preparation have reduced the incidence of wound infection from 16.6% to 7.3%. Superficial skin breakdown is not uncommon.

A rare but important aetiology of postoperative febrile morbidity is septic pelvic thrombophlebitis. Patients with spiking temperatures and tachycardia, unresponsive to antibiotics, should be suspect. Systemic heparinization results in rapid defervescence.

While the incidence of many complications such as blood loss, sepsis or cardiovascular accidents have decreased, recent reports indicate that the single most life-threatening complication is the development of a gastro-intestinal obstruction or fistula. While prolonged postoperative ileus is frequent, the risk of small bowel obstruction varies between 5% and 10% and is not related to the magnitude of the surgical procedure. Attempts to decrease this risk by 'stenting' the small bowel with a long intestinal tube have not proved helpful. There is still controversy concerning the optimal protective type of pelvic closure; however most authors agree that placing the ileum or small bowel into the pelvic defect without some type of protective covering predisposes it to a dense fibrotic reaction, increasing the risk of obstruction. In our recent report the most common factor associated with obstruction was an anastomosis in the irradiated small bowel, performed after the construction of an ileal conduit. In contrast, no patient with a transverse colon conduit and adequate pelvic closure has suffered this complication. The triad of continued obstipation, non-functioning colostomy and nausea and vomiting requires prompt management. Immediate attention to electrolyte and volume depletion, sepsis and prevention of aspiration are imperative. A small barium meal will demonstrate the point of obstruction within 30 min, and the barium will usually spill into the colon within 2 h if obstruction is not present. Management with a long intestinal tube may be preferable to surgery, especially in the light of reports in which an operative procedure in the immediate postoperative period may carry a mortality of 20% to 50%. A re-operation in an irradiated pelvis may be made extremely difficult by dense adhesions and fibrosis, increasing the risk of inadvertent enterotomies and disruption of the urinary conduit.

If surgery is necessary, controversy exists as to the appropriate operative procedure to relieve small bowel obstruction in previously irradiated small bowel. Some authors report less postoperative morbidity if the entire affected segment is resected; however after exenteration this may not be true and we have usually performed a simple bypass procedure. If at least 60 cm of small bowel can be preserved and there is no evidence of bowel necrosis, the bypass procedure can be performed with minimal morbidity or mortality.

Large bowel or rectovaginal fistulae following anterior exenteration have plagued the gynaecological oncologist. Dissection of the rectovaginal septum in the face of progressive radiation fibrosis and endarteritis probably leads to altered rectal blood supply, thereby predisposing the patient to a fistula. The development of a rectovaginal fistula after anterior exenteration is serious. The difficulty controlling cellulitis and inflammation of the pelvic defect may hinder healing. Even in patients undergoing colostomy, surgical mortality is high (33%).

Gastro-intestinal fistula involving small bowel following exenteration is associated with mortality in 30–40% of patients. The irradiated ileum is the most common site of the fistula and few spontaneous closures (less than 15%) occur despite the use of hyperalimentation. Although several authors stress the importance of obtaining a fistulogram and early intervention, the appropriate surgical procedure (bypass v. resection) to correct this fistula is not known. We have favoured intestinal resection to eliminate the risk of bowel necrosis.

Postoperative complications involving the urinary tract are serious. Subclinical urinary leaks following supravesical urinary diversion probably occur and may close spontaneously. The development of a conduit-to-cutaneous or conduit-to-pelvic defect urinary fistula is serious. Possible aetiologies include conduit necrosis secondary to compromised blood supply, disruption of the ureteral anastomosis (particularly associated with previous radiotherapy), or disruption of the distal conduit closure. As demonstrated by Symmonds (1975) and Morley (1976), the incidence decreases with increasing operative experience. Additionally, the use of the transverse colon conduit described by Nelson allows the anastomosis to be constructed in non-irradiated tissue while displacing the ureteral anastomosis away from the pelvic defect. Repair of the urinary leak is associated with significant (30–50%) mortality and should be reserved for those with life-threatening infection, deterioration of renal function or complex fistulae. Conservative management is associated with spontaneous closure in 30% of patients.

Postoperatively, depression, disorientation and occasionally frank psychosis may be encountered. Infectious, metabolic or cardiac aetiologies should be considered in these situations since correction of these abnormalities usually results in the return of a normal mental status.

The risk of operative mortality has been a significant contributor to the failure of acceptance of this operation. Operative mortality is increased with age, increased in patients undergoing total exenteration and decreased as the experience of the surgical team increases. The reported operative mortality varies between 7% and 37% (Table 7.13).

Table 7.13 Surgical mortality of patients with recurrent cervical cancer treated by exenteration

Author	Year	No. of pts	Surgical mortality
Ingersoll	1966	87	15.0
Brunschwig	1967	312	17.3
Inguilla	1967	100	37.0
Kiselow	1967	207	7.8
Ketchum	1970	90	22.0
Creasman*	1972	156	16.0
Authors	1982	128	9.6

*Includes 53 patients with radical hysterectomy

The most common causes of operative mortality are sepsis, thromboembolic phenomena and haemorrhage (Table 7.14). The first two usually constitute 50% of operative deaths and a complicated, prolonged postoperative course is the usual occurrence.

Table 7.14 Causes of postoperative deaths following exenteration

	Ketchum %	Karlen %	Authors %
Cardiac event	9.5	–	16.7
Cerebrovascular accident	–	8.3	–
Haemorrhage	14.3	25.0	8.3
Hepatitis	–	8.3	–
Ileofemoral thrombosis	–	–	8.3
Pneumonia	4.8	–	8.3
Pulmonary	–	8.3	–
Renal failure	9.5	–	–
Sepsis	42.9	33.3	33.3
Thromboembolism	19.0	8.3	25.0
Unknown	–	8.3	–

LONG-TERM POSTOPERATIVE MANAGEMENT

Psychological and social stresses are experienced by patients following pelvic exenteration. Dempsey (1975) noted the importance of the adequate preoperative contact between physician and patient and the necessity to present the nature of the recurrent tumour in a way that will prevent the patient from equating recurrence with death. Unrealistic expectations, denial and high anxiety levels appear to be detrimental to postoperative adjustment. Postoperative intervention by the physicians, nurses and stomal therapists is essential. The actual ability of the patient to accept and manage the colostomy and the conduit depends on the instructions and concerns of the health care team. The majority (80%) will return to work and are able to resume a near-normal life-style by 4 to 6 months. Reports on patients followed for longer than 3 years indicate that their overall psychological adjustment is good, suggesting that the negative reaction of many physicians to pelvic exenteration may be unfounded.

Vaginal reconstruction

Morley (1973) indicated that sexual desires may increase after recovery; however Dempsey (1975) indicated a significant loss of sexuality following exenteration. Brown (1972) indicated that while 73% of these women had no postoperative sexual interest, one experienced sensation in a phantom vagina and 26% had dreams with sexual content. The importance of the husband's attitude was demonstrated, as it was not unusual for the partner to avoid the operative site.

Rehabilitation following a sexually mutilating surgical procedure begins preoperatively. There should be discussions regarding the desirability or necessity of constructing a neovagina at the time of exenteration since half of the patients may reject an attempt at vaginal reconstruction as a second operation. The most quoted objections to another operation include lack of sexual desire, greater age, lack of marital partner or a negative attitude towards a second operation by both the patient and her husband.

The technical and psychological difficulties of a second reconstructive procedure make preoperative discussion concerning the desire and need for vaginal reconstruction at the time of exenteration important. This may require a second team to begin the vaginal reconstruction immediately following removal of the exenterative specimen.

Numerous methods of vaginal reconstruction performed initially or at an interval have been described (Table 7.15). While spontaneous epithelisation may occur, particularly in patients undergoing an anterior exenteration, it rarely results in a satisfactory vaginal vault.

Table 7.15 Methods described for vaginal reconstruction following exenteration

1. Spontaneous epithelialization
2. Split-thickness skin grafts
3. Sigmoid vaginostomy
4. Vulvovaginoplasty
5. Ileal vagina
6. Myocutaneous flaps
   a. Thigh pedicle
   b. Gluteal pedicle
7. Amnion grafts

Morley (1973) has reported satisfactory sexual function following the placement of split-thickness skin grafts performed as an interval procedure. Pregraft requirements include a good bed of granulation tissue. Care must be taken so as not to damage the gastro-intestinal tract during the second operation. Vulvovaginoplasty consists of the creation of a vaginal pouch constructed from vulvar or perineal tissue and can be performed at any time after exenteration. The resultant shallow vagina is usually in a vertical plane, requires a change in the coital position and in our experience has not been a satisfactory solution to this problem. Transposition of an ileal or sigmoid segment for use as a vaginal vault has been associated with an irritating discharge and pain and has been relegated to rare use as a method of reconstruction.

Pedicle flaps from the gluteal or thigh regions have been described and used during the past 10 years. Haemorrhage, infection, suture line breakdown and prolonged hospitalisation are potential complications. Becker's (1979) report that 95% were termed adequate for sexual function is promising despite the fact that patients with a neovagina are less orgasmic and only 65% of patients had subjectively normal sexual function.

Urinary tract and bowel complications

Long-term follow-up is important, not only to aid in psychological rehabilitation but to detect and treat the late complications of ultraradical surgery. The most common non-cancer-related indication for rehospitalisation is associated with problems in the urinary tract. especially pyelonephritis. While almost all urinary conduits are colonised with urinary pathogens, the exact significance of asymptomatic bacteriuria of the conduit is unknown. If pyelonephritis occurs repeatedly, the urinary tract should be investigated. As many as 10% of those patients rehospitalised will require revision of the urinary conduit stoma. Previously irradiated ileum is not infrequently associated with stomal stricture, leading to partial urinary obstruction.

Late unilateral ureteral obstruction or stricture, in the absence of infection or deteriorating renal function, does not necessarily require conduit revision. However, close observation and evaluation with renal scans, intravenous pyelography and serum creatinine is indicated. If deterioration of renal function is evident, the conduit should be revised.

Late non-cancer-related gastro-intestinal complications including colostomy prolapse that requires revision and small bowel obstruction occur in 10% to 15% of patients.

Observation for recurrence: long-term survival
Following exenteration, bimanual examination is difficult or impossible. Pelvic defect cytology is collected at each visit. Any unusual discharge or bleeding requires investigation, as the pelvis is the site of recurrence in over 50% of those who have recurrence. Recurrence following exenteration is associated with a mean survival of approximately 8 months.

NON-SURGICAL MANAGEMENT OF RECURRENCE

Radiation retreatment in patients with unresectable pelvic recurrence is rarely beneficial. Keettel (1968) summarised the information concerning re-irradiation for recurrent carcinoma of the cervix. That report indicated that 3% of re-irradiated patients were 5-year survivors. Brunschwig (1967) reported a 5.4% survival in 56 patients whose recurrence was treated with a second course of radiotherapy. Jones' (1970) report of patients who had failed orthovoltage radiation and were treated with maxitron or intracavitary application described little to no palliation and significant complications in patients who had early recurrent disease or persistent disease. This was particularly true of patients who had what he termed adequate initial therapy. The only patients who seemed to benefit were those with late recurrent disease (5 to 20 years) and only those who were retreated with intracavitary radium. Teletherapy was not beneficial. The extremely poor results and the risk of serious complications when utilising megavoltage radiation makes it impractical to use this method of treatment in previously irradiated patients with recurrent pelvic cancer. Intraoperative electron beam radiation as described by Goldson (1978) may prove beneficial in patients who have extrapelvic nodal spread without central pelvic recurrence or localised pelvic sidewall recurrence. Using an electron beam enables the delivery of a therapeutic dose of radiation to the lymphatic tissue without disturbing other organs. Intraoperative use allows for an accurate determination of small field size which can be visualised directly, avoiding the increased dosage to the normal structures, such as small bowel, bladder or rectum. If further studies are successful, this modality may benefit patients with localised nodal recurrences either in the pelvic sidewall or in the periaortic nodes.

Isolated pulmonary metastases may be resected with reasonable success; however pulmonary metastases are rarely isolated and treatment necessitates systemic therapy. Localised radiotherapy may be helpful in the palliative treatment of those patients with large nodal metastases obstructing the superior vena cava or the trachea. Bone metastases often respond favourably to palliative radiation with rapid relief of pain. The majority of intra-abdominal metastases are not reliably treated by radiation alone.

Central nervous system metastasis, although rare, can be palliated with whole-brain radiotherapy. Recent evidence indicates that short-time dose fractionisation schemes, i.e. 3000 rad in 2 weeks, or 2000 rad in 1 week, are as beneficial as protracted therapy, with less expense and inconvenience to the patient. Administration of steroids, which are thought to decrease cerebral oedema, probably increases the overall benefit and favours more rapid improvement.

Chemotherapy

Because the majority of patients with cervical cancer have early disease amenable to cure by either radical surgery or radical radiation therapy, the development of systemic chemotherapy has been slow. Previous radiotherapy has hampered the evaluation of chemotherapy, since pelvic fibrosis makes it extremely difficult to evaluate response rates objectively. It also decreases the blood supply thereby altering tumour perfusion and interferes with drug cycling by limiting bone marrow reserve. Additionally, pelvic recurrence may be associated with ureteral obstruction, with resultant impaired renal function and alteration of drug excretion. Few studies contain an adequate number of patients and often group patients with isolated distant metastases with those having pelvic and distant metastasis or those with advanced untreated disease. Regimens treating different histological types using different drug dosages and schedules make evaluation across drug trials difficult.

Little objective information is available on chemotherapeutic agents in the treatment of cervical cancer prior to 1976 (Table 7.16). Trials using drugs in different regimens would indicate that with the exception of Hydroxyurea, the response rates vary between 6% and 23%. These data can only be used to suggest drug activity, because they represent combined trials, often retrospective in which variable criteria for objective response and dosage were used. In general, single agent chemotherapy with these agents does not result in long-term benefit, as the average median duration of response was 4 to 6 months with little effect on survival.

Table 7.16 Single agent chemotherapy in cervical carcinoma prior to 1976 (modified from Thigpen 1981)

Drugs	Total patients		% Overall response
Alkylating	Cyclophosphamide	188	15
agents	Chlorambucil	44	25
	Melphalan	20	20
Anti-	5-Fluorouracil	140	21
metabolites	Methotrexate	77	16
Mitotic inhibitors	Vincristine	44	23
Antibiotics	Adriamycin	28	18
	Bleomycin	172	10
	Mitomycin C	18	22
	Porfiromycin	78	22
Other agents	Hexamethylmelamine	49	22
	Hydroxyurea	14	0
	6-Mercaptopurine	18	6
	Methyl CCNU	32	13
Totals		922	16.7

The Gynecologic Oncology Group (GOG) has attempted to identify new active agents in patients with recurrent or advanced squamous cell carcinoma through a systematic evaluation with defined tumour measurements and strict criteria for response (Table 7.17). Piperazinedione and cis-diamminodichloroplatinum (cis-platinum) have also been studied in non-squamous recurrent or advanced carcinoma of the cervix with respective response rates of 14% and 15%.

Table 7.17 Results of chemotherapy in GOG protocols of advanced or recurrent cervical squamous cell carcinoma (after Thigpen 1981)

Agent	No. of pts	% Response
Baker's antifol	32	16
Cis-platinum	34	38
Dianhydrogalactitol	36	19
ICRF-159	28	18
Maytansine	29	3
Piperazinedine	33	6
VP-16	30	0

The most promising single agent studied in recurrent squamous cell cancer is cis-platinum. Thigpen (1978) reported a phase 2 trial utilising 50 mg/m^2 dosage with acceptable toxicity and an objective response of 44%. Eleven per cent of patients were complete responders while 39% had stable disease. Although the overall response rates will probably decrease with widespread usage, this drug, when compared to other single agents, has a longer duration of response and improved survival.

Its activity is not confined to those patients with extrapelvic disease alone, as 43% of patients with extrapelvic disease and 33% of patients with isolated pelvic disease have an objective response. The GOG is currently studying different dose regimens to establish the presence or absence of a dose response curve.

In vitro chemotherapeutic testing has not had any predictive value in other tumours and few reports have determined its usefulness in cervical cancer. However, Cohen (1982) recently reported criteria for in vivo testing of cis-platinum. Preliminary results indicate that age, clinical stage and differentiation of the tumour do not influence the in vivo response to platinum; however, the in vivo response to a single dose may allow the physician to identify those who may benefit.

Attempts to prolong remission and increase survival rates have prompted the study of various regimens of combination chemotherapy. The most frequently used drugs are bleomycin, mitomycin C, methotrexate, cyclophosphamide, adriamycin and cis-diamminodichloroplatinum. The majority of studies involve small patient numbers with short follow-up, employ variable methods of assessment of response while utilising different doses and schedules and not allowing for comparison across studies (Table 7.18).

Miyamoto's (1978) report on a small group of patients treated with bleomycin and mitomycin C indicated a 93% response rate with 80% of patients being complete responders. However, follow-up studies have been unable to duplicate this work.

Other trials utilising mitomycin C, vincristine and bleomycin or combinations containing cis-platinum have indicated a markedly increased response frequency but to date all have failed to document the benefit of combination chemotherapy in terms of increased response duration or survival.

Theoretically, arterial infusion of chemotherapeutic drugs in recurrent cervical carcinoma should offer a distinct advantage in that higher concentration of the drug may perfuse the tumour. Unfortunately, to date reports utilising arterial infusion have not been encouraging. Morrow (1977) evaluated a continuous pelvic arterial infusion of bleomycin in 20 patients with recurrent and cervical cancer. Significant toxicity and little evidence of response was observed. Swenerton (1979) infused bleomycin, mitomycin C and vincristine with unfavourable results. Lifshitz (1978) reported a 21% rate of tumour regression in 14 patients treated with intra-arterial methotrexate and vincristine. Carlson (1981) reported a 33% response rate in patients treated with pelvic infusion of cis-platinum. Hiraoka (1980) has developed a technique for pelvic vascular bed isolation in an attempt to increase the local concentration of chemotherapy. Two patients treated with this technique utilising mitomycin C are long-term survivors.

Table 7.18 Results of combination chemotherapy in patients with advanced or recurrent cervical cancer

Author	Year	Regimen	No. of Pts	% Response
Forney	1975	CTX, ACT-D, 5-FU, VCR ARA C, MTX and BLEO	18	50
Bond	1976	ADR and BLEO	20	35
		ADR, MTX and VCR	21	48
Conroy	1976	BLEO and MTX	20	60
de Palo	1976	ADR and BLEO	15	20
		CTX and VCR	19	11
Greenberg	1977	ADR and BLEO	11	0
Haid	1977	ADR and MTX	16	12
Alberts	1978	ADR and CTX	10	10
Baker	1978	MIT-C, VCR and BLEO	115	41
Day	1978	ADR and MECCNU	31	45
Guthrie	1978	ADR and MTX	59	66
Miyamoto	1978	MIT-C and BLEO	15	93
Piver	1978	ADR and BLEO	16	6
		ADR, CTX and 5-FU	7	57
Slayton	1978	ADR and PLAT	19	32
Wallace	1978	ADR and VCR	54	17
Deka	1979	BLEO and MIT-C	20	40
Hakes	1979	MTX and VCR	29	17
Lira-Puerto	1979	BLEO, MTX and CTX	70	31
Rosenthal	1979	MTX (CF), VCR, BLEO and PLAT	7	57
Vogl	1979	MTX, BLEO and PLAT	9	89
Krebs	1980	BLEO and MIT-C	20	40
Leichman	1980	BLEO and MIT-C	19	16
Vogl	1980	MIT-C, VCR, BLEO and PLAT	13	77

ACT-D = Actinomycin D, ADR = Adriamycin, ARA-C = Cytosine arabinoside, BLEO = Bleomycin, CTX = Cyclophosphamide, 5-FU = 5 Fluorouracil, MECCNU = Methyl CCNU, MIT-C = Mitomycin C, MTX = Methotrexate, PLAT = cis-diamminedichloroplatinum, VCR = Vincristine

Alternative methods of therapeutic drug localisation utilising magnetically responsive drug-bearing microspheres have been tested in animals with some success and need further testing in humans. Chemoembolisation with sustained-release microcapsules may be beneficial in some of these patients.

Treatment of metabolic problems

Significant metabolic problems such as hypercalcaemia or uraemia are not uncommon in patients with recurrent cancer. Hypercalcaemia may be related to bone metastases or ectopic parahormone production. If the physician elects to treat this complication, initial therapy should consist of saline infusion with furosemide diuresis. Phosphate loading or steroid administration may be beneficial over the intermediate term. Calcitonin or mithramycin may be administered for long-term control. The incidence of uraemia with recurrent cancer is apparently decreasing as new radiotherapeutic regimens result in superior pelvic control. Katz (1980) recently reported a decreased incidence of uraemia from 28% to 7% over a 20-year interval. His autopsy studies suggested less extensive ureteral involvement. Over this period of observation the leading cause of death had changed from renal failure to such conditions as myocardial infarction, pulmonary thromboembolism, pneumonia, cachexia and sepsis.

The presence of ureteral obstruction, particularly if new, in patients with recurrent cervical cancer usually predicts recurrent tumour. In patients with histological confirmation of recurrence, there is no evidence that urinary diversion by conduit is beneficial as it is not associated with prolonged survival and patients often spend much of their remaining life in the hospital. However, if the stenosis is secondary to fibrosis and recurrence is not established, percutaneous nephrostomies on ureteral stents may allow recovery of renal function and time for further evaluation and consideration of permanent diversion (Fig. 7.9). Percutaneous stents may be placed without an anaesthetic and in experienced hands are associated with little morbidity.

Urinary fistulae, bowel fistulae or obstruction

Development of a late cancer-related urinary fistula is disconcerting to the patient and physician. Since simple nephrostomy diversion will not keep the patient dry, the question of a more permanent diversion by conduit should be considered. Although survival is short and morbidity and mortality is high, an occasional patient will benefit from construction of a urinary conduit. In general, only patients with a life expectancy of 4 months or more are considered for this procedure.

Cancer-related small intestinal obstruction or fistula may be relieved by a simple bypass procedure, often with significant palliation. Extensive resections are not indicated. However,because prior radiotherapy may render the ileocaecal valve incompetent, complete isolation of the fistula segment may be necessary to prevent reflux and continued fistulous drainage.

Rectovaginal fistulae may be palliated by colostomy; however utilisation of an elemental diet to effect a 'medical colostomy' might avoid the necessity for surgical intervention, especially in the near-terminal patient.

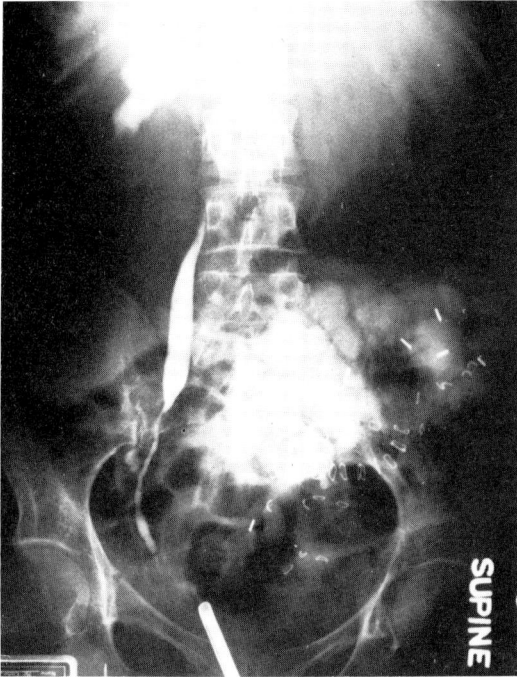

Fig. 7.9   A retrograde dye study of a 59-year-old woman demonstrating lower ureteral constriction. The contralateral kidney had no function. Intraoperative evaluation failed to demonstrate recurrent cancer and she was successfully diverted with a transverse colon conduit.

Haemorrhage

Pelvic haemorrhage is a frightening experience. If present in patients with recurrent cancer, a surgical approach is not the first line of therapy. Hypogastric artery ligation is difficult, usually morbid and rarely necessary with the advent of arterial embolisation. The decreased vascular resistance that occurs with haemorrhage results in preferential blood flow to bleeding sites and allows gelfoam or steel coil embolisation. It is important to use arteriography to identify all vessels which may contribute to pelvic bleeding as frequently vessels other than those originating from the hypogastric vessels are involved.

PAIN CONTROL — MEDICAL

Control of acute and chronic debilitating pain associated with recurrent cancer is a most difficult problem for the oncologist. Only after consideration of its location, mechanism, extent of the causative disease, the physical and mental condition of the patient and availability and practicality of the various methods of pain relief can appropriate therapy be selected. The cause of cancer-related pain is usually

Table 7.19 Aetiology of cancer-related pain

1. Compression of nerve root, trunk or plexus by tumour or tumour-related injury (i.e. fracture)
2. Tumour infiltration of nerves or blood vessels
3. Obstruction of a hollow viscus
4. Vascular occlusion by tumour with venous engorgement or arterial ischaemia
5. Infiltration and tumefaction of tissue tightly invested by fascia or other pain-sensitive structures
6. Tumour-related necrosis, infection and inflammation of pain-sensitive structures

multifactorial (Table 7.19). Careful evaluation of pain and utilisation of non-analgesic regimens such as radiation therapy for bone metastases, antibiotics for infections, agents to treat gout, surgical procedures for bowel or ureteral obstruction and chemotherapy trials are appropriate. A particular problem of lower extremity pain and oedema should be mentioned. Many would consider this problem related to lymphatic obstruction; however these patients may have primary or secondary venous thrombosis (Fig. 7.10) and are symptomatically relieved following systemic heparinisation. If no reversible component is present, then it becomes necessary to prescribe alternative analgesia (Table 7.20). It is generally agreed that the least potent analgesic agent capable of producing adequate relief should be used initially. The

Table 7.20

Mechanisms of interference with pain	Drug type
Reversal of specific pathophysiological event such as inflammation	Anti-inflammatory agents
Interference with specific chemical substance involved in pain reception peripherally	Antipyretic analgesics
Interference with conduction of pain away from affected site	Local anaesthetics
Interference with central nervous system perception of pain and development of affected responses	Narcotic analgesics
Interference with anxiety, tension or depression	Sedatives and hypnotics Phenothiazine Tranquilizers Skeletal muscle relaxants Antidepressants
Interference with consciousness	Anaesthetics

Fig. 7.10 A 53-year-old woman with pelvic recurrence had extensive right unilateral leg oedema and hip pain. A venogram demonstrated total occlusion of the venous system. She improved dramatically following 5 d of systemic anticoagulation.

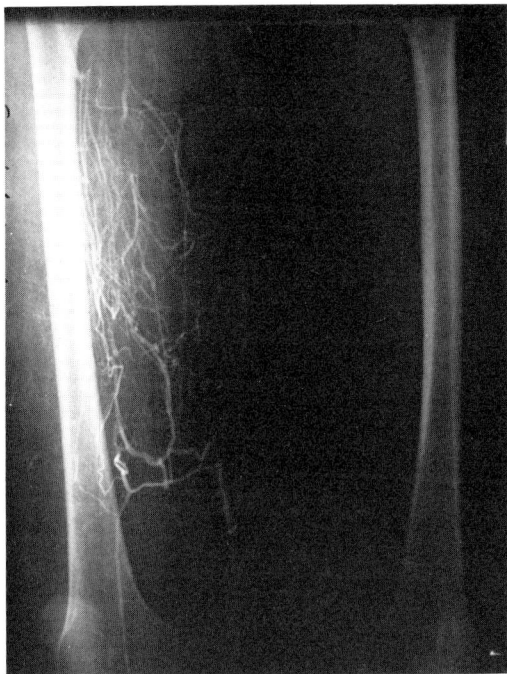

A

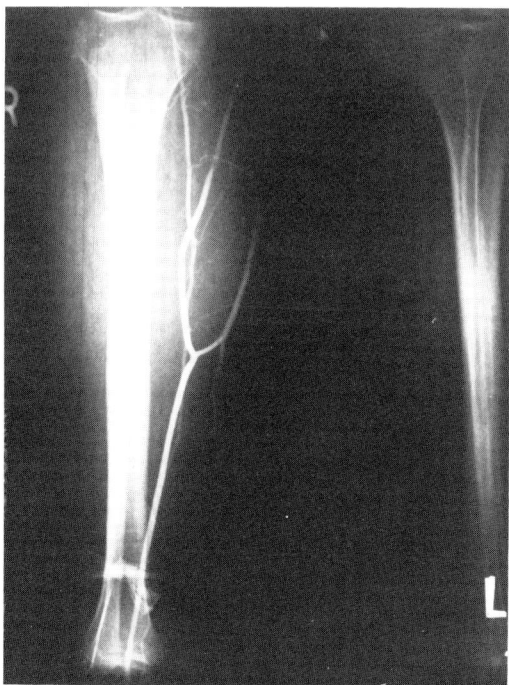

B

efficacy of narcotic analgesics for severe cancer-related pain is documented. However, premature use can result in early development of tolerance and the necessity of massive dosages to relieve pain in the later stages of disease. Aspirin results in significant relief of pain when compared to placebo and is often used initially in those patients with mild to moderate pain. Other single agents including acetominophen, codeine, mefenamic acid, pentazocine and phenacetin are superior to placebo and are used to treat mild to moderate cancer pain. Utilising a combination of drugs with different mechanisms of pain relief is the next logical regimen in patients whose pain is inadequately relieved by a single agent. Moertel (1971) has reported that drugs equianalgesic to aspirin provide superior relief for mild to moderate pain when combined with aspirin (Table 7.21).

Table 7.21 Analgesic combinations used for pain relief (after Moertel 1972)

Combinations superior to aspirin alone (mg)

   Codeine (65) + Aspirin (650)
   Oxycodone (9.75) + Aspirin (650)
   Pentazocine (25) + Aspirin (650)

Combinations *not* superior to aspirin alone (mg)

Caffeine (65)	+ Aspirin (650)
Ethoheptazine (75)	+ Aspirin (650)
Pentabarbital (32)	+ Aspirin (650)
Promazine HCl (25)	+ Aspirin (650)
Propoxyphene napsylate (100)	+ Aspirin (650)

Narcotic analgesia may be necessary for patients with intolerance to aspirin as well as for patients with severe pain. Numerous drugs with different potency, onset and duration of analgesia and side effects are available in parenteral, oral or suppository form (Table 7.22). The opioid analgesics all act centrally to relieve pain and most are less potent on a milligram for milligram dosage when given orally.

Fear of addiction and inadequate information about optimal dosage and interval often result in underprescribing pain medication. Narcotic analgesics should be offered on a regular basis, and not given 'as necessary'. This regimen not only relieves pain but reassures the patient by giving her confidence in her physician, thereby lowering the total analgesic dose by alleviating anxiety and apprehension.

The potential side effects of respiratory depression from the drugs' direct effect on the chemoreceptors of the central nervous system, the depression of the cough reflex, nausea and vomiting, decreased secretions and resulting constipation, increased smooth muscle tone of the urinary tract resulting in urinary difficulties and orthostatic

Table 7.22 Characteristics of narcotic analgesics commonly used for cancer pain relief

Analgesic	Equianalgesic milligram dose (morphine 10 mg IM)		Oral: parenteral potency	Onset of analgesia (min)	Duration of analgesia (h)	Contrasted to morphine
	IM	PO				
Morphine	10	60	0.17	30–60 (IM)	7	–
Oxymorphine (Numorphone®)	1	6	0.17	10–15 (IM)	3–6	Rapid onset; available in rectal suppository
Hydromorphone (Dilaudid®)	1.5	8	0.20	15–20 (IM or PO)	4–5	Short-acting
Levorphanol (Leov-Dromovan®)	2	4	0.50	60–90 (IM or PO)	6–8	Long-acting; high oral potency
Butorphanol (Stadol®)	2		–	30–60 (IM)	4	Nalorphine-like antagonistic properties
Heroin	5	30	0.17	–	5	Short-acting; illegal in the United States
Methadone	10	20	0.5	30–60 (IM or PO)	4–6	High oral potency
Nalbuphine (Nubain®)	10		–	15 (IM)	3–6	Rapid onset; nalorphine-like antagonistic properties
Oxycodone (Percodan®, Percoset®)	15	30	0.5	10–15 (PO)	3–6	Rapid onset; high oral potency
Alphaprodine (Nisentil®)	45		–	1–2 (IV)	0.5–1	Rapid acting; short onset
Anileridine (Heritine®)	30	50	0.6	15 (IM or PO)		Rapid onset; short acting, high oral potency
Pentazocine (Tacwin®)	60	180	0.3	20 (IM)	3	Shorter acting nalorphine-like antagonistic properties
Meperidine (Demerol®)	75	300	0.25	30–50 (IM) 40–60 (PO)	2–4	Shorter acting
Codeine	130	200	0.65	15–30 (IM or PO)	4–6	High oral potency

hypotension should be kept in mind when prescribing narcotic analgesics. Tolerance to these side effects parallels tolerance to the analgesic effects, therefore increased drug dosage to keep pace with the patient's analgesic needs carries little risk of increased toxicity.

Oral or parenteral analgesia should be adequate to control pain without interfering with the patient's mental acuity and social usefulness as long as possible. When possible, the oral or suppository route is preferable to parenteral medication, although the majority of narcotics are less potent and have more variable analgesic effects when given orally. While codeine, oxycodone and methadone have high oral to parenteral potency, continued increased dosage often results in intolerable side effects.

Brompton's cocktail, containing morphine, cocaine, alcohol, syrup flavouring and chloroform, is gaining acceptance as an oral medication allowing pain relief without undue side effects or drug dependence. Solutions without cocaine may be as effective.

Fear, apprehension, anxiety and depression accentuate cancer pain. Analgesic adjuvants such as anxiolytics or antidepressants may benefit selected patients. However these drugs have a lower potential than narcotics for controlling severe pain without producing undesired side effects. Phenothiazine derivatives when given with narcotics may produce more sedation and mental confusion than analgesia; additionally, the anticholergic and sympathomimetic effects of the tricyclic antidepressants may result in restlessness, confusion, urinary retention and visual disturbances when administered to elderly or debilitated patients.

The discovery of endogenous morphine-like polypeptides (endorphins and enkephalins) within the central nervous system holds great promise for pain control at a more fundamental level with fewer side effects and complications.

Surgical pain control

Depending on the phase of disease, life expectancy and cause of pain, there may be a place for a neurosurgical procedure for those patients whose pain is uncontrolled by conventional medical methods. Although judgment is necessary to justify postoperative morbidity and mortality, these procedures are rarely performed if expected survival is less than 3 months. Dorsal rhizotomy (sectioning of the sensory nerve roots to interrupt afferent pain fibres) may be useful when pain is localised to the sacral or perineal area. Bilateral sacral rhizotomies carry little morbidity if the sacral roots S_2 and S_3 are preserved on one side so as to prevent urinary incontinence in patients with intact bladders. Commissural myelotomy (interruption of crossing spinothalamic tracts) may also benefit those patients with sacral pain. Dysaesthesias and posterior column deficits following the procedure are transient, with satisfactory pain relief in greater than 80% of patients. Urinary incontinence and motor weakness are rare. Percutaneous cervical cordotomy is successful in more than 85% of patients; bilateral destruction of the spinothalamic tract, however, carries a significant risk of lower extremity paralysis or urinary incontinence. A phenol subarachnoid block may relieve pain in many patients with a short (less than 3-month) life expectancy.

BIBLIOGRAPHY

Adcock L L 1979 Radical hysterectomy preceded by pelvic irradiation. Gynecologic Oncology 8: 152–163
Alberts D S, Ignoffo R 1978 Adriamycin-cyclophosphamide treatment of squamous cell carcinoma of the cervix. Cancer Treatment Reports 62: 143–144
Badib A O, Kurohara S S, Webster J H, Pickren J W 1968 Metastasis to organs in carcinoma of the uterine cervix Cancer 21: 434–439
Baker L H, Opipari M I, Wilson H, Bottomley R, Coltman C A Jr 1978 Mitomycin C, vincristine and bleomycin therapy for advanced cervical cancer. Obstetrics and Gynecology 52: 146–150
Barber H R K 1969 Relative prognostic significance of preoperative and operative findings in pelvic exenteration. Surgical Clinics of North America 49: 431–447
Barber H R K, Brunschwig A 1966 Urinary tract fistulas following pelvic exenteration. Obstetrics and Gynecology 28: 754–763
Barber H R K, Brunschwig A 1967 Excision of major blood vessels at the periphery of the pelvis in patients receiving pelvic exenteration: common and/or iliac arteries and veins. Surgery 62: 426–430
Barber H R K, Jones W 1971 Lymphadenectomy in pelvic exenteration for recurrent cervix cancer. Journal of the American Medical Association 215 (12) 1945–1950
Becker D W Jr, Massey F M, McCraw J B 1979 Musculocutaneous flaps in reconstructive pelvic surgery. Obstetrics and Gynecology 54: 178–183
Bjornstahl H, Johnsson J E, Lindberg L G 1977 Hysterectomy in central recurrence of carcinoma of the uterine cervix. Acta obstetrica et gynecologica scandinavica 56: 227–231
Blythe J G, Ptacek J J, Buchsbaum H J, Latourette H B 1975 Bony metastases from carcinoma of the cervix. Cancer 36: 475–484
Bond W H, Arthur K, Banks A J, Freeman W E, Holme G M, Newsholme G A et al 1976 Combination chemotherapy in the treatment of advanced squamous cell carcinoma of the cervix. Clinical Oncology 2: 173–178
Borgelt B, Gelber R, Kramer S, Brady L W, Chang C H, Davis L W et al 1980 The palliation of brain metastases: final results of the first two studies by the radiation therapy oncology group. International Journal of Radiation Oncology, Biology, Physics 6: 1–9
Brascho D J 1980 Gynecologic malignancy. In: Brascho D J, Shawker T H (eds) Abdominal ultrasound in the cancer patient. John Wiley, New York p 209–245
Bricker E M 1980 Current status of urinary diversion. Cancer 45: 2986–2991
Brin E N, Schiff J Jr, Weiss R M 1975 Palliative urinary diversion for pelvic malignancy. Journal of Urology 113: 619–622
Brown R S, Haddox V, Posada A, Rubio A 1972 Social and psychological adjustment following pelvic exenteration. American Journal of Obstetrics and Gynecology 114: 162–171

Brunschwig A 1967 Surgical treatment of carcinoma of the cervix, recurrent after irradiation or combination of irradiation and surgery. American Journal of Roentgenology 99: 365–370

Brunschwig A, Barber H R K 1964 Extended pelvic exenteration for advanced cancer of the cervix; long survivals following added resection of involved small bowel. Cancer (October): 1267–1270

Butcher H R Jr, Sugg W L, McAfee C A, Bricker E M 1962 Ileal conduit method of ureteral urinary diversion. Annals of Surgery (October): 682–691

Carlson J A Jr, Freedman R S, Wallace S, Chuang V P, Wharton J T, Rutledge F N 1981 Intra-arterial cis-platinum in the management of squamous cell carcinoma of the uterine cervix. Gynecologic Oncology 12: 92–98

Catalano R B 1975 The medical approach to management of pain caused by cancer. Seminars in Oncology 2: 379–392

Chen S S, Kumari S, Lee L 1980 Contribution of abdominal computed tomography (CT) in the management of gynecologic cancer: correlated study of CT image and gross surgical pathology. Gynecologic Oncology 10: 162–172

Clark D G C, Daniel W W, Brunschwig A 1962 Intestinal fistulas following pelvic exenteration. American Journal of Obstetrics and Gynecology 84: 187–191

Cohen C J, Deppe G, Yannopoulos K, Gusberg S B 1982 Chemosensitivity testing with cis-platinum (II) diamminedichloride. 1. A new concept in the treatment of carcinoma of the cervix. Gynecologic Oncology 13: 1–9

Collins J A 1974 Problems associated with the massive transfusion of stored blood. Surgery 75: 274–295

Conroy J F, Lewis G C, Brady L W, Brodsky I, Kahn S B, Ross D et al 1976 Low dose bleomycin and methotrexate in cervical cancer. Cancer 37: 660–664

Copeland E M 1978 Intravenous hyperalimentation as an adjunct to cancer patient management. CA — A Cancer Journal for Clinicians 28: 322–330

Creasman W T, Rutledge F 1972 Preoperative evaluation of patients with recurrent carcinoma of the cervix. Gynecologic Oncology 1: 111–118

Creasman W T, Rutledge F 1974 Is positive pelvic lymphadenopathy a contraindication to radical surgery in recurrent cervical carcinoma? Gynecologic Oncology 2: 482–485

Cruse P J, Foord R 1980 The epidemiology of wound infection. A 10-year prospective study of 62 939 wounds. Surgical Clinics of North America 60: 27–47

Day T G Jr, Wharton J T, Gottlieb J A, Rutledge F N 1978 Chemotherapy for squamous carcinoma of the cervix: doxorubicin-methyl-CCNA. American Journal of Obstetrics and Gynecology 132: 545–548

Deckers P J, Olsson C, Williams L A, Mozden P J 1976 Pelvic exenteration as palliation of malignant disease. American Journal of Surgery 131: 509–515

Deckers P J, Sugarbaker E V, Pilch Y H, Ketcham A S 1972 Pelvic exenteration for late second cancers of the uterine cervix after earlier irradiation. Annals of Surgery 175: 48–54

Deka A C, Deka B C, Patil R B, Joshi S G 1979 Chemotherapy in recurrent or metastatic cervical cancer. Indian Journal of Cancer 16: 32–37

Delgado G 1980 Use of the automatic stapler in urinary conduit diversions and pelvic exenterations. Gynecologic Oncology 10: 93–97

Dempsey G M, Buchsbaum H J, Morrison J 1975 Psychosocial adjustment to pelvic exenteration. Gynecologic Oncology 3: 325–334

dePalo G M, Bajetta E, Beretta G, Bonadonna G 1976 Adriamycin plus bleomycin versus cyclophosphamide plus vincristine in advanced carcinoma of the uterine cervix. Tumori 62: 113–122

Deppe G, Cohen C J, Yannopoulos K, Gusberg S B 1982 Chemosensitivity testing with cis-platinum (II) diamminedichloride. II. Preliminary experience in the treatment of carcinoma of the cervix. Gynecologic Oncology 13: 10–18

Deutsch M, Parsons J A 1974 Radiotherapy for carcinoma of the cervix recurrent after surgery. Cancer 34: 2051–2055

Devereux D G, Sears H G, Ketcham A S 1980 Intestinal fistula following pelvic exenterative surgery: predisposing causes and treatment. Journal of Surgery and Oncology 14: 227–234

Dunn L J, Van Voorhis L W 1967 Enigmatic fever and pelvic thrombophlebitis. Response to anticoagulants. New England Journal of Medicine 276: 265–268

Evans S R Jr, Hilaris B S, Barber H R K 1971 External vs. interstitial irradiation in unresectable recurrent cancer of the cervix. Cancer 28: 1284–1288

Fallon R H 1962 Obstruction of the small intestine after pelvic exenteration: a preliminary evaluation of its prevention by small intestinal intubation. Surgery 51: 423–442

Forney J P, Morrow C P, DiSaia P J, Futoran R J 1975 Seven-drug polychemotherapy in the treatment of advanced and recurrent squamous carcinoma of the female genital tract. American Journal of Obstetrics and Gynecology 123: 748–752

Galante M, Hill E C 1971 Pelvic exenteration: a critical analysis of a ten-year experience with the use of the team approach. American Journal of Obstetrics and Gynecology (May 15): 180–187

Ginaldi S, Wallace S, Jing B-S, Bernardino M E 1981 Carcinoma of the cervix: lymphangiography and computed tomography. American Journal of Roentgenology 136: 1087–1091

Girtanner R E, DeCampo T, Alleyn J N, Averette H E 1981 Routine intensive care for pelvic exenterative operations. Surgery, Gynecology and Obstetrics 153: 657–659

Glover D D, Lowry T F, Jacknowitz A I 1980 Brompton's mixture in alleviating pain of terminal neoplastic disease: preliminary results. Southern Medical Journal 73: 278–282

Goldson A L, Delgado G, Hill L T 1978 Intraoperative radiation of the para-aortic nodes in cancer of the uterine cervix. Obstetrics and Gynecology 52: 713–717

Greenberg B R, Kardinal C G, Pajak T F, Bateman J R 1977 Adriamycin versus adriamycin and bleomycin in advanced epidermoid carcinoma of the cervix. Cancer Treatment Reports 61: 1383–1384

Guthrie D, Way S 1978 The use of adriamycin and methotrexate in carcinoma of the cervix. Obstetrics and Gynecology 52: 349–354

Haas T, Buchsbaum H J, Lifshitz S 1980 Nonresectable recurrent pelvic neoplasm; outcome in patients explored for pelvic exenteration. Gynecologic Oncology 9: 177–181

Haid M, Homesley H, White D R et al 1977 Adriamycin-methotrexate combination chemotherapy of advanced carcinoma of the cervix. Obstetrics and Gynecology 50: 103–105

Hakes T, Nikrui M, MaGill G, Ochoa M 1979 Cervix cancer. Treatment with combination vincristine and high doses of methotrexate. Cancer 43: 459–464

Han S Y, Laws H L, Aldrete J S 1979 How and when to use barium for diagnosis of small bowel obstruction. Southern Medical Journal 72: 1519–1523

Hiraoka O, Nakai T, Shimizu C 1980 Modified pelvic vascular bed isolation chemotherapy: theoretical basis, surgical procedure and two clinical case reports. Gynecologic Oncology 9: 135–152

Hoeg J M, Slatopolsky E 1980 Cervical carcinoma and ectopic hyperparathyroidism. Archives of Internal Medicine 140: 569–571

Hoover H C Jr, Ryan J A, Anderson E J, Fischer J E 1980 Nutritional benefits of immediate postoperative jejunal feeding of an elemental diet. American Journal of Surgery 139: 153–159

Houde R W 1980a The rational use of narcotic analgesics for controlling cancer pain. Drug Therapy (July): 41–47

Houde R W 1980b Non-narcotic alternatives for controlling cancer pain. Drug Therapy (August): 47–50

Hoye R C, Bennett S H, Geelhoed G W, Gorschboth C 1972 Fluid volume and albumin kinetics occurring with major surgery. Journal of the American Medical Association 222: 1255–1261

Ingersoll F M, Ulfelder H 1966 Pelvic exenteration for carcinoma of the cervix. New England Journal of Medicine 274: 648–651

Inguilla W, Cosmi E V 1967 Pelvic exenteration for advanced carcinoma of the cervix. American Journal of Obstetrics and Gynecology 99: 1083–1086

Issell B F, Valdivieso M, Zaren H A, Dudrick S J, Freireich E J, Copeland E W et al 1978 Protection against chemotherapy toxicity by IV hyperalimentation. Cancer Treatment Reports 62: 1139–1143

Jaffe B M, Bricker E M, Butcher H R Jr 1968 Surgical complications of ileal segment urinary diversion. Annals of Surgery 167: 367–376

Jones M A, Breckman B, Hendry W F 1980 Life with an ileal conduit; results of questionnaire surveys of patients and urological surgeons. British Journal of Urology 52: 21–25

Jones T K Jr, Levitt S H, King E R 1970 Retreatment of persistent and recurrent carcinoma of the cervix with irradiation. Radiology 95: 167–174

Judd E S 1975 Preoperative neomycin-tetracycline preparation of the colon for elective operations. Surgical Clinics of North America 55: 1325–1330

Karlen J R, Piver M S 1975 Reduction of mortality and morbidity associated with pelvic exenteration. Gynecologic Oncology 3: 154–167

Kato T, Nemoto R, Mori H et al 1981 Arterial chemoembolization with microencapsulated anticancer drug. Journal of the American Medical Association 245: 1123–1127

Katz H J, Davies J N P 1980 Death from cervic uteri carcinoma: the changing pattern. Gynecologic Oncology 9: 86–89

Keettel W C, Van Voorhis L W, Latourette H B 1968 Management of recurrent carcinoma of the cervix. American Journal of Obstetrics and Gynecology 102: 671–679

Ketcham A S, Chretien P B, Hoye R C, Harrah J D, Deckers P J, Sugarbaker E V et al 1973 Occult metastases to the scalene lymph nodes in patients with clinically operable carcinoma of the cervix. Cancer 31: 180–183

Ketcham A S, Deckers P J, Sugarbaker E V, Hoye R C, Thomas L B, Smith R R 1970 Pelvic exenteration for carcinoma of the uterine cervix, a 15-year experience. Cancer 26: 513–521

Kiselow M, Butcher H R Jr, Bricker E M 1967 Results of the radical surgical treatment of advanced pelvic cancer: a fifteen-year study. Annals of Surgery 166: 428–434

Kottmeier H L 1954 In: Meigs J (ed) The surgical treatment of cancer of the cervix. Grune and Stratton, New York

Krebs H-B, Girtanner R E, Nordquist R B, Mineau I, Helmkamp B F, Averette H E 1980 Treatment of advanced cervical cancer by combination of bleomycin and mitomycin-C. Cancer 46: 2159–2161

Lagasse L D, Johnson G H, McClure L S, Nasr M F, Byron R, Moore J G 1973 Use of sigmoid colon for rectal substitution following pelvic exenteration. American Journal of Obstetrics and Gynecology 116: 106–110

Lee R B, Weisbaum G S, Heller P B, Park R C 1981 Scalene node biopsy in primary and recurrent invasive carcinoma of the cervix. Gynecologic Oncology 11: 200–206

Leichman L P, Baker L H, Stanhope C R, Samson M K, Fraile R J, Vaitkevicius V K et al 1980 Mitomycin C and bleomycin in the treatment of far-advanced cervical cancer: a Southwest Oncology Group pilot study. Cancer Treatment Reports 64: 1139–1140 (abstract)

Lifshitz S, Debacker L J, Buchsbaum H J 1976 Subarachnoid phenol block for pain relief in gynecologic malignancy. Obstetrics and Gynecology 48: 316–320

Lifshitz S, Railsback L D, Buchsbaum H J 1978 Intra-arterial pelvic infusion chemotherapy in advanced gynecologic cancer. Obstetrics and Gynecology 52: 476–480

Lira-Puerto V M, Hidalgo I N, Morales F R, Tenorio F 1979 Bleomycin, methotrexate and cyclophosphamide in advanced squamous cell carcinoma of the uterine cervix. Proceedings of the American Society of Clinical Oncologists 20: 319

Llorens A S 1980 Chemotherapy of squamous cell carcinoma of the cervix. Obstetrics and Gynecology 55: 373–378

Long D M 1980 Relief of cancer pain by surgical and nerve blocking procedures. Journal of the American Medical Association 244: 2759–2761

Magrina J F, Masterson B J 1981 Vaginal reconstruction in gynecological oncology: a review of techniques. Obstetrical and Gynecological Survey 36: 1–9

Magrina J F, Symmonds R E, Leary F J 1979 Intentional ureteral ligation in advanced pelvic malignant disease. Obstetrics and Gynecology 53: 685–688

Mann W J Jr, Jander H P, Orr J W Jr, Taylor P T, Hatch K D, Shingleton H M 1980 The use of percutaneous nephrostomy in gynecologic oncology. Gynecologic Oncology 10: 343–349

Mann W J, Jander H P, Partridge E E, Russinovich N, Hatch K D, Taylor P T et al 1980 Selective arterial embolization for control of bleeding in gynecologic malignancy. Gynecologic Oncology 10: 279–289

Mattingly R F 1967 Indications, contraindications and method of total pelvic exenteration. Oncology 21: 241–259

Melzack R, Mount B M, Gordon J M 1979 The Brompton mixture versus morphine solution given orally: effects on pain. Canadian Medical Association Journal 120: 435–438

Meyer J E, Yatsuhashi M, Green T H Jr 1980 Palliative urinary diversion in patients with advanced pelvic malignancy. Cancer 45: 2698–2701

Miyamoto T, Takabe Y, Watanabe M, Terasima T 1978 Effectiveness of a sequential combination of bleomycin and mitomycin-C on an advanced cervical cancer. Cancer 41: 403–414

Moertel C G, Ahmann D L, Taylor W F et al 1972a Relief of pain by oral medication: a controlled evaluation of analgesic combinations. Journal of the American Medical Association 229: 55–59

Moertel C G, Ahmann D L, Taylor W F et al 1972b A comparative evaluation of marketed analgesic drugs. New England Journal of Medicine 286: 813–815

Morgan L S, Daly J W, Monif G R G 1980 Infectious morbidity associated with pelvic exenteration. Gynecologic Oncology 10: 318–328

Morley G W, Lindenauer S M 1976 Pelvic exenterative therapy for gynecologic malignancy; an analysis of 70 cases. Cancer 38: 581–586

Morley G W, Lindenauer S M, Youngs D 1973 Vaginal reconstruction following pelvic exenteration: surgical and psychological considerations. American Journal of Obstetrics and Gynecology 116: 996–1002

Morrow C P, DiSaia P J, Mangan C F et al 1977 Continuous pelvic arterial infusion with bleomycin for squamous cell carcinoma of the cervix recurrent after radiation therapy. Cancer Treatment Reports 61: 1403–1405

Morrow C P, Hernandez W L, Townsend D E, DiSaia P J 1977 Pelvic celiotomy in the obese patient. American Journal of Obstetrics and Gynecology 127: 335–339

Moss G 1981 Maintenance of gastrointestinal function after bowel surgery and immediate enteral full nutrition. II. Clinical experience, with objective demonstration of intestinal absorption and motility. Journal of Parenteral and Enteral Nutrition 5: 215–220

Mountain C F 1970 Surgical management of pulmonary metastases. Postgraudate Medicine 48: 128–132

Mullen J L, Buzby G P 1980 Nutritional assessment of the hospitalized patient — Why bother? Drug Therapy (August): 33–42

van Nagell J R Jr, Rayburn W, Donaldson E S, Hanson M, Gay E C, Yoneda J et al 1979 Therapeutic implications of patterns of recurrence in cancer of the uterine cervix. Cancer 44: 2354–2361

Nelson J H Jr 1969 Atlas of radical pelvic surgery. Appleton-Century-Crofts, New York, p 181–191

O'Leary J A, Symmonds R E 1966 Radical pelvic operations in the geriatric patient: a 15-year review of 133 cases. Obstetrics and Gynecology 28: 745–753

Orr J W Jr, Shingleton H M, Hatch K D, Taylor P T, Austin J M Jr, Partridge E E et al 1982 Urinary diversion in patients undergoing pelvic exenteration. American Journal of Obstetrics and Gynecology 142: 883–889

Orr J W, Shingleton H M, Hatch K D, Taylor P T, Partridge E E, Soong S-J 1982 Gastrointestinal complications associated with pelvic exenteration. American Journal of Obstetrics and Gynecology, in press

Papavasilion C, Angelakir P, Gouvalir P, Papakyriades L 1969 Treatment of cervical carcinoma by methotrexate combined with cyclophosphamide. Cancer Chemotherapy Reports 53: 255–261

Parker T H, O'Leary J P 1978 Effect of preparation of the small intestine on microflora and postoperative wound infection. Surgery, Gynecology and Obstetrics 146: 379–382

Partridge E E, Beasley W E, Holcomb C, Hatch K D, Shingleton H M, Austin M Jr 1979 The Swan-Ganz catheter and management of patients undergoing pelvic exenteration. Obstetrics and Gynecology 53: 253–255

Paunier J-P, Delclos L, Fletcher G H 1967 Causes, time of death, and sites of failure in squamous cell carcinoma of the uterine cervix on intact uterus. Radiology 88: 555–562

Perez-Mesa C, Spratt J S Jr 1976 Scalene node biopsy in the pretreatment staging of carcinoma of the cervix uteri. American Journal of Obstetrics and Gynecology 125: 93–95

Petrilli E S, Castaldo T W, Ballon S C, Roberts J A, Lagasse L D 1980 Bleomycin-mitomycin C therapy for advanced squamous carcinoma of the cervix. Gynecologic Oncology 9: 292–297

Photopulos G J, Delgado G, Fowler W C Jr, Walton L A 1979 Intestinal anastomoses after radiation therapy by surgical stapling instruments. Obstetrics and Gynecology 54: 515–518

Pierson R L, Figge P K, Buchsbaum H J 1975 Surgery for gynecologic malignancy in the aged. Obstetrics and Gynecology 46: 523–527

Piver M S, Barlow J J 1973 Para-aortic lymphadenectomy, aortic node biopsy, and aortic lymphangiography in staging patients with advanced cervical cancer. Cancer 32: 367–370

Piver M S, Lele S 1976 Enterovaginal and enterocutaneous fistulae in women with gynecologic malignancies. Obstetrics and Gynecology 48: 560–563

Piver M S, Barlow J J, Xynos F P 1978 Adriamycin alone or in combination in 100 patients with carcinoma of the cervix or vagina. American Journal of Obstetrics and Gynecology 131: 311–313

Powers J C, Fitzgerald J F, McAlvanah M J 1976 The anatomic basis for the surgical detachment of the greater omentum from the transverse colon. Surgery, Gynecology and Obstetrics 143: 105–106

Prudden J F 1971 Psychological problems following ileostomy and colostomy. Cancer 28: 236–238

Quindlen E A 1982 Management of pain: neurosurgical approaches. In: DeVita D T Jr, Hellman S, Rosenberg S A (eds) Cancer — principles and practice of oncology. J B Lippincott, Philadelphia

Rafla S 1971 Major surgery after radical radiotherapy. Cancer 27: 314–322

Roddick J W, Miller D H 1968 Factors affecting the management of recurrent cervical carcinoma. American Journal of Obstetrics and Gynecology 101: 53–57

Rosenthal C J, Platica O, Khulpatua N, Boyce J, Alfonso A 1979 Effective combination chemotherapy in advanced squamous cell carcinoma. Proceedings of the American Society of Clinical Oncologists 20: 371

Rutledge F N, Fletcher G H 1958 Transperitoneal pelvic lymphadenectomy following supervoltage irradiation for squamous-cell carcinoma of the cervix. American Journal of Obstetrics and Gynecology 76: 321–334

Rutledge F N, Fletcher G H, MacDonald E J 1965 Pelvic lymphadenectomy as an adjunct to radiation therapy in treatment for cancer of the cervix. American Journal of Roentgenology 93: 607–614

Rutledge F N, Smith J P, Wharton J T, O'Quinn A G 1977 Pelvic exenteration: analysis of 29 patients. American Journal of Obstetrics and Gynecology 129: 881–892

Scardino P T, Bagley DH, Javadpour N, Ketcham A S 1975 Sigmoid conduit urinary diversion. Urology VI: 167–171

Schellhas H F, Fidler J P 1975 Vaginal reconstruction after total pelvic exenteration using a modification of the Williams' procedure. Gynecologic Oncology 3: 21–31

Schlesinger R E, Berman M L, Ballon S C, Lagasse L D, Watring W G, Futoran R J et al 1979 The choice of an intestinal segment for a urinary conduit. Surgery, Gynecology and Obstetrics 148: 45–48

Schmidt J E, Buchsbaum H J, Jacobs E C 1976 Transverse colon conduit for supravesical urinary tract diversion. Urology 8: 542–546

Schmidt J E, Hawtrey C E, Buchsbaum H J 1975 Transverse colon conduit: a preferred method of urinary diversion for radiation-treated pelvic malignancies. Journal of Urology 113: 308–313

Schoenberg H W, Mikuta J J 1973 Technique for preventing urinary fistulas following pelvic exenteration and uretero-ileostomy. Journal of Urology 110: 294–295

Schwartz P E, Goldstein H M, Wallace S, Rutledge F N 1975 Control of arterial hemorrhage using percutaneous arterial catheter techniques in patients with gynecologic malignancies. Gynecologic Oncology 3: 276–288

Segaloff A 1981 Managing endocrine and metabolic problems in the patient with advanced cancer. Journal of the American Medical Association 245: 177–179

Sinclair R H, Pratt J H 1972 Femoral neuropathy after pelvic operation. American Journal of Obstetrics and Gynecology (February) 112: 404–407

Slayton R E, Mladineo J P, DiSaia P 1978 Adriamycin and cis-diamminedichloro-platinum (DDP) and recurrent and metastatic squamous cell carcinoma of the cervix. Proceedings of the American Society of Clinical Oncologists 19: 335

Sohmer P R, Dawson R B 1979 Transfusion therapy in trauma: A review of the principles and techniques used in the MIEMS program. American Surgery (February): 109–125

Steffee W P 1980 Malnutrition in hospitalized patients. Journal of the American Medical Association 244: 2630–2635

Swan R W 1974 Stagnant loop syndrome resulting from small-bowel irradiation injury and intestinal by-pass. Gynecologic Oncology 2: 441–445

Swenerton K D, Evers J A, White G W et al 1979 Intermittent pelvic infusion with vincristine, bleomycin and mitomycin C for advanced recurrent carcinoma of the cervix. Cancer Treatment Reports 63: 1379–1381

Symmonds R E, Webb M J 1981 Pelvic exenteration. In: Coppleson M (ed) Gynecologic oncology: fundamental principles and clinical practice. Churchill Livingstone, Edinburgh, vol 2

Symmonds R E, Pratt J H, Webb M J 1975 Exenterative operations: experience with 198 patients. American Journal of Obstetrics and Gynecology 121: 907–918

Tao L C, Pearson F G, Delarue N C, Langer B, Sanders D E 1980 Percutaneous fine-needle aspiration biopsy. I. Its value to clinical practice. Cancer 45: 1480–1485

Theologides A 1977 Nutritional management of the patient with advanced cancer. Postgraduate Medicine 61: 97–101

Thigpen T, Shingleton H M 1978 Phase II trial of cis-platinum in treatment of advanced squamous cell carcinoma of the cervix. American Society of Clinical Oncologists Abstracts, C-102

Thigpen T, Vance R B, Balducci L, Blessing J 1981 Chemotherapy in the management of advanced or recurrent cervical and endometrial carcinoma. Cancer 48: 658–665

Trelford J D, Silverton J S 1979 Successful plastic procedures of the perineum. Gynecologic Oncology 7: 239–247

Trope C, Johnsson J-E, Grundsell H, Mattsson W 1980 Adriamycin-methotrexate combination chemotherapy of advanced carcinoma of the cervix: a third look. Obstetrics and Gynecology 55: 488–492

Villasanta U 1979 Surgical treatment of recurrent pelvic cancer after irradiation. Maryland State Medical Journal (September): 66–68

Vogl S E, Moukhtar M, Kaplan B H 1979 Chemotherapy for advanced cervical cancer with methotrexate, bleomycin and cis-dichlorodiammineplatinum (II). Cancer Treatment Reports 63: 1005–1006

Vogl S E, Zaravinos T, Kaplan B H 1980 Toxicity of cis-diamminedichloroplatinum II given in a 2-hour outpatient regimen of diuresis and hydration. Cancer 45: 11–15

Wallace D, Hernandez W, Schlaerth J B, Nalick R N, Morrow C P 1980 Prevention of abdominal wound disruption utilizing the Smead-Jones closure technique. Obstetrics and Gynecology 56: 226–230

Wallace H J Jr, Hreshchyshyn M M, Wilbanks G D, Boronow R C, Fowler W C Jr, Blessing J A 1978 Comparison of the therapeutic effects of adriamycin alone versus adriamycin plus vincristine versus adriamycin plus cyclophosphamide in the treatment of advanced carcinoma of the cervix. Cancer Treatment Reports 62: 1435–1441

Walsh J W, Amendola M A, Hall D G, Tisnado J, Goplerud D R 1981 Recurrent carcinoma of the cervix: CT diagnosis. American Journal of Roentgenology 136: 117–122

Wang R I H 1982 Guidelines for the use of analgesics. Medstream 1: 3–11

Watring W G, Lagasse L D, Smith M L, Johnson G H, Moore J G, Berman M L 1976 Vaginal reconstruction following extensive treatment for pelvic cancer. American Journal of Obstetrics and Gynecology 125: 809–815

Webb M J, Symmonds R E 1980 Site of recurrence of cervical cancer after radical hysterectomy. American Journal of Obstetrics and Gynecology 138: 813–817

Wheeless C R Jr 1979 Avoidance of permanent colostomy in pelvic malignancy using the surgical stapler. Obstetrics and Gynecology 54: 501–505

Wheeless C R Jr, Julian C G, Burnett L S, Dorsey J H 1971 Synthetic pelvic floor sling to decrease small bowel complications after total exenteration. Obstetrics and Gynecology 38: 779–783

Willson J K V, Ozols R F, Lewis B J, Young R C 1981 Current status of therapeutic modalities for treatment of gynecologic malignancies with emphasis on chemotherapy. American Journal of Obstetrics and Gynecology 141: 81–98

Wrigley J V, Prem K A, Fraley E E 1976 Pelvic exenteration: complications of urinary diversion. Journal of Urology 116: 428–430

Yonekura M L, diZerega G S 1980 Antibiotic-associated colitis. Obstetrical and Gynecological Survey supplement 35: 743–746

Youngs D D, Wise T N 1976 Preparing a patient for surgery: consent, information and emotional support. Clinical Obstetrics and Gynecology 19: 421–448

Zenz M, Schappler-Scheele B, Neuhaus R, Piepenbrock S, Hilfrich J 1981 Long-term peridural morphine analgesia in cancer pain. Lancet (January): 91

8

Cancer complicating pregnancy

The discovery of cervical cancer in the pregnant woman has an emotional impact beyond that encountered in the non-pregnant patient. The necessity to make difficult therapeutic decisions in this environment becomes more complex when one considers the diverse opinions that exist concerning the effect of pregnancy on cervical cancer and the effect of the interaction of pregnancy and cervical cancer. Additionally, few individual institutions manage a sufficient number of these patients to determine optimal therapy.

The true incidence of pregnancy and coexisting cervical cancer is difficult to establish. The majority of these patients are treated at referral institutions, which may or may not have an obstetrical service representative of the local area. In addition, the majority of reports include those patients treated both antepartum and 2 to 18 months postpartum (Table 8.1). Depending on the patient's socioeconomic status, the hospital's referral base and the duration of study, 0.02 to 0.4% of pregnancies are complicated by coexisting invasive cervical cancer, i.e. the chance of finding an invasive cervical cancer in the pregnant woman ranges from 1 in 250 to 1 in 5000. Conversely, between 0.1 and 7.6% of cervical cancer patients are pregnant at the time of diagnosis. Depending on the duration of postpartum follow-up, it appears that postpartum patients comprise 0.03 to 6.9% of patients with cervical cancer. As expected, authors including a shorter postpartum interval indicate a lower incidence than those including longer postpartum follow-up.

DIAGNOSIS

The non-pregnant woman may neglect routine cervical cancer screening, but concern for her unborn child often increases the likelihood of a pregnant woman seeking a physician's care. The acceptance and routine use of cytological screening during prenatal care has been responsible for increasing both the number of cervical cancers

Table 8.1 Invasive cervical cancer associated with pregnancy

Author	Year	No. of pts found Antepartum	% of pregnant patients	% of cervical cancer patients	No. of pts found post partum	% of cervical cancer patients
Stander	1961	24	–	0.1	6	0.03
Lash	1961	18	–	–	–	–
Gustafsson	1962	82	–	1.1	157[c]	2.2
Cromer	1963	16	–	1.9	–	–
Waldrop	1963	48	–	0.8	132[c]	2.2
Williams	1964	12	0.02	0.7	12[a]	0.7
Van Praagh	1965	41	0.9	–	43[c]	1.0
Bosch	1966	26	–	0.9	40[c]	1.5
Prem	1966	22	–	0.2	78[g]	6.9
O'Leary	1966	18	0.02	–	–	–
Herold	1967	24	–	0.7	39[c]	1.2
Mikuta	1967	18	0.03	2.0	12[e]	1.3
Shaffer	1969	32	0.4	7.6	12[f]	2.9
Creasman	1970	48	–	3.4★	65[a]	4.6★
Wanless	1971	11	0.03	–	–	–
Fogh	1972	65	–	0.8	16[e]	0.2
Dudan	1973	23	0.05	–	–	–
Sall	1974	23	0.04	–	11[e]	0.03
Thompson	1975	41	0.05	6.0	1[b]	0.1
Sablinska	1977	63	–	0.8	264[c]	3.2
Lutz	1977	23	0.2	1.0	7[a]	0.3
Funnell	1980	10	–	3.8	7[b]	2.6
Lee	1981	21	–	2.4	20[a]	2.2

★ – % of patients age 19-49 with cervical cancer

[a]within 6 months, [b]within 3 months, [c]within 12 months, [d]excludes stage IA, [e]within 2 months, [f]within 4 months, [g]within 18 months

detected antepartum and the number of patients with early stage disease.

A vaginal speculum and bimanual pelvic examination are recognised features of good prenatal care. Cervical cytology obtained from the exocervix and endocervical canal decreases the risk of an occult lesion escaping detection. Regardless of cytology results, any suspicious cervical lesion should be biopsied even in pregnancy. The finding of parametrial induration or an enlarged cervix should increase suspicion. The responsible physician should always examine the pregnant woman who experiences vaginal bleeding, unusual vaginal discharge or pelvic pain at whatever stage of gestation, to rule out cervical cancer.

Since it is unusual for the woman of reproductive age to have cervical cancer, the physician is inclined to be less suspicious of these symptoms with a resultant delay in diagnosis and treatment. Sablinska's (1977) report of an increased rate of postpartum discovery of cervical cancer in women under 30 emphasises this problem. In the United States a cytological smear is performed at the first postpartum visit. The ectropion following delivery may be misleading; biopsies should be performed if there is any suspicion of cancer, even if the cervical cytology is negative.

Prenatal cytological screening has been associated with an increased rate of detection of invasive cancer in asymptomatic pregnant women (Table 8.2). Prior to the 1960s, the evaluation of abnormal cervical cytology in pregnancy patients included iodine staining, random punch biopsies or conisation. The first two procedures are frequently inadequate and have been replaced by colposcopically directed biopsy. While at least one author has indicated that pregnant patients might have an increased risk of complications following directed cervical biopsy, the experience at the University of Alabama in Birmingham, where 230 pregnant women have undergone cervical biopsies, indicates that while vaginal bleeding may occur, bleeding that requires transfusion is exceedingly rare. The reports of Creasman (1970), DePetrillo (1975), Lurain (1979) and Fowler (1980) substantiate this information and indicate that cervical biopsy does not increase the risk of abortion.

Hypertrophy and dilatation of the cervix associated with pregnancy usually allows adequate visualisation of the squamocolumnar junction and a satisfactory colposcopic examination. Reports by DePetrillo (1975), Talebian (1976), Tunca (1976), Ostergard (1979) and Fowler (1980), indicate that the colposcopic examination of a pregnant woman with abnormal cervical cytology can effectively limit the risk of an invasive carcinoma going undetected. No patient in this combined series (950 patients) who underwent adequate colposcopic evaluation

Table 8.2   Symptoms in patients with pregnancy co-existing with cervical cancer

Author	Year	No. of pts	Asymptomatic %	Bleeding %	Symptoms Discharge %	Pain %
Stander	1960	30	13.0	87.0	–	–
Lash	1961	18	22.2	77.8	–	–
Waldrop	1963	170	7.2	–	–	–
Williams	1964	24	20.8	58.3	8.3	4.2
Bosch	1966	66	9.0	80.0	5.0	6.0
Prem	1966	100	12.0	69.0	–	–
O'Leary	1966	18	44.4	27.8	27.8	–
Mikuta	1967	30	70.0	30.0	–	–
Shaffer	1969	11	18.2	81.8	–	–
Creasman	1970	113	3.0	5.4	13.0	–
Fogh	1972	81	1.0	77.0	21.0	1.0
Dudan	1973	23	95.0	5.0	–	–
Lutz	1977	30	[b]	26.7	–	–
Lee	1981	41	36.1	55.6[a]	–	–

[a] bleeding and discharge
[b] 'majority of patients'

had an undetected invasive cancer during the antepartum period. The necessity of conisation ranged from 1% in DePetrillo's report to 12% in Fowler's report.

The schema for evaluation of abnormal cytology in pregnant women at this institution (Fig. 8.1) has been satisfactory. In evaluating 230 patients over a 10-year period, not a single patient with invasive cancer has escaped antepartum detection. Only two patients (0.9%) have required cervical conisation.

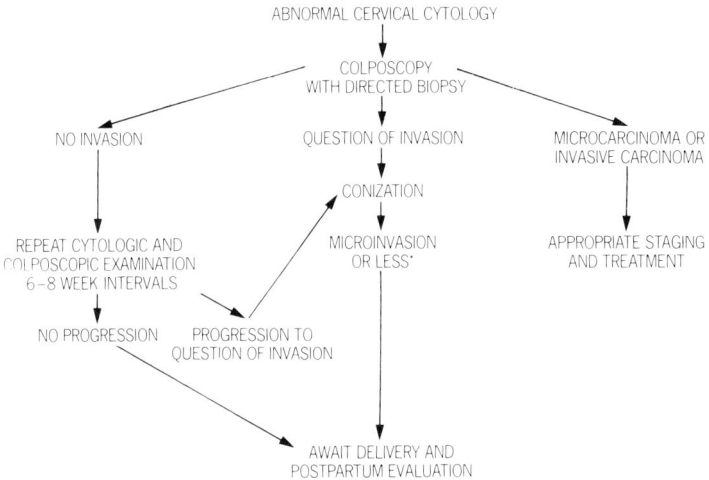

ABNORMAL CERVICAL CYTOLOGY

COLPOSCOPY
WITH DIRECTED BIOPSY

NO INVASION   QUESTION OF INVASION   MICROCARCINOMA OR
                                                    INVASIVE CARCINOMA

                     CONIZATION

REPEAT CYTOLOGIC AND   MICROINVASION   APPROPRIATE STAGING
COLPOSCOPIC EXAMINATION OR LESS*   AND TREATMENT
6–8 WEEK INTERVALS

NO PROGRESSION   PROGRESSION TO
                  QUESTION OF INVASION

AWAIT DELIVERY AND
POSTPARTUM EVALUATION

Fig. 8.1 Management flow diagram for abnormal cervical cytology.
* See Table 4.3

The indications for diagnostic conisation during pregnancy are essentially the same as those for the non-pregnant woman. Conisation is not used therapeutically in patients during pregnancy, but should be employed in any patient whose biopsy or cytological smear suggests invasive carcinoma.

Since conisation subjects the mother and fetus to complications (Table 8.3), it should not be performed without thorough review of all previous cytological and biopsy specimens. Postoperative haemorrhage complicates as many as 14% of conisations performed during pregnancy. Averette's (1970) report indicated that this risk was negligible during the first trimester, 5% in the second trimester and 10% following conisation during the third trimester. Cervical stenosis follows conisation in 3% of pregnant patients while cervical lacerations have been noted in 3% to 8% of patients who later delivered vaginally. Fear of induced abortion or prematurity is justified. The risk of abortion following conisation varies between 3% and 8% overall,

Table 8.3 Complications related to cervical conisation during pregnancy

Author	Year	No. of pts	Haemorrhage (%)	Stenosis (%)	Lacerations (%)	Infants (%)	Abortion (%)	Immature (%)	Premature rate (%)	Fetal salvage (%)
O'Leary	1966	39	2.6	–	7.7	–	7.7	–	–	–
Moore	1966	29	6.9	–	6.9	–	6.9	–	8.3	–
Rogers	1967	72	13.8	2.8	5.6	80.6	4.2	2.8	55.0	–
Smith	1968	47	8.5	–	–	–	4.5	–	4.3	–
Daskal	1968	77	10.4	–	2.6	78.4	8.1	–	12.2[e]	87.0
Stromme	1969	28	7.1	–	–	–	7.1	–	3.6	–
Shaffer	1969	20	10.0	–	–	–	–	–	–	–
Bolognese	1969	33	0	–	3.0	79.0	3.0	–	15.0	–
Averette	1970	180	7.2[a]	2.2	7.2	76.0	4.4	1.1[b]	13.0[c]	89.0
Fowler	1980	13	0	–	–	–	–	–	12.5	88.0

[a] > 500 ml
[b] Related to conisation (total of 2.2%)
[c] 79% of premature survived
[d] All prior to 20 weeks
[e] 67% of prematures survived

however if performed during the first trimester abortion rates are higher, approaching 33% to 50%. Although diagnostic conisation should not be unduly delayed, if the patient desires to continue her pregnancy it would seem prudent to avoid conisation during the first trimester. Other complications such as inadvertent rupture of the chorioamnion or intra-uterine infections are rarely reported. Despite these risks, term infants are delivered in approximately 80% of pregnancies that are complicated by the necessity of antepartum conisation. The overall fetal salvage rates approach 90%.

In contrast to conisations in the non-pregnant woman, residual disease is more likely following the procedure performed during pregnancy. This is related to the conservative nature of the cone because of the physician's fear that he may harm the pregnancy or promote premature labour. It is thus especially important that patients found to have pre-invasive or focal micro-invasive lesions during pregnancy should have repeat cytology and colposcopic evaluation later in the pregnancy. If no progression of disease is suspected by these examinations, further testing and treatment should be deferred until after delivery and involution of the uterus.

EVALUATION AND TREATMENT

Once the diagnosis of invasive cervical carcinoma is established, pretreatment studies should be performed commensurate with the stage of disease, the fetal gestational age and the patient's wishes regarding preservation of the pregnancy. It would appear that even in some patients with micro-invasive carcinoma the initiation of therapy can be safely delayed as there is apparently little risk of disease progression. The decision to initiate or delay therapy is difficult. The emotional, religious and moral needs of the mother and family become extremely important. The majority of these women are multiparous (mean parity of 4), but this decision is more complex in the primigravid patient. Any therapy delay that would predispose the mother to later treatment failure is difficult to accept.

The literature has few reports to guide the physician as to the effect of a planned delay in therapy. Thompson (1975) followed seven patients with stage IA disease (less than 3 mm of invasion), who had a mean therapy delay of 12 weeks (range 5–28 weeks). After delivery, all of the mothers were successfully treated. Prem (1966) reported five patients who had early invasive, asymptomatic stage I disease discovered between 20 and 34 weeks gestational age. A planned delay in therapy of 11 to 17 weeks did not adversely affect pregnancy outcome or cancer therapy as all of these women survived. Boutselis (1972) allowed nine patients with micro-invasion (less than 5 mm of stromal invasion), discovered during the first, second or third trimester, to complete their pregnancies. The delay was not apparently detrimental as all patients later underwent therapy. Lee (1981) recently reported eight patients (one with stage IA, two with stage IB and five with stage II) who completed their pregnancies after planned therapy delays of 1–11 weeks (mean 5 weeks). All patients gave birth to live infants and none of the patients experienced an advancement in her clinical stage.

Dudan (1973), in contrast, reported the progression of the clinical stage of disease in eight patients; although three patients who progressed had prolonged therapy delays (greater than 1 year) three other patients were said to have progressed from carcinoma in situ to invasive carcinoma after a therapy delay of only 2 to 5 months. Two additional patients with initial stage IB disease experienced an advancement to clinical stage IIA and IIIB after a 2- and 6-month delay. Lee (1981) reported one patient with a conisation diagnosis of CIS who was found to have micro-invasive disease after an 8-month delay and another patient whose invasive carcinoma was discovered in a postpartum hysterectomy specimen following a second trimester conisation which had been interpreted as negative.

In patients with clinical stage IB cancer, it may be reasonable to offer the patient a short delay in therapy in order to improve chances of fetal viability. Neonatal care in a modern high-risk nursery allows for the salvage of approximately 75% of infants delivered at 28 weeks gestational age and nearly 90% of those delivered at 32 weeks gestational age. An amniocentesis to evaluate fetal pulmonary maturity should be performed in those patients who are beyond 26 weeks gestational age and are candidates for prompt treatment, as the administration of corticosteroids may be beneficial when the lecithin:sphingomyelin ratio is immature. In patients with larger volume tumours (bulky stage IB or more advanced stages), we consider prolonged therapy delay (greater than 4 weeks) to be detrimental to the woman's chances of survival. While we prefer to deliver infants after 32 weeks gestational age, we consider infants greater than 26 weeks potentially viable and would perform an amniocentesis and proceed accordingly in these cases. Other than the problems associated with possible premature delivery, the fetus is apparently unaffected by the disease. No case of metastasis of cervical carcinoma to the fetus has been reported.

If the patient elects to coninue the pregnancy, the appropriate mode of delivery must be considered. In a literature review, Kinch (1961) noted that because of the potential of disseminating tumour cells, vaginal delivery should be avoided. Additional concerns of excessive bleeding or obstructed labour have been reported. Since that time other opinions have been expressed that maternal survival may not be significantly affected by the mode of delivery. For patients with all stages of cervical cancer, the survival (52.9%) following vaginal delivery (419 patients) is not different from that (46.1%) following abdominal delivery (115 patients) (Table 8.4). In patients with stage I disease, this collected series would indicate that following vaginal delivery 80.5% of treated patients are survivors while 71.6% of treated patients survive after abdominal delivery. Although these data cannot be adjusted for trimester of detection or volume of the tumour, they suggest that the risk of widespread dissemination of cancer following vaginal delivery may be more theoretical than real.

RECOMMENDED THERAPY

The recommended metastatic investigations prior to the initiation of treatment are the same as those for the non-pregnant woman. It should be remembered that pregnancy is associated with dilatation of the upper urinary tracts which may be present as early as 6–7 weeks gestational age and as late as the third month postpartum. These changes may mimic obstructive uropathy and should be considered before upstaging the patient. Because bimanual examination may be difficult, we would use computed tomography to aid in delineating extracervical disease (Fig. 8.2). The risk benefits of fetal radiation exposure with this (1 rad/section) and other radiological procedures should be evaluated if delayed therapy and fetal salvage is a strong consideration.

Many authors believe that early invasive carcinoma (focal micro-invasion or micro-invasion) can be treated by caesarean section combined with conservative hysterectomy. There are certain disadvantages to this form of treatment. The more conservative conisations in pregnant women are not as accurate as those in non-pregnant patients, and delay of 4–6 weeks postpartum will allow further testing before the final therapy decision is made. The risks of genito-urinary injury and bleeding following caesarean hysterectomy are higher than those of an interval total hysterectomy and because of its increased size and pliability the removal of the cervix may be more difficult in the pregnant woman. Because of these problems, we prefer to await delivery, re-evaluate the patient within 4 to 6 weeks and then institute appropriate therapy (Table 8.5). Only if the patient is unlikely to return postpartum for treatment would we consider caesarean hysterectomy. If this operation is chosen, a high vertical uterine incision is used for delivery, in order to leave the lower uterine segment and cervix undisturbed for later pathological study. Caesarean

Table 8.4 Effect of mode of delivery on cervical cancer in pregnancy

Author	Year	Stage	Abdominal delivery		Vaginal delivery	
			No. of pts	% Surviving	No. of pts	% Surviving
Kinch	1961	All stages	10	20	61	44
Barker	1963	All stages	2	100	28	36
Waldrop	1963	I	8	75	47	70
		II	7	0	48	44
		III	12	25	40	20
		IV	7	0	13	15
Van Praagh	1965	All stages	12	17	74	55
Bosch	1966	I	2	50	11	45
		II	4	0	13	38
		III	–	–	8	25
		IV	–	–	2	0
Prem	1966	I	3	67	8	63
		II	1	0	2	0
		III	1	0	2	100
O'Leary	1966	I	4	50	3	67
		II	1	100	1	0
Smith	1966	I	3	100	–	–
Mikuta	1967	All stages	5	80	11	55
Shaffer	1969	All stages	3	67	3	100
Creasman	1970	I	9	89	15	87
		II	4	50	14	64
Lee	1981	IA	2	100	1	100
		IB	10	90	10	90
		II	5	40	4	43
Totals		All stages	115	46.1	419	52.9
		I	41	80.5	95	71.6
		II	22	22.7	82	45.1
		III–IV	20	15.0	65	21.5

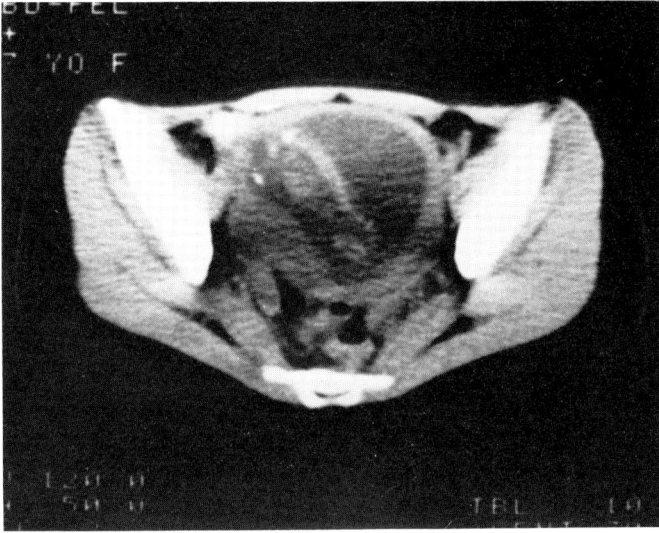

Fig. 8.2 CAT scan of a second trimester intra-uterine pregnancy in a woman with cervical cancer. This CAT scan indicated no evidence of extracervical extension and allowed appropriate surgical therapy to be instituted. (Courtesy of Dr Willie Anderson, University of Virginia, Charlottesville)

Table 8.5 Management of patients with stage 1 cervical cancer in pregnancy according to time of detection

Histological diagnosis†	Time of detection	Recommended treatment
Focal microinvasion Microinvasion	0–40 weeks	Delay therapy until viability Re-evaluate and treat postpartum
Microcarcinoma Carcinoma*	0–12 weeks 0–26 weeks 27—40 weeks	Institute therapy Consider therapy Delay until fetal viability Delay until fetal viability Deliver and institute therapy

* Avoid prolonged (>4 weeks) therapy delay in patients with clinical cervical lesions
† Refer to Table 4.3 for definitions

hysterectomy is not appropriate if antepartum evaluation has indicated carcinoma in situ. This can be treated with less morbidity after the woman delivers her child.

Although treatment of microcarcinoma and invasive cervical cancer in pregnancy can be surgery or radiotherapy, evaluation of the merits of the two modalities has been inadequate; most studies include few patients, and investigators have failed to stratify their results according to lesion size. Advocates of primary surgical therapy argue that ovarian and vaginal conservation, together with immediate therapy that can be performed safely, avoids the potential long-term complications of radiation therapy in these young women. Sall (1975) reported 23 surgically treated pregnant patients with early carcinoma of the cervix. Ninety-five per cent of these patients were 5-year survivors. While most authors describe better planes of dissection, the operative time (usually 5 h) and blood loss may be increased over procedures performed in non-pregnant women.

There appears to be little difference in survival (Table 8.6) between patients with stage IB disease treated surgically and those treated with radiation or with combined therapy. We prefer primary surgical treatment in patients who are acceptable operative risks.

The appropriate therapy for patients with stage IB cancer who are not good surgical candidates and patients with advanced stage disease is radiation. If viable, the fetus is delivered, usually by caesarean section, and therapy is begun postoperatively. Prior to viability, external teletherapy may be started. Creasman (1970) indicated that over 70% of abortions occurred prior to the patient receiving 4000 rad of external therapy; Bosch (1966) reported that 16 of 17 patients aborted spontaneously within 3 to 6 weeks. Prem (1966) stated that the time from initiation of therapy to spontaneous abortion was shorter in the first trimester (29 days) than in the second trimester (38 days). These findings would suggest no benefit of induced abortion prior to the initiation of radiotherapy.

The question of altered tissue tolerance during pregnancy has been expressed by Dudan (1973) and Thompson (1975). Both reports included a significant rate of gastro-intestinal and urinary fistulae in pregnant patients receiving radiation therapy. Reports from other institutions using radiation therapy as the primary method of treatment contain little information to confirm this hypothesis.

Some authors indicate decreased survival if detection occurs or treatment is begun in the third trimester or following delivery. However, the cited literature (Table 8.7) suggests that the clinical stage is the most important prognostic factor. Five-year survival is not significantly different in patients with stage I disease treated in the first trimester (84% survival), second trimester (89% survival), third trimester (77% survival) or postpartum (77% survival). The same is true of patients with stage II disease. However, it does appear that the third trimester or postpartum discovery of cervical cancer is associated with a more advanced clinical stage, with its corresponding decrease in survival rate.

Table 8.6 Survival of patients with stage IB cervical cancer related to the mode of therapy

Author	Year	Surgical		Radiation		Combined	
		No. of pts	% Survival	No. of pts	% Survival	No. of pts	% Survival
Stander	1960	–	–	24	83	–	–
Kinch	1961	–	–	19	68	4	50
Lash*	1961	12	92	1	0	2	100
Waldrop	1963	–	–	40	78	–	–
Van Praagh	1965	5	60	14	71	7	71
Bosch	1966	2	0	7	71	–	–
Prem	1966	–	–	58	83	–	–
O'Leary	1966	3	100	4	25	–	–
Smith	1968	5	100	1	100	–	–
Wanless	1971	3	100	2	100	–	–
Sall	1975	23	95	–	–	–	–
Thompson	1975	9	89	5	100	–	–
Lutz	1977	3	67	6	67	2	50
Funnell	1980	–	–	–	–	12	100
Lee	1981	17	93	4	80	1	100
Totals		70	89	165	87	28	82

*2-year survival

Table 8.7 Survival related to trimester of discovery and treatment

Author	Year	Stage	First trimester		Second trimester		Third trimester		Post partum	
			No. of pts	% Survival	No. of pts	% Survival	No. of pts	% Survival	No. of pts	% Survival
Kinch	1961	All stages	10	60	10	50	6	67	49	37
Lash*	1961	I	4	100	6	83	2	50	1	100
Barker	1963	All stages	2	100	2	100	1	0	27	37
Van Praagh	1965	I	71	86	–	–	4	50	15	67
		II	3	67	4	50	3	33	11	27
		III	–	–	1	0	–	–	3	0
		IV	–	–	–	–	–	–	–	–
Prem	1966	All stages	6	83	9	78	2	6	6	17
O'Leary	1966	I	2	50	1	100	5	100	60	57
		II	1	0	1	100	3	33	1	100
		III	1	0	–	–	–	–	–	–
Brown	1966	I	5	80	4	100	4	25	4	75
		II	–	–	–	–	2	50	5	40
Herold	1967	I	11	73	5	60	2	50	15	47
		II	1	0	2	50	1	0	9	33
		III	–	–	–	–	2	0	12	0
		IV	–	–	–	–	–	–	2	0
Smith	1968	I	3	100	–	–	2	100	1	100
Mikuta	1967	All stages	3	67	9	100	2	50	12	50
Creasman	1970	I	9	100	8	100	5	100	25	84
		II	5	80	9	88	2	50	21	67
Wanless	1971	All stages	4	100	2	50	4	75	–	–
Fogh	1972	I	23	80	–	–	5	80	8	100
		II	14	43	–	–	4	100	5	40
		III	2	0	–	–	3	33	2	0
		IV	1	0	–	–	–	–	1	0
Sall	1974	IB	5	100	6	100	12	92	6	100
Sablinska	1977	All stages	41	73	22	50	–	–	181	37
Lutz	1977	IB	2	100	3	100	2	0	3	100
		IIA	–	–	2	0	1	0	–	–
		IIB	–	–	–	–	1	0	–	–
		III	–	–	–	–	2	0	–	–
		IV	–	–	–	–	–	–	–	–
Totals		All stages	161	78	78	77	81	59	484	45
		I	67	84	27	89	39	77	78	77
		II	23	52	18	67	11	45.4	51	47

* 2-year survival

BIBLIOGRAPHY

Averette H E, Nasser N, Yankow S L, Little W A 1970 Cervical conization in pregnancy. American Journal of Obstetrics and Gynecology 106: 543–549

Barber H R K, Brunschwig A 1963 Gynecologic cancer complicating pregnancy. American Journal of Obstetrics and Gynecology 85: 156–164

Beecham C T, Andros G J 1960 Cervical conization in pregnancy. Obstetrics and Gynecology 16: 521–526

Berkowitz R S, Ehrmann R L, Lavizzo-Mourey R, Knapp R C 1979 Invasive cervical carcinoma in young women. Gynecologic Oncology 8: 311–316

Bolognese R J, Corson S L 1969 Cervical conization in pregnancy. Surgery, Gynecology and Obstetrics (June): 1244–1246

Bosch A, Marcial V A 1966 Carcinoma of the uterine cervix associated with pregnancy. American Journal of Roentgenology 96: 92–98

Boutselis J G 1972 Intraepithelial carcinoma of the cervix associated with pregnancy. Obstetrics and Gynecology 40: 657–666

Bowes W A, Halgrimson M, Simmons M A 1979 Results of intensive perinatal management of very-low-birth-weight infants (501 to 1500 grams). Journal of Reproductive Medicine 23: 245–250

Calanog A, Sall S, Gordon M, Sedlis A 1974 Comprehensive cytologic screening in patients undergoing voluntary abortions. American Journal of Obstetrics and Gynecology 118: 102–105

Covell L M, Disciullo A J, Knapp R C 1977 Decidual change in pelvic lymph nodes in the presence of cervical squamous cell carcinoma during pregnancy. American Journal of Obstetrics and Gynecology 127: 674–676

Creasman W T, Rutledge F N, Fletcher G H 1970 Carcinoma of the cervix associated with pregnancy. Obstetrics and Gynecology 36: 495–501

Cromer J K, Hawken S W 1963 Cancer of the cervix and pregnancy. Obstetrics and Gynecology 22: 346–351

Daskal J L, Pitkin R M 1968 Cone biopsy of the cervix during pregnancy. Obstetrics and Gynecology 32: 1–5

DePetrillo A D, Townsend D E, Morrow C P, Lickrish G M, DiSaia P J, Roy M 1975 Colposcopic evaluation of the abnormal Papanicolaou test in pregnancy. American Journal of Obstetrics and Gynecology 121: 441–445

Dillon W P, Egan E E A 1981 Aggressive obstetric management in late second-trimester deliveries. Obstetrics and Gynecology 58: 685–690

Dudan R C, Yon J L Jr, Ford J H Jr, Averette H E 1973 Carcinoma of the cervix and pregnancy. Gynecologic Oncology 1: 283–289

Fogh I 1972 Cancer colli uteri and pregnancy. Cancer 29: 114–116

Fowler W C Jr, Walton L A, Edelman D A 1980 Cervical intraepithelial neoplasia during pregnancy. Southern Medical Journal 73: 1180–1185

Funnell J D, Puckett T G, Strebel G F, Kelso J W 1980 Carcinoma of the cervix complicating pregnancy. Southern Medical Journal 73: 1308–1310

Gustafsson D C, Kottmeier H L 1962 Carcinoma of the cervix associated with pregnancy. Acta obstetrica et gynecologica scandinavica 41: 1–21

Hacker N F, Berek J S, Lagasse L D, Charles E H, Savage E W, Moore J G 1982 Carcinoma of the cervix associated with pregnancy. Obstetrics and Gynecology 59: 735–746

Herold J 1967 Cancer of the uterine cervix in pregnancy, after delivery and after miscarriage. Acta Universitatis Carolinae Medica 13: 189–205

Jacobs J P 1965 Pregnancy complicating carcinoma of the cervix. Postgraduate Medicine (August): 178–182

Jones E G, Schwinn C P, Bullock W K, Varga A, Dunn J E, Friedman H Jr et al 1968 Cancer detection during pregnancy. American Journal of Obstetrics and Gynecology 101: 298–307

Kiguchi K, Bibbo M, Hasegawa T, Kurihara S, Tsutsui F, Wied G L 1981 Dysplasia during pregnancy: a cytologic follow-up study. Journal of Reproductive Medicine 26: 66–72

Kinch R A H 1961 Factors affecting the prognosis of cancer of the cervix in pregnancy. American Journal of Obstetrics and Gynecology 82: 45–51

Kistner R W, Gorbach A C, Smith G V 1957 Cervical cancer in pregnancy. Review of the literature with presentation of thirty additional cases. Obstetrics and Gynecology 9: 554–560

Kopelman A E 1978 The smallest preterm infants. American Journal of Diseases of Chidren 132: 461–462

Lash A F 1961 Management of carcinoma of the cervix in pregnancy. Obstetrics and Gynecology 17: 41–45

Lee R B, Neglia W, Park R C 1981 Cervical carcinoma in pregnancy. Obstetrics and Gynecology 58: 584–589

Lurain J R, Gallup D G 1979 Management of abnormal Papanicolaou smears in pregnancy. Obstetrics and Gynecology 53: 484–488

Lutz M H, Underwood P B Jr, Rozier J C, Putney F W 1977 Genital malignancy in pregnancy. American Journal of Obstetrics and Gynecology 129: 536–542

Mikuta J J 1967 Invasive carcinoma of the cervix in pregnancy. Southern Medical Journal 60: 843–847

Moore J G, Wells R G, Morton D G 1966 Management of superficial cervical cancer in pregnancy. Obstetrics and Gynecology 27: 307–318

Morrow C P, DiSaia P J, Mangan C F et al 1977 Continuous pelvic arterial infusion with bleomycin for squamous cell carcinoma of the cervix recurrent after radiation therapy. Cancer Treatment Reports 61: 1403–1405

Nebel W A, Shingleton H M, Swanton M C 1967 Cold knife conization of the cervix uteri. Surgery, Gynecology and Obstetrics 125: 780–784

O'Leary J A, Munnell E W, Moore J G 1966 The changing prognosis of cervical carcinoma during pregnancy. Obstetrics and Gynecology 28: 460–468

Orr J W Jr, Grizzle W E, Huddleston J F 1982 Squamous cell carcinoma metastatic to placenta and ovary. Obstetrics and Gynecology 59: 81S–83S

Ostergard D R, Nieberg R K 1979 Evaluation of abnormal cervical cytology during pregnancy with colposcopy. American Journal of Obstetrics and Gynecology 134: 756–758

Park R C, Duff W P 1980 Role of caesarean hysterectomy in modern obstetric practice. Clinical Obstetrics and Gynecology 23: 601–627

Phelan J T 1968 Cancer and pregnancy. New York State Journal of Medicine 68: 3011–3017

Philip A G S, Little G A, Polivy D R, Lucey J F 1981 Neonatal mortality risk for the eighties: the importance of birth weight/gestational age groups. Pediatrics 68: 122–130

Prem K A, Makowski E L, McKelvey J L 1966 Carcinoma of the cervix associated with pregnancy. American Journal of Obstetrics and Gynecology 95: 99–108

Roddick J W Jr, Crossen P S 1966 Invasive carcinoma of the cervix complicated by pregnancy. Southern Medical Journal 59: 417–423

Rogers R S III, Williams J H 1967 The impact of the suspicious Papanicolaou smear on pregnancy. American Journal of Obstetrics and Gynecology 98: 488–496

Sablinska R, Tarlowska L, Stelmachow J 1977 Invasive carcinoma of the cervix associated with pregnancy: correlation between patient age, advancement of cancer and gestation, and result of treatment. Gynecologic Oncology 5: 363–373

Sall S, Rini S, Pineda A 1974 Surgical management of invasive carcinoma of the cervix in pregnancy. American Journal of Obstetrics and Gynecology 118: 1–5

Shaffer W L, Merrill J A 1969 Carcinoma of the cervix associated with pregnancy. Southern Medical Journal 62: 915–921

Smith C J 1967 Clinical problems. American Journal of Obstetrics and Gynecology 98: 425–427

Smith M R, Figge D C, Bennington J L 1968 The diagnosis of cervical cancer during pregnancy. Obstetrics and Gynecology 31: 193–197

Stanhope C R, Smith J P, Wharton J T, Rutledge F N, Fletcher G H, Gallager H S 1980 Carcinoma of the cervix: the effect of age on survival. Gynecologic Oncology 10: 188–193

Stewart A L, Reynolds E O R, Lipscomb A P 1981 Outcome for infants of very low birthweight: survey of world literature. Lancet (May): 1038–1041

Stromme W B 1969 Preclinical carcinoma and dysplasia of the cervix associated with pregnancy. American Journal of Obstetrics and Gynecology 105: 1008–1014

Swenerton K D, Evers J A, White G W et al 1979 Intermittent pelvic infusion with vincristine, bleomycin and mitomycin C for advanced recurrent carcinoma of the cervix. Cancer Treatment Reports 63: 1379–1381

Talebian F, Krumholz B A, Shayan A, Mann L I 1976 Colposcopic evaluation of patients with abnormal cytologic smears during pregnancy. Obstetrics and Gynecology 47: 693–696

Thompson J D, Caputo T A, Franklin E W III, Dale E 1975 The surgical management of invasive cancer of the cervix in pregnancy. American Journal of Obstetrics and Gynecology 121: 853–863

Tunca J C, Franklin E W III, Clark J C 1976 Colposcopic management of abnormal cervical cytology during pregnancy. Southern Medical Journal 69: 705–707

Van Praagh I G L, Harvey M H, Vernon C P 1965 Carcinoma of the cervix associated with pregnancy. Journal of Obstetrics and Gynaecology of the British Commonwealth 72: 75–80

Villasanta U, Durkan J P 1966 Indications and complications of cold conization of the cervix. Observations on 200 consecutive cases. Obstetrics and Gynecology 27: 717–723

Waldrop G M, Palmer J P 1963 Carcinoma of the cervix associated with pregnancy. American Journal of Obstetrics and Gynecology 86: 202–212

Wanless J F 1971 Carcinoma of the cervix in pregnancy. American Journal of Obstetrics and Gynecology 110: 173–179

Wharton J T, Rutledge F N 1980 Adjunctive surgical procedures with irradiation therapy for carcinoma of the cervix. In: Fletcher G H (ed) Textbook of radiotherapy. Lea and Febiger, Philadelphia, p 783–789

Williams T J, Brack C B 1964 Carcinoma of the cervix in pregnancy. Cancer 17: 1486–1491

9

Social, psychological and sexual aspects

To the patient and her family, the diagnosis of cancer evokes a bleak image of physical pain, suffering, debility and untimely death. Although confrontation with death is the main issue for many patients, for others the struggle to survive assumes equal importance (Fig. 9.1).

Reaction and adjustment to the diagnosis of cancer is a somewhat accelerated version of the phases of dying described by Kuebler-Ross (1969). Initially, the woman may deny the seriousness of her symptoms and consequently delay seeking professional help. When she does report the symptom(s) to her physician, her anxiety may be further heightened because she is aware of delay and may wonder if this has compromised her opportunity for cure. The shock and disbelief that she experiences after hearing the diagnosis may compromise her understanding of the physician's statements concerning treatment and prognosis. Anger and hostility may follow as the woman feels betrayed by her body, guilty because of her delay and frightened about the future. The physician, referring or primary, as the bearer of bad news, may become the target of her rage. Bargaining is evident in those women who co-operate fully with the health care provider, the unspoken expectation being that they will be cured in exchange for their good behaviour. Disappointment over the loss of physical well-being is to be expected and may be followed by depression. The treating physician, therefore, must follow

Table 9.1 Disclosure of the diagnosis of cancer

1. The physician, the nurse, the patient and the patient's mate or family member should participate

2. The setting must be quiet, private and comfortable

3. In an unhurried discussion, the patient is asked to state her understanding of the situation and is encouraged to guide the conversation with her questions

4. The physician should be factual, optimistic within reason and alert to cues

5. After the physician leaves, the nurse can repeat, reinforce or expand the key elements of the discussion

6. Instructions concerning the initiation of treatment must be clear, concise and preferably in writing

210

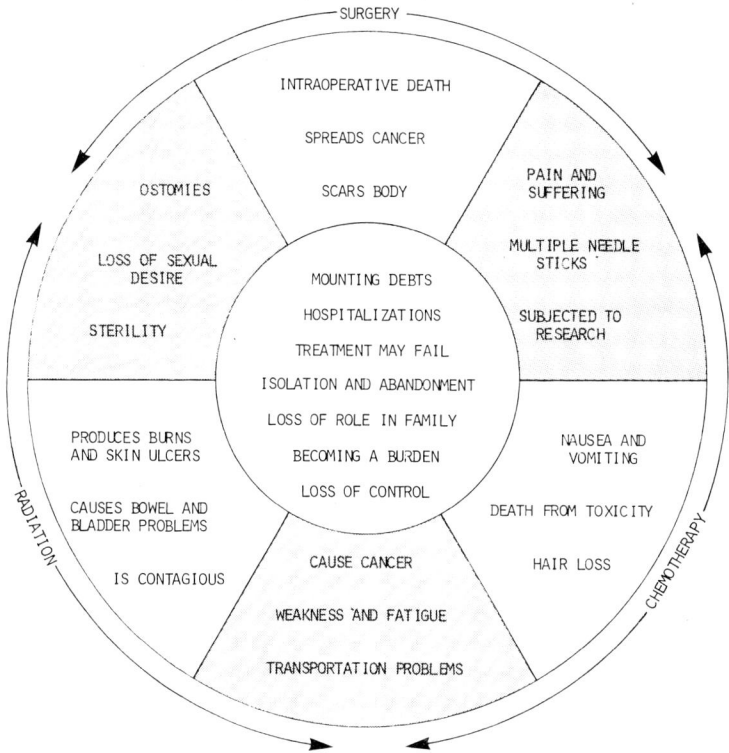

Fig. 9.1 Patient fears and concerns about cervical cancer and its treatment

certain steps (Table 9.1) to calm the patient and her family, to dispel the gloom and hopelessness, and to ensure that they understand the nature of the illness and its treatment.

Some patients' reactions are more understandable in terms of their previous history. The relationship between squamous cell carcinoma of the uterine cervix and sexual behaviour is well established and accounts for a number of fears and anxieties. A woman who develops cervical cancer after having experienced an abortion, an extramarital affair, or a venereal infection is likely to interpret her disease as punishment for sin or wrongdoing. The compliant, passive woman who endures treatment as if 'she is getting what she deserves' may be a candidate for special assistance, including counselling. The highly anxious or guilt-ridden patient often cannot process information effectively and may appear unco-operative when in fact she needs intervening supportive psychotherapy. The genital site of origin mandates that the physician discuss the effect of the disease on each woman in terms of her self-image and sexuality.

Not only the patient must be considered. Her life, full of activities, responsibilities and interdependent relationships, has been invaded. She has feelings for and responsibilities to her children, her spouse, her parents and other people. She may be working and active in a church, a club, or other professional, political or social organisations. Her creativity may be expressed in homemaking, childrearing as well as in outlets such as producing an income or providing a service as a member of the work force. As one cannot separate the body from the mind, neither can a woman be severed from her family and society at large.

Cancer disrupts an individual's daily activities and makes great demands on her ability to cope with stress. Previously successful defence mechanisms are threatened, anxiety is generated and self-esteem may be lost. The goal of medical or surgical intervention must be to eradicate the cancer with minimal physical and psychological trauma, in order that the individual can resume her normal life.

If cure is not a realistic expectation, the cancer patient must be assisted in functioning and coping for the duration of her illness. Fundamental to achieving this goal is an understanding of what the disease means to the individual patient and the development of a sense of rapport and trust among the health care team, the patient and her family.

Attention is usually focussed on the effect of cancer on the psyche, yet psychological factors as a cause of cancer have received attention in the literature for centuries. While one can correlate certain personality characteristics with the development of cancer, any actual causative effect remains unproven. Severe emotional trauma, such as the loss of a spouse or child, with its attendant grief and depression, has been implicated in both the development and acceleration of the course of cancer. It has been suggested that cancer patients can utilise this relationship between psyche and cancer to their advantage, shifting the effect in a positive way. Some patients visualise the destruction of cancer cells by their own white blood cells. While the scientist would obviously dismiss the validity of this approach in controlling the disease, the benefit in terms of the patient's perception of control of her own body is evident.

SURGICAL TREATMENT

When hysterectomy is part of the treatment for cervical cancer, familiarity with the psychological implications of the procedure is important. The attendant anatomical and physiological changes are obvious to the clinician but not so readily apparent to the patient.

Many women believe that the uterus is the source of their femininity and strength and, consequently, feel 'less of a woman' without it. Well-meaning friends and family members are often sources of misinformation. The woman facing hysterectomy or other cancer treatment may be told that the loss of the uterus will lead to premature aging, senility, and even insanity. Such misunderstandings can often be clarified during a preoperative session which includes questions such as (1) What does your uterus mean to you? (2) How will hysterectomy change your life? (3) What is the most important function of your uterus? (4) What are your thoughts about losing your uterus? Details of the operative procedure can be described at the same time. The effects of oöphorectomy, including loss of libidio, reduction of vaginal lubrication, and decreased sensation in the lower genital tract may be disruptive. She should be told that many of these symptoms may be alleviated by the administration of oestrogen. Young women can be told that the ovaries, if normal, may be conserved.

The loss of control that accompanies anaesthesia and surgery makes many women feel helpless and defenceless. The unspoken fears of 'never waking up' and of intolerable pain are often present. The importance of addressing these fears in a preoperative counselling session with the patient cannot be over-emphasised.

In premenopausal women, the cessation of menses and loss of fertility caused by the hysterectomy must be addressed. Women who view their menses as a cleansing function are less likely to accept this change than are the women who dislike the process or who have experienced significant menstrual discomfort. Knowing that contraception is absolute allows some women to feel relief and to experience increased sexual enjoyment. Others feel a loss of identity associated with loss of the ability to reproduce.

If surgery is perceived as mutilating, it is likely to become damaging rather than restorative. The woman who expects hysterectomy to decrease her sexual excitability or enjoyment often exhibits a self-fulfilling prophecy when she experiences decreased libido postoperatively. Women who depend upon their gynaecological illness to secure relief from sexual commitments to their husbands may develop anxiety if they believe the removal of the presumed source of their symptomatology will lead to the expectation that they will become more responsive sexually. Thus, surgery may constitute a threat to the marital relationship in opposing ways.

Many patients and spouses believe that genital cancer is contagious, therefore, whatever sexual relationship that previously was experienced may cease. Guilt associated with prior sexual activity and a belief that this may have caused the cancer becomes a deterrent to positive adjustment and recovery. Marital discord and abandonment of the woman by her mate is common. In general, however, the single most significant factor in postoperative sexual behaviour is pre-treatment sexual adjustment. The woman who experienced a satisfying sexual relationship prior to surgery is likely to resume such a relationship postoperatively, while those with sexual dysfunction preoperatively are likely to continue or worsen following surgery.

The resection of the proximal vagina may present problems for some women in terms of sexual function, particularly in the early months after surgery. Most women can be assured that the shortening of the vagina will not necessarily affect sexual activities. Postoperative dyspareunia may be lessened by a change in coital position that limits penetration by the male, i.e. female astride or 'legs together' which gives the impression of greater depth.

The interruption of sensory nerve pathways to the vagina and perineum by pelvic operations may result in decreased sensation and, in rare cases, lack of orgasm. The tendency toward depression in such cases is not surprising.

To alleviate sexual dysfunction, one might encourage extended foreplay and stimulation of the clitoris, since clitoral orgasm may be possible in the absence of vaginal orgasm. Other expressions of affection, such as fondling or oral-genital sex, may be helpful in reassuring the woman that she is still a sexual being with the ability to love and be loved in a physical way. If successful, her increased feelings of self-worth will serve to combat the depression.

Bladder dysfunction frequently complicates the course of recovery for some patients after radical hysterectomy. While the catheter is in place, many women fear that others will notice the catheter, and will hesitate to leave home because of embarrassment. Some women become excessively preoccupied with voiding, measuring and recording residual urine, thereby becoming so anxious that they delay their postoperative recovery. The postoperative use of sophisticated urodynamic testing equipment may make voiding trials unnecessary with a resultant decrease in anxiety levels. A more serious difficulty is encountered in the occasional patient who has persistent bladder dysfunction that requires intermittent self-catheterisation. This may be viewed by the woman as humiliating and as disabling in terms of gainful employment. The involuntary loss of urine that may occur after surgery presents another set of social, personal and medical problems. Most women can be assured, however, that bladder sensation will ultimately return to normal and that there is little risk of serious long-term problems.

Many patients have difficulty relinquishing the 'sick' role. The patient who enjoyed the love and concern that others expressed during her treatment may suddenly be without this support when she is pronounced well. She fears recurrence and may attribute every ache and pain to cancer. Cancer patients realign their life goals toward survival. Once it appears that this goal will be achieved, they may again be faced with many of the problems they experienced before the diagnosis was made. In effect, they have focussed all their energies on enduring the ordeal of cancer and its treatment only to find that the cure returned them to a previous existence in which unhappiness may have prevailed. They receive no sympathy from friends and relatives who tell them to be grateful, and their sense of isolation may become intolerable.

RADIATION TREATMENT

It is important to discuss the patient's ideas about radiotherapy before it is begun and to make the effects of radiation clear to them. Many patients think that radiotherapy can cause cancer and that not only cancer, but radiation itself is contagious, i.e. exposure to her irradiated body may harm others. Others have difficulty in viewing radiation therapy as first-line treatment, believing that it is in actual fact the last resort since the tumour could not be removed surgically. The physician should always be prepared to answer the question, 'Why can't you operate?' It is human nature to want the diseased organ removed so that the whole idea of cancer can be dismissed and forgotten. The time element can also be stressful. Radiation therapy is usually delivered over a 5- or 6-week interval, compared to an operation which can be performed in one day. In addition, an immediate statement of the likelihood of a successful result cannot be provided to patients who are treated by radiation, whereas surgically treated patients are relieved when told, 'The cancer is out and had not spread'.

Radiotherapy as primary treatment for cervical carcinoma is associated with a variety of symptoms and disturbances of body functions. As curative doses of radiation are delivered to the pelvis, the normal tissues of the bladder and rectum are affected, and the patient may experience haematuria, urinary urgency, frequency, dysuria, nocturia, tenesmus, diarrhoea, or rectal bleeding. These effects and the associated fatigue, anorexia, nausea and vomiting lead some patients to perceive the treatment as damaging, or harmful. Since most people seek medical attention to feel better or to obtain relief, thay may lose sight of the long-term goal of cure as long as symptoms persist.

The likelihood of transient skin changes in the radiation field, such as desquamation and ulceration, should be mentioned. Subcutaneous fibrosis, increased pigmentation and hair loss may develop in the radiation fields and patients should be warned of these possibilities. Such changes are often of little significance medically, but may be of major importance to the patient, who feels disfigured and senses a loss of sexual attractiveness. These skin changes represent tangible evidence that she is indeed different and acceptance by her partner of them is quite important.

The anatomical and functional alteration of the vagina following radiation therapy can be a major problem for many women. While the effects are more pronounced for the first few weeks after completion of treatment, many symptoms persist for years or even for a lifetime. The epithelium thins, the vagina shortens and may become stenotic, inelastic or completely obliterated. Lubrication does not occur with sexual excitement. Vaginal bleeding, discharge, and dyspareunia may accompany attempts at vaginal intercourse. Exogenous oestrogen replacement, topical or systemic, may improve the elasticity of the vaginal epithelium. Vaginal dilatation during and following completion of the treatment programme may promote patency. If this cannot be accomplished by sexual intercourse, use of a mechanical device (obturator) may be helpful. Many women may equate the use of such a dilator with masturbation, a practice which may not be acceptable. When sexual intercourse has been abandoned, the reasons for abstinence should be explored with the patient and her spouse. If a woman suspects a link between sexual intercourse and the development of her cancer, she may logically avoid that activity to prevent recurrent disease. Post-coital bleeding or discharge, with or without dyspareunia, may raise fears of recurrence since these often were the symptoms the woman experienced prior to diagnosis and treatment.

Patients should be made aware of the safety precautions employed during intracavitary radiation placement, especially those that restrict visiting rights of family and friends. Such preparation lessens the sense of isolation that might otherwise be experienced.

The duration of radiation treatment may make other demands on the patient and her family. The financial burden of transportation to a treatment facility, time away from home, loss of income, expense of child care, and cost of meals and lodging can be overwhelming. The support of a governmental or charitable agency may be needed since many of these women are from low-income families.

ULTRARADICAL SURGERY FOR RECURRENT CANCER

The choices of further therapy for the woman who has persistent or recurrent cancer are somewhat limited. The majority of women who have recurrent or persistent tumour are incurable. The only hope for survival in those women who have recurrences limited to the central pelvis is pelvic exenteration, a radical operation which in itself is life-threatening. Since the operation usually requires urinary and faecal diversions and removal of the vagina, the woman's lifestyle is completely changed. The alternative to the surgery is death within 1 to 2 years. The woman must, with the help of her physicians and family, carefully assess the quality of her life and decide if she is willing to accept the risks and the changes in order to survive. Most women will choose surgery as they desire to remain a part of their families and their communities as long as possible. Some are not willing to endure more pain and they should not be coerced into accepting the surgery as they are likely to be dissatisfied with the results. The physician must decide if the patient can benefit from the procedure based on the potential for resection of the tumour, and the general medical and psychiatric health of the woman.

It has been suggested that some women with a previous or current psychiatric problem are not candidates for an exenteration due to their marginal ability to cope with their environment. There is no psychological test available to predict the effect of surgery on the psyche, and in our experience a number of such patients have done well following exenterations. It is important to allow the psychiatrist who is familiar with the patient to participate in the decisions both before and after the surgery.

Many times the physician is concerned that the exenteration candidate does not fully comprehend the extent and effects of the surgical procedure. This may be due to a limited educational background, to use of defence mechanisms such as denial, or to a sense of well-being achieved through religious beliefs. If the patient can give a reasonably accurate description of the extent of the operation, the physician has met his responsibility of informed consent. Many patients require time to make their decisions. Repetition of the previous information may be necessary to ensure understanding by the patient and her family. A family united in favour of the decision will serve as a source of support for the patient postoperatively. However the final decision ultimately rests with the woman, even though this may be contrary to the wishes of her family.

The loss of the vagina following exenteration is a major threat to women who are sexually active, particularly to those who are accustomed only to vaginal intercourse. Women who have utilised other forms of sexual expression will find loss of the vagina less of an assault to their sexuality. In contrast, the patient who indicates that sexual activity is not important to her may be denying her sexuality to her physician for fear of embarrassing herself or her 'rescuer', may be expressing an inability to deal with any issue beyond survival, or may be responding to fear of an additional surgical procedure aimed at interval vaginal reconstruction. This problem may be minimised by the surgeon's willingness to perform exenteration and concurrent vaginal reconstruction, and his recognition of the need for the woman to express her sexuality in a physical way following the surgery.

An important factor in the decision relating to patient acceptance of exenteration revolves around the woman's role in the family. If she is employed outside the home, important income may be lost and other members of the family may not be able or willing to assume her responsibilities. This is particularly true if she has young children. However, to allow these considerations to postpone the surgery for very long would be shortsighted, since without the surgical procedure, she has a very limited chance of survival. The social worker can be a valuable member of the health care team in identifying resources available to the family during the absence of the woman from her family environment.

Postoperative adjustment to exenteration depends on the severity of the physical insult, the duration of convalescence, preoperative concept of self, previous ability to cope with crises, the availability of family support, and the relationship with the physician and other health professionals. It is clear that a complicated recovery is more stressful to all concerned. Patients who are doing well medically in the early postoperative period nonetheless suffer an emotional decline and physical deterioration; grieving is an appropriate response to loss of body parts, separation from home and loved ones, and disruption of an independent life-style. Excessive anxiety and depression, however, may indicate that the physical changes related to the operation have exacerbated a pre-existing identity problem. Alternatively, if the patient's preoperative concept of self was based on internal values more than external physical factors, she will better tolerate the postoperative changes in her body. Some women may feel that their body image is threatened if they perceive themselves as less than complete; others, however, are acutely aware of their diseased parts and may experience an improved sense of self-image following successful removal of the cancerous tissues.

An essential component of the exenteration patient's ability to recover her self-image is her attitude toward the urinary and faecal diversions. The need for radical surgery is not always clear to some women as the organs removed may have caused few, if any, symptoms. In addition, the creation of the ostomies is associated with a new set of problems, real or imagined. The patient must learn new skills to manage leakage, odour, gas and excoriation of the peri-stomal skin in addition to new patterns of clothing selection. A period of trial and error in the utilisation of ostomy equipment follows surgery, during which persistence, flexibility, attention to detail and a sense of humour can be the patient's best defences against frustration. The whole idea of soilage or faecal contamination is respulsive to some women who feel that it is not socially acceptable for one to eliminate faeces through an opening in the abdominal wall. Many patients live in relative isolation without disclosing information about the ostomies to even their closest friends. The support of an enterostomal therapist is mandatory in preoperative selection of stoma sites, assistance in psychological rehabilitation, and in teaching the patient how to contain and manage waste. A visit by a rehabilitated exenteration patient is very helpful to the early postoperative patient in establishing a goal of recovery, that is, an image of ability instead of the perception of disability that may be the patient's fantasy. Later, participation in ostomy groups can be beneficial in overcoming isolation and fears of social embarrassment.

Depression is the most common psychopathology encountered postoperatively. Beyond a given point in the normal grieving process, depression becomes counter-productive and constitutes a real threat to recovery. Sleep disturbances, failure to eat, and reluctance to ambulate or participate in self-care activities impede progress and can precipitate major physical complications. Individuals with a previous history of depression are more likely to experience postoperative depression, though patients who have never been clinically depressed before usually exhibit some symptoms. Psychiatric intervention and antidepressants may be necessary if the patient is to successfully negotiate this part of the rehabilitation process.

Every individual has patterns of coping with stress that have been developed through trial and error. It is helpful to identify those patterns preoperatively so that their use may be encouraged following surgery. For example, the woman whose hobby is needlepoint should be encouraged to begin again as soon as possible, particularly if it is an activity that has provided relaxation or release of tension. The individual who copes by being in charge and controlling her environment must be given as many opportunities as possible for making choices and maintaining control. For instance, if she prefers to bathe in the evening, arrangements should be made so that this can be accomplished according to her wishes.

Personal support is vital following an exenteration. The husband is the key figure in most instances, but a parent, child or sibling may play the central role. Because the husband is so significant, he must be included in teaching, planning, and in gauging progress following surgery. In the absence of a family, alternate figures assume more importance. Close friends or nurses can attach themselves more closely to the patient. The individual who actually assists the patient in her struggle toward recovery is not important as long as someone is available for such assistance.

Occasionally, patients may have difficulty escaping from the dependent role imposed by exenteration. Some women enjoy the attention they receive and feel special in contrast to their preoperative feeling of isolation. Others may lack the courage to risk failure in their attempts to regain independent functioning. Another group may have been dependent even without the imposed physical disability. A preoperative assessment of the value the patient assigns to her own independence may be helpful after the surgery.

The ideal relationship between the physician and patient is one of trust, warmth and closeness. The physician who remains emotionally distant loses considerable advantage in influencing the patient's recovery. The satisfaction and positive adjustment evidenced by the patients in a study such as Dempsey's (1975) is an excellent example of what can be accomplished in an atmosphere of physician interest and assurance.

CHEMOTHERAPY

Chemotherapy is the only alternative available for those women who have received tolerance dosages of irradiation and are not candidates for pelvic exenteration. Administration of chemotherapy in patients with cancer of the cervix excludes cure as a realistic objective. Palliation, with reduction in tumour mass, relief of symptoms, and extended survival is the goal. For those patients whose best response to chemotherapy is stable disease, it is often difficult to say whether tumour growth has been contained, or whether chemotherapy had any effect at all.

Continued treatment, in the absence of measurable response, does have positive psychological effects as the patient feels something is being done to help her, and continues to hope for a more tolerable existence or for a miracle. She does not yet assume that the best days of her life are past, that she will never feel any better or that the medicines have failed. There is an element of specialness in the treatment process as the patient is the subject of conferences and the object of attention by the entire health care team. These women may also enjoy the attention showered upon them by friends and family and an intense caring relationship with the physician and the oncology nurse.

Women who demand all that medical science has to offer are likely to find their needs met as the clinician usually responds to the challenge. In contrast, women who are not assertive may be denied aggressive management. Obviously, treatment should be offered to all if it is likely to help, and should not be dependent on the demands or lack of demands on the part of the patient or her family.

Few individuals decline participation in clinical trials. Some patients genuinely want to contribute to the advancement of knowledge, and in a sense, to make their deaths more meaningful in that way. Others are fearful of being involved in these investigational protocols and may not understand the benefit of such programmes. It is important that the physician assure the patient entered in a protocol study that her participation is valuable. It is one of few opportunities in medicine to enhance or reinforce the feeling of self-worth of a patient.

The patient who accepts treatment with a chemotherapeutic agent must be informed and must agree to the risks of possible side effects of a particular regimen. The toll these drugs exact is significant, including the real possibility of death secondary to toxicity. Hair loss caused by many of the agents is upsetting to some women, not only because it changes their appearance but also because it is tangible evidence that a serious problem exists. It prevents the simplest of tasks: personal grooming. The price these women pay for hope is high; some women, however, are quite willing to accept any bodily insult to remain alive.

It is important that the physician consider the chemotherapy patient's plight. She is subjected to a form of therapy that may not be helpful but will usually produce unwanted symptoms. The outcome of the disease and the effect of the therapy are equally unknown to her. A financial burden ensues that aggravates her sense of guilt as she is no longer able to provide for her family. At every visit she fears, yet must be prepared for, the words that indicate treatment failure. Family members, including her partner, may begin to withdraw as her suffering becomes too great for them to bear, and they begin the process of separation that will culminate in her death.

The patient and her family need help in dealing with this extraordinary amount of stress. The oncology nurse is a key individual in assisting the patient and her family. The social worker has the ability to tap community resources to meet specific needs in a given set of circumstances. The minister or priest can give spiritual guidance, assist the family in setting priorities, and help keep hope alive. Nonetheless, involvement of the physician remains at a premium.

THE DYING PATIENT

In spite of all efforts, a significant number of cancer patients do not respond to treatment. When all forms of therapy have failed, the focus must change to preparation for the death of the patient. The physician may share the patient's sense of failure but must reassure the patient that she will not be abandoned. The goals of treatment are to keep the patient pain-free and comfortable, to assist the patient in remaining functional for as long as possible and to keep the family informed so that shared time is well spent. The physician, the patient and her family must accept each small victory over a symptom or a complaint while acknowledging a loss of control over the disease process.

Communication is important in the care of the terminal patient. It is of utmost importance that all health care professionals understand the goals and objectives in regard to any given patient. The patient and her family may ask the same question (how long?) in different ways to many people, hoping to get a promising reply. In their distress and denial, the family may insist that a given piece of information has never been provided them when, in fact, it simply was not heard. The spokesman for the family usually comes forward and makes his or her presence known to the clinician. This individual can be an ally and should be regarded as such. Communicating with numerous members of the family separately is not advised and is often disruptive. The physician meets his responsibility best in encouraging family members to communicate with each other at this time of great pain.

It is very important at this time to determine where the death will occur. For many patients and families, death at home is viewed as comforting, because this provides an opportunity for the patient and family to have uninterrupted time together. Even if death at home is chosen, the link between the patient and the treatment centre needs to be maintained. During times of stress, the family and the patient need a person to contact who can advise them and provide the medical supplies and medication required. Special hospital beds may be made available through community agencies, and visiting nurses can assist with care on an interval basis.

Hospital admission for terminal care and death will be chosen by some, often due to the inability to provide the nursing care required in the home, due to young children in the home, etc. The medical staff must be available in order to arrange admission at the appropriate time.

The concept of hospice care for the terminally ill originated in England and is used in some metropolitan areas in the United States. In Great Britain, these patients are admitted to facilities with a home-like atmosphere and whenever possible, patients are allowed to return to their homes if they become functional and pain-free. Caring for the patients in their own home has been the focus of the American hospice movement. The key elements of hospice care include pain control with scheduled drug administration without impairment of the patient's mental faculties, increased involvement of family members in patient care with the support of a professional nursing staff and development of the remaining capabilities of the patient. The nurses also work with family members to aid their adjustment to the loss, both before and after the death of the patient. The hospice adds a dimension of compassion to care of the dying patient.

Patients nearing death have been described as passing through several phases of dying, i.e., denial, hostility, bargaining, depression and acceptance. Denial is a useful tool for managing stress unless it prohibits rational intervention. The physician's need to implement a particular treatment plan may be an expression of his anxiety about his own death and his frustration in being unable to cure the patient. As a rule, denial will not be overcome until the patient feels and expresses a readiness to proceed with treatment. It is the responsibility of the health care professional to be alert for the cues that demonstrate that the patient is willing to move to another phase.

Hostility or anger is often an expression of frustration at the perceived loss of control and may be evident at any time in the treatment process. The anger of the terminally ill patient results from a failure to find an answer to the question, 'Why me?' The providers of health care must not react to this hostility, since anger on their part further alienates the patient.

Bargaining is apparent when patients make statements such as 'When I am well again, I will work for the church' or 'I've just got to get my children educated.' The bargains involved are that she will dedicate her life to the church if the doctor will cure her or, in the second instance, she is prepared to die if given time to raise her family. Such statements may be made by women who are model patients, as though co-operation on their part will improve their chances of cure. If the bargain is accomplished, a new one may surface to replace it. These patients should be encouraged to discuss their expectations and should not be given false encouragement.

Distress manifests itself as depression in many patients treated for cancer and may appear at repeated intervals at any of the diagnostic and therapeutic phases of the treatment process. It is more likely to occur in those individuals who have previously experienced such feelings of despair. Depression should be carefully assessed as the depressed patient with a chronic illness may respond to treatment differently from one with an acute depressive episode. The symptoms of inability to sleep, change in eating patterns, and lack of energy may be secondary to the disease and its sequelae, not to depression. If present, correction of metabolic disturbances may benefit the patients but will not help depression based on guilt, self-reproach, or feelings of worthlessness. In the latter group, the use of tricyclic antidepressants is encouraged and may provide considerable improvement in the quality of life in these patients.

Acceptance of impending death occurs when prolonged suffering is viewed as inescapable, or in some cases when the patient comes to terms with her own philosophy and fears of death. During that time, plans for burial are made, wills are revised and appropriately witnessed, and long-standing conflicts with loved ones are resolved. Many patients never reach this phase of acceptance, while others alternate between acceptance and denial. Vascillation among all the stages is common and should not invite the disapproval of the health care professional. The physician, the patient and the family are often out of phase in the stages of the dying process. For example, the physician may be accepting, the patient depressed, and the family hostile or denying.

Acceptance may come late, or take unusual forms. One patient who at an early age witnessed her father's death due to a haemorrhage was terrified that she would die in the same manner. She was overwhelmed by her feeling of helplessness, and could not imagine anything more horrifying than bleeding to death. In the final phase of her illness she experienced a number of episodes of bleeding. During one such event, she slowly lost consciousness. She later described this as a comforting and reassuring experience; thereafter, she no longer feared haemorrhage as a cause of death, or death itself, since she had foreseen the peaceful nature of it.

BIBLIOGRAPHY

Abitbol M M, Davenport J H 1974 Sexual dysfunction after therapy for cervical carcinoma. American Journal of Obstetrics and Gynecology 119: 181–189
Adelusi B 1980 Coital function after radiotherapy for carcinoma of the cervix uteri. British Journal of Obstetrics and Gynecology 87: 821–823
Amias A G 1975a Sexual life after gynaecological operations. I. British Medical Journal (June 14): 608–609
Amias A G 1975b Sexual life after gynaecological operations. II. British Medical Journal (June 21): 680–681
Bahnson C B 1975 Psychologic and emotional issues in cancer: the psychotherapeutic care of the cancer patient. Seminars in Oncology 2: 293–309
Becker D W Jr, Massey F M, McCraw J B 1979 Musculocutaneous flaps in reconstructive pelvic surgery. Obstetrics and Gynecology 54: 178–183
Bronner-Huszar J 1971 The psychological aspects of cancer in man. Psychosomatics 12: 133–138
Brown R S, Haddox V, Posada A, Rubio A 1972 Social and psychological adjustment following pelvic exenteration. American Journal of Obstetrics and Gynecology 114: 162–171
Capone M A, Westie K S, Good R S 1980 Sexual rehabilitation of the gynecologic cancer patient: an effective counselling model. Frontiers of Radiation Therapy and Oncology 14: 123–129
Capone M A, Good R S, Westie K S, Jacobson A F 1980 Psychosocial rehabilitation of gynecologic oncology patients. Archives of Physical and Medical Rehabilitation 61: 128–132

Craig T J, Abeloff M D 1974 Psychiatric symptomatology among hospitalized cancer patients. American Journal of Psychiatry 131: 1323–1327

Davis K 1981 Helping the gynecologic cancer patient and her partner. Sexual Medicine Today (July): 6–13

Decker W H, Schwartzman E 1962 Sexual function following treatment for carcinoma of the cervix. American Journal of Obstetrics and Gynecology 83: 401–405

Dempsey G M, Buchsbaum H J, Morrison J 1975 Psychosocial adjustment to pelvic exenteration. Gynecologic Oncology 3: 325–334

Dennecstein L, Wood C, Burrows G D 1977 Sexual response following hysterectomy and oophorectomy. Obstetrics and Gynecology 49: 92–96

Donahue V C, Knapp R C 1977 Sexual rehabilitation of gynecologic cancer patients. Obstetrics and Gynecology 49: 118–121

Drellich M G, Bieber I, Sutherland A M 1956 Adaptation to hysterectomy (Paper). 9th Annual Cancer Symposium of the James Ewing Society: 88–94

Dunphy J E 1976 Annual discourse. Caring for the patient with cancer. New England Journal of Medicine 295: 313–319

Goldberg R J 1981 Management of depression in the patient with advanced cancer. Journal of the American Medical Association 246: 373–376

Hinton J M 1963 The physical and mental distress of the dying. Quarterly Journal of Medicine New Series 32: 1–21

Jackman S 1980 Anxieties about the body which hinder sexual intimacy. Medical Aspects of Human Sexuality (June): 15–28

Kuebler-Ross E 1969 On death and dying. Macmillan, New York

Labrum A H 1976a Psychological factors in gynecologic cancer. Primary Care 3: 811–824

Labrum A H 1976b Psychological factors in the etiology and treatment of cancer of the cervix. Clinical Obstetrics and Gynecology 19: 419–430

Lamont J A, DePetrillo A D, Sargeant E J 1978 Psychosexual rehabilitation and exenterative surgery. Gynecologic Oncology 6: 236–242

LeShan L 1959 Psychological states as factors in the development of malignant disease: a critical review. Journal of the National Cancer Institute 22: 1–18

Peck A, Boland J 1977 Emotional reactions to radiation treatment. Cancer 40: 180–184

Pitkin R M, Bradbury J T 1975 The effect of topical estrogen on irradiated vaginal epithelium. American Journal of Obstetrics and Gynecology 92: 175–182

Plumb M M, Holland J 1977 Comparative studies of psychological function in patients with advanced cancer. I. Self-reported depressive symptoms. Psychosomatic Medicine 39: 264–276

Polivy J 1974 Psychological reactions to hysterectomy: a critical review. American Journal of Obstetrics and Gynecology 118: 417–426

Schmale A H, Iker H 1971 Hopelessness as a predictor of cervical cancer. Social Sciences and Medicine 5: 95–100

Seibel M M, Freeman M G, Graves W L 1980 Carcinoma of the cervix and sexual function. Obstetrics and Gynecology 55: 484–487

Simonton O C, Matthews-Simonton S, Sparks T F 1980 Psychological intervention in the treatment of cancer. Psychosomatics 21: 226–233

Surawicz F G, Brightwell D R, Weitzel W D, Othmer E 1976 Cancer, emotions and mental illness: the present state of understanding. American Journal of Psychiatry 133: 1306–1309

Surawicz F G 1977 Women, cancer and emotions. Journal of the American Medical Women's Association 32: 18–29

Sutherland A M 1981 Psychological impact of cancer and its therapy. CA — A Cancer Journal for Clinicians 31: 159–171

Vasicka A, Popovich N R, Brausch C C 1958 Postradiation course of patients with cervical carcinoma. Obstetrics and Gynecology 11: 404–414

Vincent C E, Vincent B, Greiss F C, Linton E B 1975 Some marital-sexual concomitants of carcinoma of the cervix. Southern Medical Journal 68: 552–558

Index